Writing Grant Proposals in Epidemiology, Preventive Medicine, and Biostatistics

Securing research funds in epidemiology, preventive medicine, and biostatistics is highly competitive, and, at the same time, the grant application and review process at such agencies at the National Institutes of Health (NIH) has undergone substantial revisions. *Writing Grant Proposals in Epidemiology, Preventive Medicine, and Biostatistics, Second Edition* targets effective grant proposal writing in this highly competitive and evolving environment. Covering all aspects of the proposal writing process, the updated second edition

- Includes new chapters on Fellowship Grants and Career Development Awards designed for graduate students, postdoctoral fellows, and early-career faculty
- Provides strategies to highlight the "overall impact" of the grant, one of the most important aspects determining NIH funding in a new chapter on Significance and Innovation
- Provides step-by-step guidelines for grant structure and style alongside broader strategies for developing a research funding portfolio
- Explains how to avoid common errors and pitfalls, supplying critical dos and don'ts that aid in writing solid grant proposals
- Illustrates key concepts with extensive examples from successfully funded proposals

Written by an established NIH reviewer with inside knowledge and an impressive track record of funding, this book is an essential cookbook of the appropriate ingredients needed to construct a winning grant proposal. The text is not only relevant for early-stage investigators including graduate students, medical students/residents, and postdoctoral fellows but also valuable for more experienced faculty, clinicians, epidemiologists, and other health professionals who cannot seem to break the barrier to obtain NIH funds for their research.

T0171927

Writing Grant Proposals in Epidemiology, Preventive Medicine, and Biostatistics
Second Edition

Lisa Chasan-Taber

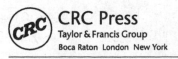

CRC Press
Taylor & Francis Group
Boca Raton London New York

CRC Press is an imprint of the
Taylor & Francis Group, an **informa** business

A CHAPMAN & HALL BOOK

Second Edition published 2022
by CRC Press
6000 Broken Sound Parkway NW, Suite 300, Boca Raton, FL 33487-2742

and by CRC Press
4 Park Square, Milton Park, Abingdon, Oxon, OX14 4RN

© 2022 Lisa Chasan-Taber
First Edition published by CRC Press 2014
CRC Press is an imprint of Taylor & Francis Group, LLC

ISBN: 978-0-367-72530-3 (hbk)
ISBN: 978-0-367-72232-6 (pbk)
ISBN: 978-1-003-15514-0 (ebk)

DOI: 10.1201/9781003155140

Typeset in Times
by Deanta Global Publishing Services, Chennai, India

Contents

Preface to 2nd Edition

The first edition of this book was published in 2014, eight years ago. Since that time, there have been substantive changes to NIH grant submission guidelines and review criteria. More importantly, it has become clear in these competitive times that graduate students, medical students/residents, postdoctoral fellows, and early-career faculty need additional support launching their careers. This is even more critical in light of new NIH guidelines that allow only one resubmission of any grant application. It is imperative, therefore, for early-stage investigators to learn "grantsmanship" and have the ability to construct competitive grant applications.

The primary goal of this second edition is to present concise, useful information about common errors, research plan dos and don'ts, template examples of grant sections, and many other strategies for success that may assist any first-time candidates for these awards. The most strategic approach is to focus on grants targeted for their career stage. Therefore, this second edition includes two new chapters, Chapter 18, "Fellowship Grants," and Chapter 19, "Career Development Awards." These chapters not only provide step-by-step strategies and examples but also include tips for success and pitfalls to avoid.

This text is not only highly relevant for early-stage investigators but also valuable for more experienced faculty, clinicians, and epidemiologists. In light of NIH's increased focus on the "overall impact" of the grant, this edition now includes Chapter 8, "Significance and Innovation," as these concepts are the most important aspects determining funding. Similarly, Chapter 11, "Study Design and Methods," has been updated to reflect NIH's call for applicants to enhance reproducibility through rigor and transparency. Chapter 17, "Submission of the Grant Proposal," has been substantially revised to incorporate current NIH required components.

All of the chapters have been updated and re-ordered to follow best practices for grant proposal writing from "soup to nuts" starting with the new Chapter 2, "Setting Up a Time Frame," through Chapter 3, "Identifying a Topic and Choosing the Right Funding Source," and continuing through the grant proposal section by section. The text culminates with chapters on the submission and resubmission process. New examples are included throughout.

I had, as usual, invaluable support from the publisher, CRC Press/Taylor & Francis Group. I especially want to thank Vaishali Singh and Rob Calver for their interest in my work and their encouragement in the project.

Adding to the list of people who gave valuable input to the first edition of the book, I also want to thank Dr. Rebecca Spencer and Dr. Peter Lindenauer, who contributed their expertise on grant writing for fellowship grants and career development awards. Many thanks also to Drs. Serena Houghton and Nicole VanKim for sharing their experiences and to the students in my course, *Scientific Writing for Thesis, Dissertation, and Grant Proposals in Epidemiology*, for making this work possible.

Author Bio

Lisa Chasan-Taber is Professor of Epidemiology and former Associate Dean for Research in the School of Public Health & Health Sciences at the University of Massachusetts Amherst. Chasan-Taber has had a history of continual funding from NIH and national foundations throughout her research career. She has been a standing member on National Institutes of Health (NIH) review panels, a mentor on NIH Research Career Development Awards, and the Principal Investigator of mentoring grants designed to provide early-career faculty with successful grant-writing strategies. For more than 20 years, she has taught a class on grant proposal writing for graduate students which formed the basis for this textbook. Chasan-Taber has been recognized for her research through the Chancellor's Medal, the highest recognition bestowed to faculty by the university. She received her postdoctoral and doctoral training in epidemiology at the Harvard School of Public Health.

Ten Top Tips for Successful Grant Proposal Writing

1

If I were asked to distill my grant proposal writing advice down to the ten most important tips, the following would be my list. Graduate students, postdoctoral fellows, and early-career faculty hear a lot about grant-writing **'pitfalls to avoid'** and common **mistakes** that can be made. Instead, I believe it's more useful to focus on tips for **successful** grant-writing.

1.1 TIP #1: START SMALL BUT HAVE A BIG VISION

It is critical to have a big vision. Each small grant—be it a seed grant, a postdoctoral fellowship, or an early-career award—should be viewed as providing preliminary data for one or two of the specific aims of your ultimate larger grant. Typically, large grants are funded by the NIH R01 mechanism. Chapter 3, "Identifying a Topic and Conducting the Literature Search," provides step-by-step strategies for identifying research gaps, critical for success in grantsmanship.

Therefore, early on in the process, with the help of a mentor, try to envision your ultimate large project. For example, let's assume that a typical large grant (i.e., an NIH R01) contains three to five specific aims. Once you are able to envision these aims, your next steps become clear: Step by step, you start *biting off* small chunks of this larger grant through writing small grants designed to support *one or two* of these ultimate aims. These small grants should not be designed to provide the definitive answer to these aims but instead to show that the aims are feasible and/or provide preliminary data in their support. These small grants will be limited by smaller sample sizes and budgets, but will be able to show proof of principle—that you can *pull it off* (see Tip #5: Show That You Can Pull It Off). This approach pays off as grant review panels often see a large grant as the culmination of a growing body of work progressing from small seed grants to larger and larger awards in a cumulative fashion. Chapter 10, "Pilot Grants: Reproducibility and Validity Studies," provides examples of validation studies, typical for a first pilot grant.

Finding a mentor   A key factor in developing a vision of your ultimate large grant will be the advice of your mentor(s). If you do not currently have a mentor, ask your department chair if they can assign you one. It is also usually considered acceptable to seek out your own mentor. Indeed, many early-career faculty will assemble a *mentorship team*, each member of which can provide guidance in different career aspect (i.e., a teaching mentor, a research mentor, and a work–life balance mentor). Consider both on-site and off-site faculty as potential mentors.

In this age of virtual communication, I often find that I communicate more with my off-site mentors than with those directly down the hall. You can use web-based resources such as Research Gate (https://www.researchgate.net/) and NIH RePORTER (https://reporter.nih.gov/) to help locate a potential mentor by searching on your topic and identifying a list of principal investigator (PI) names. Then view their NIH grant-funding track record. Ask yourself if their pathway matches up with your grantmaking goals—if

DOI: 10.1201/9781003155140-1

so, they are likely a good choice of mentor. In contrast, PIs who have not received a large NIH grant, as indicated by NIH RePORTER, may not be the best choice.

1.2 TIP #2: FOCUS ON SMALL GRANTS TARGETED TO EARLY-CAREER INVESTIGATORS

Early-career faculty want to be successful and are often tempted to make a big impact by quickly *landing a big grant* even in the absence of a track record of smaller grant funding. Others are under pressure from their institutions and department chairs to immediately apply for a large grant (e.g., an NIH R01). In my experience as an NIH review panel member, this approach is almost certainly destined to fail. As noted in Tip #1: Start Small but Have a Big Vision, review panels often see a large grant as the culmination of a growing body of work. They want to see evidence of this stairway to success, and it's your job to demonstrate that you have been on this stairway. You do this by showing your successful procurement and management of previous smaller grants, as well as the translation of these grants into publications. A desirable grant-funding history starts from small seed grants progressing to larger and larger awards in a cumulative fashion (Figure 1.1). Chapter 4, "Choosing the Right Funding Source," provides example plans for a steady trajectory of grants from small to large.

There are certainly some exceptions to this rule. For example, you may be an early-career faculty member within a research team that already has a track record in your area. If so, consider serving as a **coinvestigator** on a grant led by one of your more senior colleagues while launching your own **independent** research. Including senior researchers as co-PIs can help shore up the "research team." For example, their preliminary data become the *team's* preliminary data in your application.

Alternatively, you may take advantage of more senior expertise by writing a multiple PI (MPI) proposal. The MPI approach requires that each PI brings substantive expertise to complementary components of the proposal. In other words, the goal is to encourage collaboration among *equals* when that is the most appropriate way to address a scientific problem. Therefore, care should be taken with the MPI approach as these grants are not designed to be mentored grants such as Fellowship Grants or Career Development Awards (see Chapter 18, "Fellowship Grants," and Chapter 19, "Career Development Awards").

Ultimately, however, as described in Chapter 20, "Review Process," and Chapter 21, "Resubmission of the Grant Proposal," one of the key criteria upon which a grant is scored is the expertise of the PI. When you are submitting an application as the sole PI, the reviewers will be looking for your track record in managing a large grant and translating that work into publications. So, remember not to go-it-alone with a big grant submission too early.

Therefore, starting early in your career and capitalizing upon the advantages of having an "early-career faculty status" has never been as important as it is now.

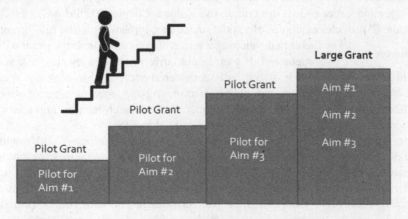

FIGURE 1.1 Each small grant provides preliminary data for your large grant.

1.2.1 Early-Career Awards and Postdoctoral Granting Mechanisms Provide the Highest Chances for Success

These mechanisms typically do not require significant preliminary data. Instead, funding decisions rely most heavily on your promise and potential as a candidate: your training to date, your mentors, and the importance of your topic.

This potential is indicated by three items:

- Your education to date (including prior publications and project-related experience)
- The mentors with which you have surrounded yourself
- The public health importance of your topic

Another key advantage of these funding mechanisms is that, unlike larger grant awards, you will be competing against a smaller pool of people, all of whom are at a comparable stage in their careers. This avoids the risk of competing against senior investigators who already have established track records. As a senior investigator once said to me, "Avoid competing against the 'big boys and girls' as long as you can!" Remember that this advantage will quickly be over after several years pass by and you find yourself no longer eligible for these awards—so seize this opportunity while it lasts.

Therefore, if you are a graduate student, seek out grant mechanisms designed for graduate students such as the National Institutes of Health (NIH) predoctoral (F31) and postdoctoral (F32) fellowship awards (see Chapter 18, "Fellowship Grants"). If you are an early-career faculty member, look for grants designed for early-career faculty members such as the K series awards (see Chapter 19, "Career Development Awards"). These may also include small seed money grants provided by your university (e.g., Faculty Research Grants) or foundation grants targeted for career development (e.g., the American Diabetes Association Junior Faculty Development Award and the Minority Junior Faculty Development Award, the American Heart Association Career Development Award, the March of Dimes Starter Scholar Research Award). Chapter 4, "Choosing the Right Funding Source," provides an in-depth discussion of how to locate these opportunities.

At the same time, always be on the lookout for opportunities to collaborate as a coinvestigator on applications where the principal investigator (PI) is a senior, established investigator. These grants will require a somewhat reduced effort on your part (in comparison to being PI). In addition, because ongoing projects were underway before you joined, you can also anticipate an earlier payoff in terms of published manuscripts. Joining an established research project also provides you with the opportunity to apply for an NIH Research Supplement (i.e., funds added to an existing grant to increase the participation of scientists from underrepresented groups in health-related research that builds upon the aims of these ongoing grants).

All this being said, developing your own independent line of research is important. Indeed, one criterion for tenure and promotion at many research institutes is movement away from the area of your dissertation work and development of independence in your own research aims. If the work of your departmental colleagues does not relate to your area, then other collegial relationships and sources of grant data can be found in many locations—be they across campus or even across the state or country.

1.2.2 Putting Tips #1 and #2 into Action: An Example

By way of example, let's say your overall vision is to understand the impact of diet on psychosocial status. You meet with your mentor and decide that an interesting and novel topic for an ultimate large grant application would be to study the impact of vitamin D on risk of depression. You sketch out a plan for an R01 to conduct a large prospective study of vitamin D intake and risk of depression (Figure 1.2).

The next step is to work together to outline potential specific aims (Figure 1.3). Each of these specific aims is going to serve as the topic of a smaller grant (Figure 1.4).

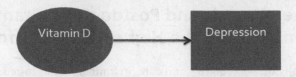

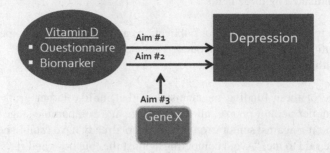

FIGURE 1.2   Example overall grantsmanship goal.

FIGURE 1.3   Example specific aims figure.

The specific aims corresponding to this example would be the following:

- *Overall Grantsmanship Goal*:
  - To obtain an R01 grant to conduct a large prospective study of vitamin D intake and risk of depression.
- *Specific Aims of the R01*
  - Aim #1: To evaluate the association between **self-reported vitamin D** and risk of depression.
  - Aim #2: To evaluate the association between a **biomarker of vitamin D** and risk of depression.
  - Aim #3: To evaluate whether the impact of vitamin D on depression risk is stronger among those with **gene x** as compared to those without the gene.

Example small grant proposals   Now, for each of these aims, you develop plans for small grant proposals (Figure 1.4). Reproducibility and validity studies and pilot feasibility studies are typical small grant projects as they have clearly defined parameters and aims and are feasible to conduct.

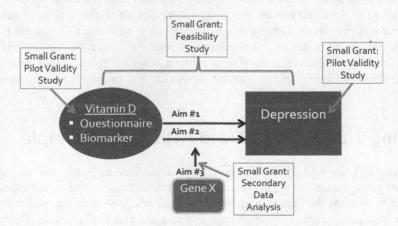

FIGURE 1.4   Example small grant proposals corresponding to specific aims.

Aim #1 could be supported by a small grant proposal to conduct a reproducibility and validity study of the vitamin D questionnaire against an objective measure of vitamin D. This small grant would support the validity of your measurement tool for your exposure of interest.

Aim #2 could be supported by a small grant proposal to conduct a reproducibility and validity study of the depression questionnaire against a clinical diagnosis of depression. This small grant would support the validity of your measurement tool for your outcome of interest.

Aim #3 could be supported by a small grant proposal to analyze the influence of gene x on the association between vitamin D and depression using an existing publicly available dataset. While this small grant would not be conducted in your population of interest, findings from this project could support your proposed association between vitamin D, gene x, and depression.

Aim #4 could be supported by a small grant proposal to conduct a pilot/feasibility study of recruiting a prospective cohort study at the proposed study site. This small grant would generate recruitment and retention rates and provide measures of the variability of your exposure and outcome of interest in the study population. These findings would support the power and sample size calculations for the larger grant.

All of these small grants will support your skills as a Principal Investigator. In other words, they will provide evidence that you have experience in writing grant applications and managing the logistics of grant projects and can translate these grants into publications.

Example Small Grant Proposals and the Corresponding Utility of Their Findings

- **Small Grant Proposal to Support Aims #1 and #2**: Reproducibility and validity study of vitamin D questionnaire.
  - **Results**: Degree of measurement error and ability to correct for this error; validity and reproducibility scores.
- **Small Grant Proposal to Support Aims #1 and #2**: A reproducibility and validity study of the depression questionnaire.
  - **Results**: Degree of measurement error and ability to correct for this error; validity and reproducibility scores.
- **Small Grant Proposal to Support Aim #3**: Analyze the influence of gene x on the association between vitamin D and depression using an existing publicly available dataset.
  - **Results**: Findings of a suggested impact of gene x in another dataset provides proof of principle for evaluating this in your proposed study.
- **Small Grant Proposal to Support Aims #1, 2, and 3**: A pilot/feasibility study of recruiting a prospective cohort study at the proposed study site.
  - **Results**: Eligibility, recruitment, and retention rates as a basis for power and sample size calculations.
  - **Results**: Participant satisfaction surveys: Acceptability of the study.
- **From All Three Pilots**
  - **Results**:
  - Principal investigator skills:
    - Write grant applications
    - Manage the logistics of grant projects
    - Translate these grants into publications

1.2.3 A Pitfall to Avoid: Interdependent Aims

In earlier, more economically advantaged times, it was considered acceptable for a large NIH R01 grant to include pilot studies within its aims. However, in the current climate, reviewers do not look favorably upon this approach. They naturally ask, "What if the pilot study finds that the methods are not successful? How would the investigator accomplish the subsequent aims of the project?" For example, consider if Specific Aim #1 proposes to conduct a validation study of the questionnaire to be used in Specific Aims #2 and #3. If Specific Aim #1 subsequently fails to find that the questionnaire is valid, then how can the remainder of the project proceed? These are termed interdependent aims, and reviewers often consider such aims to be a fatal flaw of a proposal. In Chapter 6, "Specific Aims," I describe how to create a strong set of study aims, avoiding this as well as other pitfalls.

1.2.4 Plan for More Than One Potential Funding Pipeline

Given the challenges of securing grant funding, the only way to ensure grant success is to have several proposals in the pipeline and/or under review **at the same time** (Figure 1.5). For example, you could take the "Small Grant Proposal to Support Aim #1" above and submit it for an internal seed grant at the same time that you submit the "Small Grant Proposal to Support Aims #1, 2, and 3" to NIH as an R03. Because all these initiatives fit within your overall grantsmanship goal, in the wonderful event that all are funded, they can all serve as pilot data for your larger R01-type grant.

Another strategic approach is to consider multiple funding options for the *same* application. In this vein, I always advise my mentees to take the same or similar grant application and submit it to multiple potential funders. For example, the **Small Grant Proposal to Support Aim #1**, "a reproducibility and validity study of the proposed vitamin D questionnaire against an objective measure," could be submitted for (1) an internal seed grant if your institution offers such faculty research grants as well as to (2) a small foundation and (3) to NIH for a smaller grant mechanism.

On the highly unusual chance that you obtain funding for this grant from more than one source, you will simply be faced with the luxury of declining one of these grants. Most often, the grant submission requirements differ between these funding agencies, such that you will already have made modifications between each version of the proposal. The **key** here is that you are being efficient by taking the same small grant topic and shaping it to apply to several granting mechanisms.

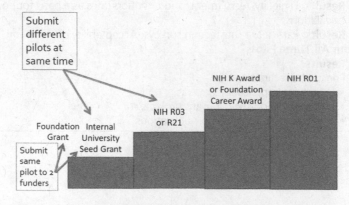

FIGURE 1.5 Plan for more than one potential funding pipeline.

1.3 TIP #3: LOOK AT WHO AND WHAT THEY FUNDED BEFORE YOU

Funding agencies typically post a list of prior grant **awardees** online; if not, your own institution's grants office can provide you with a list of faculty on your campus who have obtained these same grants. For example, NIH posts the full Project Summary/Abstracts of both active and prior awards (e.g., NIH RePORTER http://projectreporter.nih.gov/reporter.cfm). This list is critical, as it shows the interest (or lack of interest) of the agency in funding your area of research. For example, some funding agencies simply don't have the interest or track record in funding epidemiologic research and instead limit their funding to laboratory studies. It would be a high-risk proposition to write a grant for a foundation that has never funded an application in your area of expertise before. It is reasonable to consider asking successful fundees to share their applications with you, particularly if you, or your mentors, recognize any names on the fundee list or see that they are from your institution. Reassure these successfully funded investigators that you are simply seeking a model for the appropriate scope and depth of the research plan, not the actual content of their aims. When framed in this manner, people are typically willing to share.

Funding agencies may also post a list of prior and current grant **reviewers** and their affiliations online. Ask yourself if the expertise of these reviewers overlaps with your study aims and methodology. For example, are any of these investigators population health researchers? Are any from similar departments/divisions to yours? It would be a higher risk proposition to write a proposal for a foundation that does not include investigators in epidemiology and preventive medicine on their review panels.

1.4 TIP #4: SPEND HALF YOUR TIME ON THE SPECIFIC AIMS AND PROJECT SUMMARY/ABSTRACT

The Specific Aims page should be the first item that you write when you "set pen to paper," well before writing your Research Strategy section (e.g., Significance, Innovation, and Approach). Writers of successful grant applications typically report that 50% of their time was spent on revising and rewriting their specific aims (Figure 1.6). Send this one-page sketch to your mentor and coinvestigators early in the grant-writing process with the goal of kicking off an iterative process of rewriting, revising, and re-review. In Part I of this text, "Preparing to Write the Grant Proposal," Chapter 2, "Setting Up a Time Frame," provides suggested timelines to set you up for success. In addition, it is critical that these aims be understandable by anyone with a scientific background. Chapter 6, "Specific Aims," and Chapter 7, "How to Develop and Write Hypotheses," discuss strategies and writing conventions for developing specific aims and hypotheses including exercises and annotated examples and tips.

Another excellent resource is the NIH RePORTER (http://projectreporter.nih.gov/reporter.cfm) as mentioned above. This site can be invaluable in helping you to formulate the scope of your grant. This

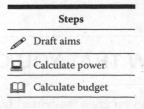

Steps
✎ Draft aims
💻 Calculate power
📖 Calculate budget

FIGURE 1.6 The first three steps in grant proposal writing.

site lists abstracts, referred to as *Project Summaries*, and can give you a critical sense of what has been successful in your research area. Such aspects as the number of specific aims and the typical range of sample sizes will provide you with key insights as to what has "worked" for your targeted grant funding agency/research institute. Because these awards have all successfully been funded, they serve as excellent examples. Viewing funded Project Summary/Abstracts can help you answer the following questions: "How many aims did the investigators include?" and "What was their sample size?" You can limit your search to particular key terms as well as particular grant mechanisms (e.g., smaller and larger awards). The output, in addition to listing the Project Summary/Abstract, will also provide the name of the review panel and the NIH institute. Therefore, *surfing* NIH RePORTER is useful not only for both the smaller grant mechanisms but also for envisioning the ultimate larger grant.

One reason that specific aims are so critical is the nature of the peer review process described in more detail in Chapter 20, "Review Process." Because only three to four reviewers are typically assigned as primary and secondary reviewers of your grant, the majority of the reviewers on the panel will only have read your Project Summary/Abstract. Therefore, the aims must not only provide a clear snapshot of the entire study but also convey what is novel about your application. Chapter 16, "Project Summary/Abstract," provides tips and strategies for how to write, and what merits inclusion, in this section. See Figure 1.1.

After drafting your aims, the second step in this process is to calculate your statistical power to achieve these aims. This will help you to answer the question, "Will your sample size provide you with sufficient power to detect a difference between groups, if there is truly a difference?" If you are basing your grant upon a preexisting dataset, your sample size is typically fixed, and the question of whether or not you have adequate power can be answered quickly. A negative answer, while disappointing, can quickly and efficiently result in a change in study aims.

If instead you are proposing to launch a new study and recruit participants, you can choose the sample size you need to achieve sufficient power. However, in this case, progressing to Step #3 and calculating your budget will be critical. A common pitfall of new investigators is to be too ambitious—proposing a larger sample size than they have the budget and experience to handle. Chapter 13, "Power and Sample Size," provides user-friendly approaches to power and sample size calculations, available software, and annotated examples with strategies and tips.

Therefore, the third step is to evaluate whether your budget can afford your required sample size. The number of participants will have an immediate impact on the costs of conducting your study. Such costs include the number of assays, interviewer time for recruitment and follow-up, as well as the cost of participant incentives. Also, ask yourself whether your study site can feasibly provide this number of participants. For example, does the hospital actually see that number of patients per day/week/year? Are that many patients likely to be eligible *and* agree to participate? Such questions of feasibility can be answered by your own preliminary work, by that of your coinvestigators, or by other investigators at your proposed study site. Alternatively, if you are proposing a pilot grant, you can clearly state that the goal of your pilot is to assess recruitment and eligibility rates to calculate power for a larger grant submission. Chapter 9, "Preliminary Studies," describes this approach in greater detail.

Now, in light of everything you have learned from Steps 1, 2, and 3, and incorporating your mentors' and colleagues' feedback, go back and refine the aims and start the process over again. Once you have settled on the aims, you will find that writing the rest of the application will flow easily. As described in Part II of this text, "The Grant Proposal: Section by Section," each section of a well-written grant proposal flows directly from, and mirrors, the components of the specific aims.

1.5 TIP #5: SHOW THAT YOU CAN PULL IT OFF

Showing that you can feasibly conduct your grant is a critical factor for reviewers. If you are an early-career faculty, if possible, collaborate with senior investigators who have conducted similar grants in similar populations. Their involvement on your grant will be a key factor supporting your potential for success.

Capitalize upon your coinvestigators Don't let coinvestigators appear in name only. Show established working relationships with them via co-authored publications, co-presentations, and/or an established mentoring relationship (e.g., as part of a training grant, fellowship grant, or career development award). List grants on which you are **both** listed as investigators or consultants. Of course, much of this information will appear in your biosketches but you cannot rely upon the reviewers to connect the dots between you and your coinvestigators. Make it easy for the reviewers by clearly noting these prior collaborations in your "Preliminary Studies" section. Specific examples of this grantsmanship strategy as well as others are discussed in detail in Chapter 9, "Preliminary Studies."

Lastly, present evidence that you have conducted smaller feasibility studies as mentioned in Tip #1: Start Small but Have a Big Vision and Tip #2: Focus on Small Grants Targeted to Early-Career Investigators. These show proof of principle and provide reassurance to reviewers that you, as a principal investigator, will be able to conduct your proposed aims and ideally translate this work into publications. These studies can provide preliminary data necessary for calculating power and sample size for your larger grants. Participant satisfaction surveys administered in a feasibility study can provide data on the acceptability of your methods. Validation studies of your proposed methods (as described in Chapter 10, "Pilot Grants: Reproducibility and Validity Studies") can provide assurance that a study based upon these methods will work. In summary, your goal is to show proof of principle.

1.6 TIP #6: YOUR METHODS SHOULD MATCH YOUR AIMS AND VICE VERSA

Include methods that address each of your study aims while taking care not to include additional methods that do not correspond to any aims. The latter is a great temptation among early-career faculty who are often driven to impress reviewers with how many questions their research project will be able to answer. In actuality, this approach often back-fires, and an *overly ambitious* application is one of the most common *fatal flaws* of an early-career application. It is one of the most common reasons for reviewers to give an application a poor score (or to triage the application, as described in Chapter 20, "Review Process"). Instead, it is more impressive to exercise restraint and have a focused plan with a data analysis section directly tied to your specific aims.

For mentored fellowship grants and career development awards, this mistake is typically attributed to the mentor—either to the failure of the mentor to spend time to adequately review your proposal or to their inability to detect this problem at all. It may be viewed as reflective of the future amount and content of mentorship that you would be receiving over the course of the grant period if awarded.

All that being said, there are some specific situations where it may be reasonable to mention additional methods that do not correspond to the proposed aims. For example, in a small grant proposal (e.g., a seed grant), it is often acceptable to state that some data will be collected solely to support subsequent grant applications. However, this is only considered appropriate when it is highly efficient in terms of both study design and participant burden to collect this information in real time, as opposed to returning to participants at a later point in time. See the below example.

Example Methods That Do Not Correspond to Specific Aims
While we are not including genetic aims within this proposal, these stored samples will be available to support the investigation of future hypotheses. Similarly, placentas will be collected and stored for future hypotheses.

In this example, it is clear that trying to collect biologic samples from participants at a later point in time would not be feasible, either because the participants would no longer be readily available or because disease may have already occurred and thereby influenced levels of these biomarkers. For these proposed aims, a data analysis plan is not typically included.

So, moving forward, there are several ways to ensure that your methods are tied directly to your aims and vice versa. The most traditional approach (and the approach that is most kind to your reviewer) is to copy your aims verbatim from the specific aims page and repeat them, in italics, in the data analysis section. Below each italicized aim, insert the relevant statistical analysis designed to achieve this aim. Alternatively, format the structure of the proposal sequentially such that Aim #1 is immediately followed by its methods; Aim #2 is followed by its methods, etc. This approach is only efficient when each aim has a distinct methodological and data analysis plan. Otherwise, you run the risk of repetition of similar methods and wasteful use of precious space. In Chapter 11, "Study Design and Methods," and Chapter 12, "Data Analysis Plan," I describe tips for efficient writing of methods and data analyses sections corresponding to study aims.

1.7 TIP #7: A PROPOSAL CAN NEVER HAVE TOO MANY FIGURES OR TABLES

The more figures and tables in a grant application, the better. As compared to dense text, figures and tables make it easy for the reviewers to quickly grasp your proposal. In addition, the act of creating these figures and tables will help you to crystallize your specific aims and study methods. Figures and tables can save space—reducing the text—critical to meeting the page limitations of most grants.

One general rule is to consider having *a figure or table on almost every page* of your proposal. The inclusion of figures and tables is relevant for every section of a grant application. For example, a figure showing how the specific aims interrelate is always appreciated by reviewers (see Chapter 6, "Specific Aims"). Another key figure displaying your anticipated results can be placed in the Significance or Approach sections (see Chapter 8, "Significance and Innovation"). This helps reviewers envision the value/results/products of your proposal. Other examples include study design figures, tables listing study variables, and statistical power displays. The grant application often ends with a timeline figure—showing each study activity and the quarters during which it will be conducted. Chapter 11, "Study Design and Methods," shows examples of key tables and figures that can be used throughout the proposal.

1.8 TIP #8: SEEK EXTERNAL REVIEW PRIOR TO SUBMISSION

The same person cannot write a grant and review it for clarity. Regardless of how carefully you write and reread your grant, simply by virtue of your familiarity with the material, you will miss gaps and errors. Follow the guidelines for clear and direct writing as outlined in Chapter 5, "Scientific Writing." Then, ask your colleagues to read the application. Even a generalist reviewer will be able to assess (1) whether your goals are clearly stated, (2) how the grant extends prior work in the field (i.e., its innovation), and (3) the impact of your potential findings on the field. These aspects are often the most critical in the score you receive for an application. In Chapter 8, "Significance and Innovation," I outline tips for making these points clear. Chapter 20, "Review Process," describes how these sections are considered in the review process.

In fact, it may be preferable for some of your readers not to have expertise in your area at all, given that not all members of the grant review panel will have expertise in every aspect of your proposal. As noted earlier, at NIH your grant will only be assigned to three to four reviewers. While one reviewer may have a specific background in your area, some others will be assigned based on their expertise in the proposed methodology (e.g., epidemiology), and others are assigned to review the statistical analysis section. For example, a grant designed to identify risk factors for infertility may be assigned to the following three reviewers: (1) a physician who has a track record of publications on *in vitro* fertilization techniques, (2) an epidemiologist who has conducted prospective cohort studies among infertile women, and (3) a statistician. It is even possible that the physician or the epidemiologist will not have direct experience with infertility but are instead more generalist reproductive or perinatal epidemiologists.

It is also generally acknowledged that a local mock review panel can double your chances of funding. For example, mock NIH review panels simulate the grant review process by relying upon faculty at your university who have NIH experience to play the role of reviewers. Similarly, "Chalk-Talk" seminars are also highly effective—these are informal opportunities to discuss your ideas and/or specific aims with your departmental colleagues early in the process to get immediate feedback. If your department does not currently offer Chalk-Talk seminars, suggest that they start to.

Both Chalk-Talk seminars and Mock NIH Study Sections are described in more detail in Chapter 2, "Setting Up a Time Frame."

Some departments will fund early-career faculty to attend local and national grant-writing workshops and will compensate outside experts on your proposed topic to review and critique your grant proposals. Your office of grants and contracts may sponsor a grantsmanship seminar series or brown bag lunch session in which you can participate. Lastly, many departments will enlist the services of a grant writer. By helping you concisely convey your specific aims, significance, innovation, and approach, the best grant writers will help you to best convey the potential impact of your findings.

Real-world (not mock) submission and resubmission processes are carefully described in a step-by-step manner with accompanying strategic tips in Part III of this text, "Submission and Resubmission," in Chapter 17, "Submission of the Grant Proposal," Chapter 20, "Review Process," and Chapter 21, "Resubmission of the Grant Proposal."

1.9 TIP #9: BE KIND TO YOUR REVIEWERS

A happy reviewer should be one of your top goals. Reviewers are typically burdened with an onerous number of applications to read—in addition to their own responsibilities as a researcher themselves. The most effective way to make a reviewer happy is to help them complete their review forms. Do this by using the grant review criteria as subheadings in your application.

1.9.1 Subheadings Should Match Review Criteria

Every reviewer, regardless of the funding agency, is required to use a structured critique form. For example, NIH reviewers are required to write bullet points on the strengths and weaknesses of the overall impact, significance, investigators, innovation, approach, and environment. However, the formatting requirements of NIH grant applications do not require clearly labeled sections for each of these criteria. Therefore, the first way to be *kind* to your reviewers is by using these key terms as subheadings in your application.

For example, reviewers typically have to complete a section on "Innovation." You may think that the innovative aspects of your application are obvious. This is risky. Not only may the reviewer not find your application as clearly innovative as you do, but they may not deduce its innovation at all. A clearly labeled subsection on "Innovation" not only saves the reviewer time but gives you the opportunity to "educate" the reviewer on innovative aspects they may not have recognized on their own. In Chapter 8, "Significance and Innovation," I describe tips for writing the innovation section.

1.9.2 Highlight Key Sentences

A second key kindness is to bold, or otherwise highlight, one key sentence in each paragraph of the Significance and Innovation section. Indeed, choosing what sentence to highlight will ensure that each paragraph does indeed have a key point. With space at a premium in grant proposals (e.g., current limits for the research strategy for smaller NIH grants can be as low as six pages), each paragraph needs to count.

Another way to be kind to the reviewers is in the Preliminary Studies section. The description of each preliminary study should end with a sentence specifying the rationale for why it is relevant to the current proposal. This summary sentence removes the burden on the reviewer. It is your job to connect the dots between your preliminary work and how it relates to or supports your proposed aims. The act of creating these summary sentences also serves a dual purpose of ensuring that you are not including extraneous preliminary findings not relevant to your aims. Examples of such summaries are provided in Chapter 9, "Preliminary Studies."

Another kindness to the reviewer is to insert a brief summary paragraph at the very beginning of the Methods section that encapsulates all the key features of the study design. This paragraph would give the sample size, study population, study design (e.g., prospective cohort case-control study, cross-sectional study), the key assessment tools to be used (e.g., self-reported questionnaire, biomarkers, medical record data), and any other key features of your study methods. This will help the reviewer to concisely present your study to the review panel. Examples of such summaries are provided in Chapter 11, "Study Design and Methods."

In summary, the underpinning of all of these kindnesses is to remember that it is not the job of the reviewer to justify the importance of your proposal but instead your job. Indeed, making their job as easy as possible is the recipe for a happy reviewer.

1.10 TIP #10: IF AT ALL POSSIBLE, CHOOSE A TOPIC THAT YOU FIND INTERESTING!

There is nothing less conducive to your future success and day-to-day productivity than choosing a topic that you don't find interesting. Having several grants in the pipeline and under review at the same time can help stack the deck in your favor.

It is even more preferable if these initiatives fit within an overall research theme (as discussed in Tip #1: Start Small but Have a Big Vision) so that, in the wonderful event that all are funded, they can all serve as pilot data for your larger R01-type grant.

In summary, it is my hope that these ten top tips for successful grant proposal writing will help launch you on your career!

PART I

Preparing to Write
the Grant Proposal

Setting up a Time Frame

2

2.1 HOW TO VIEW THE SUBMISSION PROCESS OVERALL

A colleague of mine once described the grant submission process as a marathon. You should arrive at the finish line completely exhausted but holding aloft your completed grant application with your last iota of strength. The grant represents your absolute best efforts. You hand it in and then collapse. Thus, your advance preparation for the "race" and your support team are critical.

2.2 GETTING STARTED

Back in the days when NIH pay lines were higher and multiple resubmissions of the same grant proposal were allowed, some investigators used their first grant submission as a way of *testing the waters*. This first review would indicate if the reviewers *liked* the topic and put the onus on the reviewer to identify the proposal's limitations. The investigator would then address these concerns in their second submission, knowing full well that they had a third submission to address any final issues.

This approach was a saving grace for procrastinators who like to wait till the deadline nears or those spontaneous investigators who respond to NIH Requests for Application (RFAs) at the last minute.

However, this old approach is no longer likely to be effective, given the current limitation of only one resubmission for the same grant proposal, as well as fairly strict NIH funding pay lines.

There are also two other reasons why this approach is problematic.

First, it is difficult to recover from a low first submission score. First impressions matter, and the reviewers assigned to your resubmission may be the same as those assigned to your first submission. Even if they are not, the new reviewers will be provided with a copy of the original reviewers' comments and typically defer to them.

Second, time is precious and the effort involved in any single submission is enormous—both on your part, on the part of your co-investigators, and your grants and contracts office.

In this current economic climate, investigators not only need to perfect the application down to the finest detail before submitting but also need to choose among their ideas and only submit their **best work**. The onus is now on the investigator to find their own study limitations and to present alternative strategies.

To be best prepared for this first submission, I always recommend starting the grant proposal writing process **four to six months in advance** of the due date depending upon the type of grant. I lean closer to four months for research grants and more toward six months for mentored grants, given the additional career development forms required. This provides time:

- To adequately review the prior literature such that the research gap can be identified
- To revise your specific aims if you find you have insufficient power
- To obtain advance feedback and incorporate the comments of your co-investigators, consultants, and mentors

DOI: 10.1201/9781003155140-3

- To consider alternatives and limitations
- To complete final fine-tuning and editing

Most importantly, this timeline allows for **iterative versions of the specific aims** such that you can incorporate your colleagues' comments and then have time for re-review and revision. The majority of the review panel will only read these aims and therefore they are the most critical portion of the grant submission (see Chapter 20, "Review Process," and Chapter 6, "Specific Aims," for how to write strong aims).

After writing your draft aims, an early stab at your power and sample size calculations avoids the last-minute panic of discovering that you have insufficient power, given your budget. Instead, it allows for a consideration of alternatives and limitations. The four-month timeline also allows for a final evaluation to see whether submission should be delayed to the next cycle to allow for the conduct of small pilot studies or the accumulation of more preliminary data to support the proposed aims.

Lastly, the timeline comfortably incorporates time for a final fine-tuning such that reviewers don't become frustrated with inconsistent table references/titling and other typographical errors, omissions, or lack of adequate citations. These small errors can significantly reduce a reviewer's enthusiasm.

2.3 TIMELINE FOR SUBMISSION OF AN NIH GRANT

Standard NIH submission due dates are three times per year (termed cycle I, cycle II, and cycle III), typically corresponding to winter, spring, and fall time periods (https://grants.nih.gov/grants/how-to-apply -application-guide/due-dates-and-submission-policies/due-dates.htm). Creating a timeline for your grant submission process will help you to meet these deadlines. Table 2.1 provides a suggested timeline for the submission of an NIH *Research* grant (i.e., R-series) that can be modified depending on the requirements of your granting agency or the type of grant. See Chapter 18, "Fellowship Grants," and Chapter 19, "Career Development Awards," for timelines specific to those types of applications.

2.4 GET INSTITUTIONAL HELP

If your institution provides you with the services of a **pre-award** grants manager or an **office of grants and contracts**, meet with these personnel early in the process and determine how they can assist you with the submission. Often, such personnel can complete many of the non-scientific forms required for the submission (see Chapter 17, "Submission of the Grant Proposal").

In addition, if you are an early-career faculty, try to involve **graduate students** (e.g., research assistants or other mentees) in the submission process. This will help you while at the same time provide the students with exposure to grantsmanship and the nuts and bolts of the submission process—critical for their own careers.

2.5 BEGIN TO ASSEMBLE THE RESEARCH TEAM EARLY

2.5.1 How to Choose Collaborators

If you are an early-career faculty, try to enlist the participation of more senior investigators with a track record of funding by your funding agency. Keeping your proposed topic in mind, determine the expertise needed to strengthen your research study team (e.g., individuals, collaborating organizations, and/or their

TABLE 2.1 Timeline for Submission of an NIH Research (R-Series) Grant Application

Four months to submission deadline
- Identify the *funding agency* (see Chapter 4, "Choosing the Right Funding Source")
- Confirm *eligibility requirements* with the funding agency Program Director
- Write *Specific Aims* (see Chapter 6, "Specific Aims")
- Calculate *power* (see Chapter 13, "Power and Sample Size")
- Assemble the *research team*
- Send specific aims/power to co-investigators, consultants, and mentors to get *feedback*
- Meet with your *research office/grants manager* to draft budget and review timeline and responsibilities

Three months to submission deadline
- Request relevant *non-scientific forms* from co-investigators and consultants (e.g., biosketches, letters of collaboration, and subcontracts)
- Revise and recirculate *Specific Aims*
- Write *Project Summary/Abstract* and send to co-investigators, consultants, and mentors (see Chapter 16, "Project Summary/Abstract")
- Start work on *Research Strategy* (i.e., Significance, Innovation, and Approach) (see Chapters 8 through 16)

Two months to submission deadline
- Complete *Research Strategy* and send to co-investigators, consultants, and mentors
- Work on *References* while research strategy is out for review
- Meet with *research office/grants manager* to finalize budget and budget justification
- Work on remainder of *scientific forms* and *non-scientific forms* (Chapter 17, "Submission of the Grant Proposal")
- Write *Project Narrative*
- Update your *Biosketch*

One month to submission deadline
- *Incorporate comments* from co-investigators, consultants, and mentors
- Send revised *final grant proposal* to co-investigators, consultants, and mentors and make final edits two weeks prior to submission
- Review all *non-scientific forms* to ensure consistency across the application
- Meet with *research office/grants manager* to incorporate any final changes to budget
- Final update to *Biosketch* (include any last-minute publications)

One week to submission deadline
- Submit application to your *research office/grants manager*
- *Research office/grants manager* submits the grant to NIH

After submission
- Start collecting *pilot data* in anticipation of a rejection
- *Resubmission* (see Chapter 21, "Resubmission of the Grant Proposal")

accompanying resources). Collaborators can fill gaps in your own expertise and can assure reviewers of the competence of your proposed team. In addition, NIH looks favorably upon interdisciplinary collaborations as they can lead to a more novel proposal with greater impact. You will find that many NIH PAs and RFPs emphasize the importance of interdisciplinary teams.

For grant-writing in epidemiology and preventive medicine, reviewers often look for a doctoral-level epidemiologist and/or statistician on the research team.

2.5.2 Common Pitfalls to Avoid

Failure to include such a *card-carrying* statistician (unless you are one yourself) is a common reason for a lower score. Enlist a statistician early in the grant-writing process right after the research question is elucidated. Collaborate closely with them on the methods, data analysis, and power/sample size sections. Be open to concerns they may have.

Similarly, be sure that your research team includes at least one clinician who is an expert in the particular health outcome of interest. Also, consider enlisting at least one co-investigator who is an expert in the main exposures of interest, even if the dataset is already built. On the other hand, be mindful of not including too many co-investigators, particularly those with no clear ties to your aims! In other words, co-investigators should not appear in name only. Reviewers will carefully watch for the inclusion of too many collaborators—otherwise known as "padding the application."

Example Research Team

Consider that you are planning to submit a grant proposal designed to prospectively identify genetic and environmental risk factors for prostate cancer. Your research team should ideally include (1) an **oncologist** who has a track record of publications on prostate cancer, (2) a **cancer** epidemiologist who has designed and led studies on prostate cancer or a related cancer, (3) a **genetic epidemiologist**, and (4) a **statistician** with expertise in genetic analyses, ideally in the cancer field.

2.6 CONSIDER A MULTIPLE PRINCIPAL INVESTIGATOR MODEL

If an interdisciplinary approach to your proposal is appropriate, consider the option of a multiple principal investigator (MPI) model. This approach is useful when your project spans multiple domains. For example, an R21 project proposing a methodology grant to validate a pregnancy physical activity questionnaire using objective measures could include three PIs: the first with expertise in the epidemiology of pregnancy physical activity, the second a kinesiologist with expertise in methods for objective monitoring of physical activity, and the third a statistician with expertise in physical activity.

An MPI model can also be particularly helpful to shore up the experience of your research team when you are an early-career faculty and have a limited track record. For example, if you are proposing a larger project that might be considered ambitious by some reviewers (e.g., an R01). Let's say you have a publication track record in the area of prostate cancer using secondary data sources. However, the proposal involves the de novo recruitment and follow-up of a relatively large sample of participants—a new area for you. In this case, consider a second PI with a track record of expertise in conducting large prospective follow-up studies.

The format, peer review, and administration of applications submitted under the MPI model have some significant differences from the traditional single principal investigator model that will need to be taken into consideration as you plan. Therefore, if you are considering an MPI model, then you will want to contact the relevant NIH program official (listed on the relevant FOA) early in the grant preparation process to discuss whether this model would be appropriate for that mechanism.

2.7 ESTABLISH WORKING RELATIONSHIPS WITH COINVESTIGATORS BEFORE SUBMISSION

Whenever possible, your grant application should demonstrate that you have established working relationships with your co-investigators. If you are early in your career, you may be concerned that you do not yet have these established relationships. However, consider the following list of options—which will provide reassurance to the reviewers of such a relationship:

- Co-authored publications (or submitted publications under review)
- Co-presentations
- An established mentoring relationship (e.g., as part of a training grant)
- Other grant applications on which you are both investigators or consultants

A pitfall to avoid   Don't rely upon the reviewers to connect the dots between you and your co-investigators. It may be obvious to you that you've co-authored publications with your collaborators, but the reviewer is unlikely to cross compare the publications in your biosketch with those in your collaborators' biosketches. Instead, make it easy for them by clearly stating your prior collaborations at multiple points in the application. These include:

- The preliminary studies section (see Chapter 9, "Preliminary Studies," for examples)
- The *Personal Statement* in their Biosketch and in your Biosketch
- In their *Letters of Support*
- The *Personnel Justification* section within the budget justification

See Part II of this text, "The Grant Proposal: Section by Section," for relevant strategies for each of these individual sections.

2.8 SPEND HALF YOUR TIME ON THE SPECIFIC AIMS AND PROJECT SUMMARY/ABSTRACT

As noted in Chapter 1, "Ten Top Tips for Successful Grant Proposal Writing," the Specific Aims should be the first item that you write when you *set pen to paper*, prior to writing your Research Strategy (i.e., Significance, Innovation, and Approach) section. Indeed, writers of successful grant applications typically report that 50% of their time is spent on revising and rewriting their specific aims (Figure 2.1). Once a draft is ready, send it to your mentor and co-investigators with the goal of kicking off an **iterative process of rewriting, revising, and re-reviewing**.

After drafting your aims, the **second step** in this process is to calculate your statistical power to achieve these aims. This will help you to answer the question, "Will your sample size provide you with sufficient power to detect a difference between groups, if there truly is a difference?" If you are basing your grant upon a preexisting dataset, your sample size will typically be fixed, and the question of whether or not you have adequate power can be answered quickly. A negative answer, while disappointing, can quickly and efficiently result in a change in study aims.

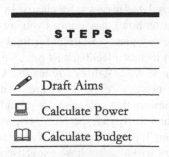

STEPS

✏ Draft Aims

🖥 Calculate Power

📖 Calculate Budget

FIGURE 2.1   The first three steps in grant proposal writing.

If instead you are proposing to launch a new study and recruit participants, you can choose the sample size that you need to achieve sufficient power. In this case, progressing to Step #3 of calculating the budget will be critical. A common pitfall of new investigators is to be too ambitious in this regard—proposing a larger sample size than they have the budget and experience to handle.

Evaluate if your budget can afford your required sample size. Such costs include the number of assays, interviewer time for recruitment and follow-up, as well as the cost of participant incentives. Also, ask yourself whether your study site can feasibly provide that number of participants. For example, does the hospital actually see that number of patients per day/week/year? Are that many patients likely to be eligible *and* agree to participate? Such questions of feasibility can be answered by your own preliminary work, by that of your co-investigators, or by other investigators at your proposed study site. Alternatively, if you are proposing a pilot grant, you can clearly state that the goal of your pilot is to assess recruitment and eligibility rates to calculate power for a larger grant submission.

Now, in light of everything you have learned from Steps 1, 2, and 3 and incorporating your mentors' and colleagues' feedback, go back and refine the aims and start the process over again. Once you have settled on the aims, you will find that writing the rest of the application will flow easily and fit within the rest of your time frame.

2.9 SOLICIT THE NON-SCIENTIFIC FORMS EARLY IN THE PROCESS

Unlike the rest of the application (e.g., the scientific component), these are the sections that you are relying primarily upon others to complete in a timely fashion. Examples of such items include mentor letters and letters of recommendation (if a training/mentored grant), co-investigator biosketches, and letters of collaboration.

Similarly, if your co-investigators are located at other institutions, you will need their subcontract forms (e.g., consortium/contractual arrangements, scope of work, facilities, and budget) signed off by their institution's office of grants and contracts. Given that you need all these materials in hand before submitting the grant to your own grants and contracts office for review, it is key to start requesting these forms early. Remember to factor in time for your own review of these external forms to ensure consistency across the application.

2.10 SOLICIT EARLY INFORMAL FEEDBACK ON YOUR GRANT PROPOSAL

The same person cannot write a proposal *and* review it for clarity. In other words, regardless of how carefully you reread your grant, and no matter how conscientious you are, simply by virtue of your familiarity with the material, you will not be able to review your grant for final clarity.

Therefore, it is always best to get as much feedback as possible, as early in the process as possible, when there is still time to make changes. We call this early feedback *low stakes*. The more feedback you can receive from your colleagues and mentors—even if they are not experts on your topic—the less likely that you will hear concerns from reviewers that you have not already addressed. The more rigorous the comments, the better, as it is more than likely that the NIH reviewers would have the same comments. Remember, as noted in Chapter 1, "Ten Top Tips for Successful Grant Proposal Writing," it is likely that some of your assigned grant reviewers will also not have expertise in your area of interest. This is why a well-written application should be readable and understandable by anyone with scientific knowledge.

Even a generalist reviewer will be able to assess (1) whether your goals are clearly stated, (2) whether your proposal clearly justifies what is new and how it extends prior work in the field, (3) what is innovative about your proposal, as well as (4) the *overall impact* of your potential findings on public health and clinical practice. In recent years, this last point has become one of the most critical factors that reviewers consider in assigning your score for an application.

Allow time for all co-investigators and consultants to review the complete proposal. At a minimum, it is customary to provide your co-investigators with a complete copy of the draft of your proposal at least 1 month before it is due. In this way, they will have two weeks to read the proposal, and then you have time to incorporate their comments and to follow-up with a revised draft or requests for clarification. Even better if you've already incorporated the co-investigator feedback much earlier in the process with their review of your specific aims. There is nothing more inconsiderate of a colleague's time than to ask for their comments at the last minute—it implies either that they do not have competing responsibilities or that you will not be incorporating their comments. This is not to say that you cannot disagree with this preliminary feedback, but that you should always leave time for a substantive discussion of suggestions that you chose not to incorporate. Then, allow plenty of time for the redrafting process.

2.11 ALLOW TIME FOR EXTERNAL REVIEW PRIOR TO SUBMISSION

In addition to asking your co-investigators to read your grant application, the use of other external reviewers will substantially increase your odds of success. The **bottom line** being that the more comments you can obtain prior to submission, the fewer comments you are likely to receive from the actual grant review panel. Given that many granting agencies provide only one opportunity for resubmission, this is critical. It is difficult to be able to improve from a poor score on a first submission to a fundable score on a second submission. Therefore, factor in time for this early review.

Your mentor should be able to assist you in identifying and recruiting external reviewers with expertise in your proposed topic area. Some departments will compensate these outside scientists or will provide funding for a grant-writing consultant. By encouraging you to convey the study aims and methods as clearly as possible, the best grant-writing consultants will help you to further refine your specific aims and convey the potential impact of your findings.

2.11.1 Chalk-Talk Forums

Another useful way to get constructive feedback on your grant proposal is to participate in a *chalk-talk forum*. These consist of informal seminars in your department where you could present your draft specific aims or research ideas to your fellow faculty members—early in the process—prior to writing a full proposal. If your department does not currently offer such a forum, suggest that they start one.

Example Description of a Chalk-Talk Forum
Chalk-talk forums will bring the department faculty together on a monthly basis to discuss grant proposals generated by early-career faculty. To maximize the utility of the session, the early-career faculty will submit a "press release" one week prior to the chalk-talk forum outlining their specific aims and corresponding public health significance. Mentors will be encouraged to assist their faculty mentee in crafting their press release. At the session, the faculty will provide feedback.

2.11.2 Mock NIH Study Sections

One of the most useful, albeit the most time-intensive, ways to get constructive feedback on your grant proposal is to participate in a *mock NIH study section*. Mock study sections simulate real NIH review panels (termed *study sections*) by following the NIH grant proposal review process as closely as possible. It is generally acknowledged that a local mock study section review can double your chances of funding by providing you with substantive feedback on your proposal prior to submission to NIH. If your department or college does not currently provide such a review panel, encourage them to start one.

Example Procedures for Conducting a Mock Study Section
Early-career faculty will submit a proposal for review using the NIH submission guidelines. The review panel will be made up of senior faculty who have served on NIH study sections, are familiar with the area of study, and have a track record of mentorship. Each proposal will be reviewed by three panel members. Faculty will receive the written reviews of their proposals and the NIH scoring system will be applied.

To provide even greater mentorship, a mock NIH study section can be modified from a true NIH study section in two key ways. First, the study section could invite the "applicants" to sit in on the mock study section as silent observers. While it may be stressful to watch the reviewers discuss your proposal, in this manner you will gain firsthand experience of the dynamics of study section deliberations—and the proposal review process begins to become demystified. You will learn to look at proposals through the eyes of a reviewer, one of the most valuable ways to learn how to write fundable grants.

Second, the study section can incorporate a short **debriefing period** after the session, during which you could talk directly with your reviewers and ask them follow-up questions. This differs substantively from a true study section in which you will only receive written comments from the reviewers. For more about the NIH review process, see Chapter 20, "Review Process."

2.12 ANTICIPATE BEING REJECTED

In your timeline, anticipate having your first submission rejected. A colleague of mine shares the rule of thumb that out of every ten grant applications submitted, you should only expect to get one successfully funded. Even the most famous scientists have had their grant proposals rejected. Reviewers like to make their mark on your application; by asking you revise and resubmit, they can see how responsive you are to their concerns and suggestions. Therefore, Chapter 21, "Resubmission of the Grant Proposal," focuses on resubmission of the grant proposal.

Identifying a Topic and Conducting the Literature Search

3

The importance of conducting a literature review early in the grant proposal writing process cannot be understated. Unlike literature reviews that you may have conducted in the past, the literature review for a grant proposal is your opportunity not only to clarify the gap in the prior research for yourself but also to clarify it for the reviewer. Showing that your proposal will extend this prior literature by filling, at least in part, this **research gap** is critical in justifying your research and obtaining funding. It is one of the key aspects on the reviewers' critique forms in their sections on "Significance" and "Innovation."

Therefore, in this chapter, I describe a three-step process for conducting a literature search designed to best justify the need for your study. This process begins with drafting a literature review outline, which in turn drives the collection of literature. The process then culminates with the completion of a summary table—a critical component to have in place before writing. These methods are key not only for grant proposals but also for journal articles. To this day, I follow the process as outlined below whenever I write a grant proposal.

The first step—creating a literature review outline—describes the process of going from your hypotheses to an outline that will serve as a roadmap for your literature search.

The second step—conducting the literature search—describes techniques for the collection of literature and goes over how to locate relevant research articles.

The third step—organizing the literature: summary tables—describes how to analyze, synthesize, and evaluate the articles in an efficient manner with the goal of clarifying and/or further refining the **research gap**.

The summary table that you create will be your guide to writing the Research Strategy (i.e., Significance, Innovation, and Approach) as described in Part II of this text, "The Grant Proposal: Section by Section."

3.1 HOW DO LITERATURE REVIEWS FOR GRANT PROPOSALS DIFFER FROM LITERATURE REVIEWS FOR JOURNAL ARTICLES?

The process of conducting the literature review for a grant proposal is essentially the same as the process of conducting the literature review for a journal article. For a journal article, the literature review is found in the Introduction section of the article. It is typically brief and usually consists of the first *one to two paragraphs* of the article. It is designed to provide the rationale for the research questions—that is, to describe the current state of literature in the topic area and clarify how the article is designed to **extend this prior research**. Similarly, the literature review for a grant proposal is found in the "Significance and Innovation" section of the proposal. The space for this section is usually limited but is typically longer

DOI: 10.1201/9781003155140-4

than a journal article depending on the granting agency's requirements (from one to two paragraphs to one to two pages). It is through this section that you assure the reviewer that the proposed study will **fill a research gap and extend prior research** in the area.

Highlighting the research gap is one of the most important components in a grant application and directly addresses the National Institutes of Health (NIH) call for applications to address the **rigor of the prior research**. Specifically, NIH Grant application instructions and the criteria by which reviewers are asked to evaluate the scientific merit of the application include components that describe the following:

- A careful assessment of the rigor of the prior research that serves as the key support for a proposed project helps to identify weakness or gaps in a line of research. NIH expects applicants to describe the general strengths and weaknesses in the rigor of the prior research that serves as the key support for the proposed project. https://grants.nih.gov/policy/reproducibility/guidance.htm.
- The strengths and weaknesses in the rigor of the prior research as the key support for the proposed project.

In summary, writing a literature review for a proposal has three main goals:

1. Provide a comprehensive and up-to-date **review of the topic**.
2. Identify the **research gap**.
3. Clarify how the proposed work will **extend the prior literature**.

3.2 HOW BIG A RESEARCH GAP DO I NEED TO FILL?

All literature reviews, whether written for a journal article or grant proposal, are designed to identify a research gap.

The research gap needs to be clearly elucidated and be of scientific importance in direct proportion to the size of the grant. The size of this research gap will vary according to the type of proposal—smaller for a pilot or feasibility study and larger for an R01 award.

In my experience, graduate students and early-career faculty are sometimes dissuaded by the presence of even one prior study that evaluated their hypothesis. They worry that there is no longer a research gap and that their hypothesis of interest has already been answered. However, recall that the **Bradford Hill criteria** (i.e., the group of minimal conditions necessary to provide adequate evidence of a causal relationship between an exposure and a disease) include *consistency*. Consistency refers to repeated observations of a similar association across different study populations using different study designs. Clearly, one prior study is not going to be sufficient to conclude *consistency*. In other words, in epidemiology and preventive medicine, it is important to remember that causality can only be determined by a multiplicity of studies of varying designs in varying study populations. As indicated in Table 3.1, there are many other possible research gaps even in the face of a large body of prior literature.

TABLE 3.1   Example Research Gaps

Prior Literature Is ...
Limited to particular study designs
Limited to particular methodology
Limited sample size
Conflicting findings
Limited control for confounding factors
Limited to particular study populations
Limited number of prior studies

For example, consider if your hypothesis is that antioxidant use will reduce the risk of Alzheimer's disease. Even as many as 20 prior epidemiologic studies on this topic can be considered insufficient if, for example, their findings have been conflicting, or if few of them used your proposed study methods, or if few utilized a prospective study design or were conducted among an at-risk study population.

3.3 THE LITERATURE REVIEW IS AN ITERATIVE PROCESS

Writing the literature review should be viewed as iterative. In other words, after searching for and reviewing the literature in the area, you may find that your aims and hypotheses need to be revised in order to convincingly extend the prior literature. The process of the literature search will often lead to a refining or even, at times, a redefining of your topic and research questions.

The key point to keep in mind, therefore, when conducting your search is that it is best to not become too wedded to your initial aims and hypotheses and to be flexible in response to what you learn in the literature search.

3.4 STEP #1: CREATING A LITERATURE REVIEW OUTLINE

The process of conducting a literature search starts with creating an outline of the literature review. The outline will directly relate to and be driven by your specific aims and hypotheses. Having an outline in hand when you start to search the literature will be invaluable in keeping you focused and avoid the common pitfall of becoming overwhelmed by the literature. Without an outline, much time can be misspent collecting literature that does not directly relate to an aspect of the proposal; or alternatively, omitting to collect literature that does relate to an aspect of the proposal. In general, all the literature collected should directly support one of the specific aims/hypotheses.

For proposals in epidemiology and preventive medicine, the literature that you will collect will typically address the areas outlined in Table 3.2.

Your first step is to create an outline. The below example specific aims and hypotheses will be used to demonstrate how to create a literature review outline:

TABLE 3.2 Example Significance and Innovation Outline

I. Significance and Innovation
  A. Importance of the topic
    i. Public health impact of the outcome
      a. Prevalence and incidence of the outcome
      b. Sequelae of the outcome
      c. Established risk factors for the outcome
      d. Prevalence and incidence of the exposure (optional)
    ii. Physiology of the exposure–outcome relationship(s)
    iii. Epidemiology of the exposure–outcome relationship(s)
  B. How previous research is limited (research gap)
  C. The overall goal of your proposal and how it will fill this research gap

Example Specific Aims and Hypotheses
Specific Aim #1: We propose to assess the relationship between menopausal hormone therapy and Alzheimer's disease in the Phoenix Health Study.
  Hypothesis #1a: Menopausal hormone therapy will be inversely associated with Alzheimer's disease.
Specific Aim #2: We propose to assess the relationship between antioxidants and Alzheimer's disease in the Phoenix Health Study.
  Hypothesis #2a: Antioxidant use will be inversely associated with Alzheimer's disease.

Corresponding Outline
A. Importance of the topic
   i. Public health impact of the outcome
       a. Prevalence and incidence of Alzheimer's disease
       b. Sequelae of Alzheimer's disease
       c. Established risk factors for Alzheimer's disease
       d. Prevalence of menopausal hormone therapy and antioxidant use
   ii. Physiology of the exposure–outcome relationships
       a. The physiologic relationship between menopausal hormone therapy and Alzheimer's disease (Hypothesis #1a)
       b. The physiologic relationship between antioxidants and Alzheimer's disease (Hypothesis #1b)
   iii. Epidemiology of the exposure–outcome relationships
       a. The prior epidemiologic studies on the relationship between menopausal hormone therapy and Alzheimer's disease (Hypothesis #1a)
       b. The prior epidemiologic studies on the relationship between antioxidants and Alzheimer's disease (Hypothesis #1b)
B. How previous research is limited (research gap)
C. The overall goal of your proposal and how it will fill this research gap

3.5 STEP #2: SEARCHING FOR LITERATURE (DOS AND DON'TS)

Now that you have your outline in hand, you are ready to start searching for literature. Remember that you will only be searching for articles that directly relate to Section i (public health impact of the outcome), Section ii (physiology of the exposure–outcome relationship), and Section iii (epidemiology of the exposure–outcome relationship). As you retrieve articles, group them in these categories. Within each category, you may want to additionally organize by topics and subtopics and in chronological order.

3.5.1 Choosing a Relevant Database

For proposal writing in epidemiology and preventive medicine, the literature review will focus on empirical research reports. These are original reports of research found in academic journals and constitute the primary sources of published information. As such, these articles provide detailed methods, results, and discussion of findings. These details will be critical in helping you justify the research gap. In contrast, secondary sources of data (e.g., textbooks, newspaper articles) provide a global description of results with few details on methods and should be avoided or used as a source of last resort.

The first step is identifying the correct database to search. Typically, for proposals in epidemiology and preventive medicine, PubMed which encompasses the MEDLINE database is the primary choice (https://www.ncbi.nlm.nih.gov/pmc/about/intro/). PubMed is a free resource supporting the search and retrieval of biomedical and life sciences literature. PubMed facilitates searching across several National Library of Medicine (NLM) literature resources including MEDLINE. The PubMed database contains more than 32 million citations and abstracts of biomedical literature. It does not include full-text journal articles; however, links to the full text are often present when available from other sources, such as the publisher's website or PubMed Central (PMC). For some epidemiologic studies that involve a psychosocial exposure or outcome, the database PsycINFO may also be relevant. Google Scholar or Lexus/Nexus may also be useful. Refer to your library's website for a description of the searchable databases to which your institution has access or contact a reference librarian for further assistance.

3.5.2 What Type of Literature to Collect for Each Section of the Literature Review Outline

Using the example above, I will describe the type of literature to collect for each section of the literature review outline.

3.5.2.1 i. Public Health Impact of the Outcome

a. Prevalence and incidence of the outcome

The goal of this section of the grant proposal is to describe the public health significance of your outcome of interest (e.g., Alzheimer's disease). Search for literature that shows the current **prevalence and incidence rates** of Alzheimer's disease, changes in incidence rates over time, and how many people are affected by this disorder. If your grant will be conducted among a particular subpopulation, collect literature that not only provides national rates but also provides specific rates in your subpopulation (e.g., postmenopausal women) or the geographic region where the study will be conducted if these rates are available. The goal is to start broad and then drill down as closely as possible to rates in your proposed study population.

Depending on your study outcome, these data can be found on such websites as the Centers for Disease Control and Prevention (CDC) and Surveillance, Epidemiology, and End Results (SEER) Program or in published findings from large surveillance studies such as the *National Health and Nutrition Examination Survey*. Another efficient way to locate such incidence/prevalence data can be found by carefully reading the introductions of journal articles that you included in Section iii (epidemiology of the exposure–outcome relationship) below. A well-written introduction to a journal article will cite current rates and provide a corresponding citation. By obtaining these cited articles, you can get a head start on identifying sources of such data.

b. Sequelae of the outcome

The second important way to support the public health importance of your outcome of interest is to collect literature that describes the **sequelae of your outcome/disease**. Does your outcome (e.g., Alzheimer's disease) lead to significant future morbidity and/or mortality?

c. Established risk factors for the outcome

Thirdly, collect literature that demonstrates the **established risk factors** for your outcome of interest. Locate studies (or a review article) that describe established risk factors for your outcome (e.g., Alzheimer's disease).

d. Prevalence and incidence of the exposure (optional)

Finally, the public health impact of your proposal can be further enhanced by collecting literature that describes the prevalence and incidence of your exposure. In terms of the example above, studies showing a high and/or increasing prevalence of menopausal hormone therapy would be relevant. In other words, the more the people exposed, the greater the potential public health impact of your proposal.

3.5.2.2 ii. Physiology of Exposure–Outcome Relationship

The goal of this section of the grant proposal is to describe the physiologic or behavioral rationale for a potential relationship between your exposure and your outcome (Figure 3.1). In other words, your job in this section is to demonstrate that there is a feasible mechanism by which your exposure may impact your disease. In terms of our example, search for literature that describes the physiologic mechanisms by which menopausal hormone therapy could impact Alzheimer's disease.

It is easy to go astray in this section by collecting literature which only focuses on the physiology of your **outcome** in isolation. In doing so, you'll inadvertently fail to identify literature that describes the potential mechanism by which your exposure may influence your outcome. Using our example above, avoid only collecting literature on the physiology of Alzheimer's disease—its symptoms, signs, and impact on the body. Instead, focus on literature that describes the **mechanism** by which hormones may impact Alzheimer's disease. Certainly a basic knowledge of how Alzheimer's disease develops is key to understanding how it could be impacted by exposures such as hormones. However, failure to cite literature which addresses the **link** between menopausal hormone therapy and Alzheimer's disease is failure to justify your specific aim.

A pitfall to avoid A similar pitfall to avoid is collecting literature that only focuses on the physiology of your **exposure** variable in isolation. Using our example above, collecting literature that simply describes the general impact of menopausal hormone therapy on the body would not be sufficient. Instead, after a brief description of how hormones function, locate literature that shows how menopausal hormone therapy could influence the occurrence of Alzheimer's disease.

Remember that reviewers are expected to have a general scientific knowledge. So, in light of your page limitations, focus on the causal mechanisms between your exposure and your disease (see Figure 3.1).

3.5.2.3 iii. Epidemiology of Exposure–Outcome Relationship

The goal of this section of the grant proposal is to summarize the findings of prior epidemiologic studies that evaluated the association between your exposure and outcome. Search for epidemiologic studies that included, using our example, an evaluation of the relationship between menopausal hormone therapy and risk of Alzheimer's disease.

A pitfall to avoid For this section, collect prior studies **regardless of whether the studies found positive, negative, or null results**. It will be important for you to describe the full state of the science on this topic and not to omit anything that does not support your findings. It can be reassuring to note that a common "research gap" is the simple fact that the prior literature has observed contradictory findings. Also, consider the fact that some of the reviewers will be authors of these contradictory or null papers and would not appreciate having their paper omitted from your summary.

What not to include: When searching through the prior epidemiologic literature, articles that only provide information on the prevalence of your exposure without also evaluating the relationship between your exposure and your outcome would not merit inclusion in this section. For example, a paper that just

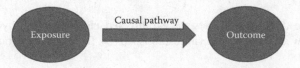

FIGURE 3.1 The causal pathway between an exposure and an outcome.

gave incidence rates of Alzheimer's disease would be very useful for Section i.a. (prevalence and incidence of the outcome), but unless it also gave **measures of association** between menopausal hormone therapy and Alzheimer's disease, it is not relevant for this epidemiology section. Instead, look for studies that present measures of association (e.g., relative risks [RRs], odds ratios, correlation coefficients, or mean differences in levels of the outcome) between exposed and unexposed groups.

3.5.3 Should You Collect Epidemiologic Literature That Only Secondarily Evaluated Your Exposure–Outcome Relationship?

Sometimes an epidemiologic study will have evaluated your exposure and outcome relationship but only as an ancillary analysis in the context of a larger topic on which they are primarily focused. Using our example, let's consider that a prior published study evaluated the association between stress, as the exposure variable, and its impact on Alzheimer's disease. However, in their tables, the authors also included findings on the impact of menopausal hormone therapy on Alzheimer's disease. Perhaps they conducted this *sidebar* analysis to assess menopausal hormone therapy as a potential confounder of stress.

Even though your exposure–outcome relationship of interest was not the prior publication's relationship of interest, if their tables provide measures of association between your exposure and outcome variables, then it is still relevant to include this article. At the same time, it is also important to note that these findings are often unadjusted for potential confounding factors. That is, they simply show the unadjusted relationship between your exposure (e.g., menopausal hormone therapy) and your outcome (Alzheimer's disease). Most likely, you will be improving upon these prior findings!

3.5.4 Collecting Literature for an Effect Modification Hypothesis

You may also wish to evaluate whether the relationship between your exposure and disease of interest differs within the strata of your population. In other words, you might hypothesize that the relationship will be different among one particular subgroup of people as compared to another. Subgroups could be groups of differing sex, gender, races, ethnicities, ages, or other factors. This is classically termed effect modification or interaction. If this is of interest, include this question as a hypothesis. By including this hypothesis *a priori* (i.e., before the research has been initiated), you will minimize reviewer concerns that you are simply *data dredging* or on a *fishing expedition*.

Using our example above, let's say that you found physiologic studies that suggested that the impact of menopausal hormone therapy on Alzheimer's disease might be stronger among women with obesity; in other words, that there may be some type of synergy between obesity and menopausal hormone therapy. If so, it would be reasonable to assume a different physiological association between menopausal hormone therapy and Alzheimer's disease among women with obesity than among women without obesity. This hypothesis must also be addressed in the outline (see Table 3.3).

The example below uses our same proposed study as earlier, but now adds an effect modification aim. For simplicity, I've removed the second specific aim evaluating the impact of antioxidant use on Alzheimer's disease from this example:

Example Effect Modification Specific Aims and Hypotheses
> Specific Aim #1: We propose to assess the relationship between menopausal hormone therapy and Alzheimer's disease in the Phoenix Health Study.
>> Hypothesis #1a: Menopausal hormone therapy will be inversely associated with Alzheimer's disease.
>> **Hypothesis #1b: There will be a stronger inverse association between menopausal hormone therapy and Alzheimer's disease among women with obesity as compared to women without obesity.**

$\begin{array}{l} e \\ \text{example} \end{array}$ **Corresponding Outline**

A. Importance of the topic
  i. Public health impact of the outcome
    a. Prevalence and incidence of Alzheimer's disease
    b. Sequelae of Alzheimer's disease
    c. Established risk factors for Alzheimer's disease
    d. Prevalence of menopausal hormone therapy and antioxidant use
  ii. Physiology of the exposure–outcome relationship(s)
    a. The physiologic relationship between menopausal hormone therapy and Alzheimer's disease
    b. The physiologic relationship between menopausal hormone therapy and Alzheimer's disease among women with obesity and among women without obesity
  iii. Epidemiology of the exposure–outcome relationship(s)
    a. The prior epidemiologic studies on the relationship between menopausal hormone therapy and Alzheimer's disease
    b. The prior epidemiologic studies on the relationship between menopausal hormone therapy and Alzheimer's disease among women with obesity and among women without obesity
B. How previous research is limited (research gap)

TABLE 3.3   Example Significance and Innovation Outline Including an Effect Modification Aim

I. Significance and Innovation
A. Importance of the topic
  i. Public health impact of the outcome
    a. Prevalence and incidence of the outcome
    b. Sequelae of the outcome
    c. Established risk factors for the outcome
    d. Prevalence and incidence of the exposure (optional)
  ii. Physiology of the exposure–outcome relationship(s)
    a. The physiologic relationship between the exposure and outcome
    b. *How the above* physiologic relationship differs among strata of an effect modifier [optional—if proposing an effect modification hypothesis]
  iii. Epidemiology of the exposure–outcome relationship(s)
    a. The epidemiologic relationship between the exposure and outcome
    b. *How the above epidemiologic relationship differs among strata of an effect modifier* [optional—if proposing an effect modification hypothesis]
B. How previous research is limited (research gap)

To support this new effect modification aim, you will now need to locate literature suggesting that there is a different physiologic association between menopausal hormone therapy and Alzheimer's disease in women with obesity.

Secondly, check each of the epidemiologic studies that you already collected as part of Section iii (epidemiology of the exposure–outcome relationship) to see whether those authors also evaluated the same effect modification hypothesis. Summarize their findings to inform the reviewers how this work extends the prior literature.

3.5.5 How to Start the Search

First, consider which section of the outline that your search is aiming to fill. For the epidemiology section, adding the key term *epidemiology* along with your other keywords to the search box will help to limit your search to population-based studies and not bench science.

Once you identify relevant articles, check their **reference lists** for additional relevant citations. Start with the most recent article and work backward using the reference list of each article. At some point, you will have reached a saturation point where you see that each manuscript is pointing to another one that you already have in hand.

Another good first step is to start with a **review article** on your topic. This can be done by limiting the search to "review articles" using the filter option. However, caution should still be taken. Although review articles provide you with a comprehensive reference list, you will still need to search for articles published since the review. In addition, often review articles are on a similar, but not identical, topic to yours—therefore requiring more searching on your part. Also, I cannot emphasize enough that it is not sufficient to abstract information on the individual studies as presented in review article. Instead, obtain copies of each relevant article referenced in the review. Review articles rarely present the level of detail that you will require and you want to avoid relying on the author of the review article for the accuracy of their abstracted information.

3.5.6 What to Do When Your Search Yields Thousands of *Hits*

Search engines such as PubMed make the search process easier but have the associated hazards of retrieving too many *hits*. Imagine the shock faced by a faculty member proposing to evaluate the association between coffee and bladder cancer when they find 30,000 hits after entering the key terms *coffee* and *bladder cancer*, many of which will not be directly relevant to their proposal.

Therefore, the first step is learning how to carefully limit the search. Consider your choice of key search terms. As noted in the example above, inserting the term "**epidemiology**" will help to limit the search to epidemiologic studies. In addition, restricting where the search term must appear (e.g., **title or title/abstract**) will also limit the number of hits. In PubMed, such a limit can be set using the *filter* option.

Another approach is to limit the search to **key journals** in your field. For example, a search limited to *American Journal of Epidemiology* will ensure that you start out with some key epidemiology articles in your area. To do this in PubMed, enter the standard journal abbreviation *Am J Epidemiol* in the search box along with your key terms.

In a similar vein, consider limiting the search to a specific time frame. Typically searches are limited to the **past 5–10 years**. If the techniques/methodology for studying your topic have changed, it would be perfectly reasonable to limit the search to the years since these advances. Share this rationale with your reviewer so that they aren't concerned if an older paper, of which they are familiar, is not included.

If you are proposing to conduct a study of a particularly design, for example, a clinical trial, then it would be reasonable to limit your search to prior clinical trials. In this manner, your summary table will help you to clearly articulate how your study advances the prior clinical trial research in this area.

3.5.7 What to Do If There Are Too Few Hits

Conducting a search that yields no, or few, hits can be a particular concern. In an area that is little studied, you may be forced to go back several decades to obtain the relevant work on your topic. Even if a study is older, if it is the only evidence available on a given topic, then it is important to include. It is also reasonable to include a landmark or classic study in the area whose inclusion helps to understand the evolution of a research technique.

If you determine that there is no literature with a direct bearing on one or more aspects of your topic, this should be cautiously viewed as good news. That is, you may have identified a research gap. However, at the same time, you need to assure the reviewers that your proposed hypotheses are reasonable. There are two approaches to address this:

1. Search for studies with *same exposure* as yours, but a *different, albeit physiologically related, outcome*.

2. Search for studies with *same outcome* as yours, but a *different, albeit physiologically related, exposure*.

In terms of the first approach, the concept is to choose an outcome similar to your own, so that a reasonable reviewer would consider it possible that a similar mechanism might link your exposure to your outcome. See the example below.

Example of How to Proceed if There Is Sparse Literature on Your Topic
Search on a physiologically similar *outcome*:
Consider a proposal to study the association between prenatal depression and risk of gestational diabetes mellitus (defined as diabetes that develops during pregnancy). You conduct a search for epidemiologic studies on this topic using PubMed but find no studies. Therefore, you select a physiologically similar outcome—searching instead on prenatal depression and **type 2 diabetes** (outside of pregnancy). You find a plethora of studies supporting an association. In your proposal, you argue that if depression impacts diabetes, then it is reasonable to assume that it also impacts prenatal depression.

In terms of the second approach, select an exposure similar in nature to your exposure. Again, the criteria for including such studies should be to bolster up a reasonable physiologic mechanism for your proposed, but clearly novel, association.

Example of How to Proceed if There Is Sparse Literature on Your Topic
Search on a physiologically similar *exposure*:
Consider a proposal to study the association between prenatal depression and risk of gestational diabetes mellitus (defined as diabetes that develops during pregnancy). You conduct a search for epidemiologic studies on this topic using PubMed but find no studies. Therefore, you select a physiologically similar exposure—searching instead on **stress/anxiety** and gestational diabetes. You find a plethora of studies supporting an association. In your proposal, you argue that if stress/anxiety impacts risk of gestational diabetes, then it is reasonable to assume that depression also impacts risk of gestational diabetes.

3.5.8 How to Retrieve Articles (Hits)

Most universities provide their faculty with access to online versions of most journal articles. These are often immediately available to you via your university library's subscriptions or after requesting an interlibrary loan which will also be sent to you electronically. As noted earlier, PubMed does not include full-text journal articles. However, links to the full text are often present when available from other sources, such as the publisher's website or PubMed Central (PMC). If you cannot locate the complete text of a journal article in this manner, it is also acceptable to email the corresponding author of the article.

3.5.9 How to Scan Articles for Relevance

Once you retrieve articles, the first step is to quickly scan the:

- Abstract
- Last paragraph of the Introduction
- Tables
- First and last paragraphs of the Conclusion

In scanning the article, your goal is simply to identify whether this article will provide key substantive findings that will support the key sections of your literature search outline as delineated above. The **Abstract** will, in 200–250 words, encapsulate the key aspects of the paper including the goals/purpose, study design, study methods, highlights of the results, and primary conclusions. The last paragraph(s) of the **Introduction** is important as this is where the authors will have summarized the relevant prior literature. Cross check their citations with yours to ensure you aren't missing any. The Introduction will also articulate the research gap and the specific aims and hypotheses of the article. Then go directly to the **tables** to see whether they provide relevant measures of association between your exposure and your outcome. The first and last paragraphs of the **Conclusion** are also key because this is where the author will reiterate the major findings of the article.

3.5.10 Evaluating Your References for Completeness

At this point, you should now have collected articles that relate to Section i (public health impact of the outcome), Section ii (physiology of the exposure–outcome relationship), and Section iii (epidemiology of the exposure–outcome relationship). Ensure that your list is complete and up to date. The *Significance and Innovation* section of your grant proposal will need to demonstrate that it represents the latest work done in the subject area. Grant reviewers or journal reviewers are selected based on their expertise in the field. Imagine their concern if they are assigned to review your proposal and see that you did not cite their relevant publications.

3.6 STEP #3: ORGANIZING THE EPIDEMIOLOGIC LITERATURE—SUMMARY TABLES

A summary table is an invaluable tool for organizing the epidemiologic literature collected for Section iii (epidemiology of exposure–outcome relationship). You are probably familiar with summary tables as they are included in review articles as an efficient way to present the key aspects of the published studies in an area. Indeed, the process of creating a summary table will be one of the most valuable activities in helping you to identify the major trends or patterns in the literature and thereby identifying the **research gap**—one of the most critical aspects looked for by reviewers in scoring an application.

3.6.1 What Data Should I Include in a Summary Table?

Summary tables are flexible and can be customized to best highlight your research gap (Table 3.4). Standard column headings include the **Author/Year**. Order the studies chronologically.

The **Study Design** column includes the name of the study design (e.g., prospective cohort, cross-sectional, case-control, and ecologic/correlational or subvariations of these studies).

The **Study Population** column typically includes the sample size and the study location. If you are proposing to conduct your study within a particular subpopulation (e.g., Black/African American or children), also list the percentage of people in these subgroups in this column to further highlight a research gap.

The **Exposure Assessment** can include up to four or more columns that concisely describe the *tool* used to measure your exposure; the *timing* of assessment (e.g., at six-month post intervention or at baseline); how this variable was *parameterized* (e.g., as a dichotomous variable, a categorical variable, or a continuous variable); and whether it was *validated*. For example, using our prior example, this column would state how menopausal hormone therapy was assessed (e.g., self-reported questionnaire, medical record abstraction).

TABLE 3.4 Example Summary Table for Organizing the Epidemiologic Literature

AUTHOR, YEAR	STUDY DESIGN	STUDY POPULATION	EXPOSURE		OUTCOME	EFFECT	ESTIMATE
			TYPE OF PHYSICAL ACTIVITY	WHEN ASSESSED	BIRTH WEIGHT		
Jones, 2021	Prospective cohort	500 prenatal patients; NYC	Occupational	Once at 20 weeks gestation	Medical record abstraction	⟵	1.60 (95% CI 1.10–1.90)
Smith, 2020	Prospective cohort	3000 prenatal patients; Utah	Total	Once at 23–26 weeks gestation	Birth certificates	⟶	0.75 (95% CI 0.45–0.92)
Tyler, 2019	Prospective cohort	250 prenatal patients; Australia	Occupational, household	Each trimester at 17, 28, and 36 weeks gestation	Medical record abstraction	⟷	Nonsignificant mean differences
Frank, 2017	Prospective cohort	800 prenatal patients; Sweden	Recreational	Each trimester	Medical record abstraction	⟶	0.61 (95% CI 0.48–0.85)

The **Outcome Assessment** can include up to four or more columns that concisely describe the *tool* used to measure your outcome; the *timing* of assessment (e.g., at six-month post intervention or at baseline); how this variable was *parameterized* (e.g., as a dichotomous variable, a categorical variable, or a continuous variable); and whether it was *validated*. For example, using our prior example, this column would state how Alzheimer's disease was assessed (e.g., proxy questionnaire, medical record abstraction).

The **Results** column should concisely provide findings on your association of interest. Provide the actual magnitude of association (e.g., RRs, odds ratios, correlation coefficients) between your exposure and outcome as opposed to simply listing *p*-values.

Other potential columns to consider include a **Covariates** column that lists all the adjustment factors and an **Exclusions** column.

3.6.2 Tips to Make Your Summary Table Most Useful

Be consistent across studies in the type of data that you present. In other words, if you provide the age range for one study, then do it for all the studies in the table.

Many articles will have assessed **multiple exposures and outcomes**. Don't list exposures and outcomes that you won't be assessing in your study, regardless of whether the authors evaluated them. Similarly, only list those that provide the results for the associations that you'll also be evaluating in your proposal. Remember that the reviewer can always access their complete journal article. Instead, this is a summary table designed for you to identify research gaps in your specific area. The summary table should be *lean and mean*.

If you have **several outcome variables**, it is preferable to create separate tables for each outcome type. Similarly, if you have one outcome variable but **several exposure variables**, you may want to create separate tables for each exposure type. In both of these situations, the same papers may be included in both tables; however, key measurement columns as well as Results columns will differ, and you will find it useful to have the entire details of these studies in both tables.

The Results column: A pitfall to avoid Be as specific and concise as possible in the Results column. Present the actual numerical findings showing the *magnitude of association* between your exposure and outcome, as opposed to quoting a narrative of the text of the findings. For example, "OR = 3.2, 95% CI 2.1–3.5" is more concise than a statement like *The authors found a positive association between physical activity and risk of low birth weight*. The latter sentence is not only cumbersome to read, but it does not provide key information on the magnitude of association nor the variability of the findings. Based on this sentence alone, the reviewer would not know if the authors found only a 10% increased risk or a fourfold increased risk.

Always try to insert a *measure of variation* (e.g., confidence intervals, standard deviations), instead/in addition to text. Instead of using phrases like "significantly different," insert the actual findings and confidence intervals. The same holds true for findings that were not statistically significant—present those associations and measures of variation too. It is just as important to include studies with null findings as studies with statistically significant findings in your summary table. One could argue that it is even more important as it points out a potential research gap that your study could fill. For example, perhaps the methods used in those prior studies faced more measurement error than yours will, which led to their failure to observe an association.

Even more simply, consider inserting arrows in the Results column, that is, up arrows for positive associations, down arrows for inverse associations, and cross arrows for null associations. In this manner, you can quickly scan across this column to assess the overall thrust of prior study findings.

Lastly, be sure that the results you provide correspond to the list of Exposure and Outcome measures in the earlier columns. For example, be careful not to list an exposure in the exposure column without saying how it's related to the outcome in the Results column.

3.6.3 Reviewing the Table to Identify Research Gaps

As mentioned earlier, your goal in creating the table is not only to summarize the prior literature but also to **make the research gaps clearly evident**. In reviewing the table, make note of trends (weaknesses) across studies. For example, looking down the *Study Design* column, ask yourself questions such as "Are the majority of studies cross sectional?" "Are the majority of studies based on small sample sizes?" Look at the characteristics of the participants and note if any groups at high risk of your outcome are not included. These are *research gaps*.

Continue to examine the table and note whether study findings in the **Results** column differ according to the study designs or measurement techniques used. For example, ask yourself, "Do all studies that support a certain conclusion use one method of measurement, while those that support a different conclusion use a different method?" "Do all studies that support a certain conclusion control for key confounding factors?"

Now that you have examined the summary table with this goal in mind, you may want to make modifications to the table. This may involve adding column headings, or column content, to make the research gaps most apparent. For example, if you will be the first to use a new measurement technique, you'll want to be sure that your **Exposure Assessment** column lists the measurement techniques used by each study. In this way, a scan of that column will make it evident that no or few prior studies used your proposed measurement technique. If your study is the first study to adjust for body mass index (BMI), you'll want to include a **Covariates** column that lists all the adjustment factors. In this way, a scan of that column will make it clear that no or few prior studies evaluated BMI. For example, in a proposed study of physical activity and low birth weight, I included a column titled **Validated Exposure Assessment**. The response under this column for each study was *no*, making it clear that no prior study had used a measure of physical activity validated in pregnant women—a key research gap.

If your study will be filling these research gaps, then you'll want to highlight these facts when writing the Significance and Innovation sections of the grant (as described in Chapter 8, "Significance and Innovation"). Having this summary table in hand when you start the writing process will make this process go much more smoothly. It is also reasonable at this point to consider altering your hypotheses in light of your findings. Remember if it is not clear to you that you will be extending the prior literature, then it certainly will not be to your reviewers.

Example Identification of Research Gaps from a Summary Table
Consider that you are proposing to evaluate the association between physical activity during pregnancy and birth weight. After reviewing the summary table (Table 3.4), you note two themes: (1) few studies measured physical activity each trimester of pregnancy and (2) only one study measured total activity (e.g., occupational + household + recreational). Indeed, the one study that measured physical activity in each trimester did **not** measure the total activity. Therefore, you revise your proposal to measure *total physical activity at all three trimesters* of pregnancy—becoming the first study to date to do so.

3.6.4 Should I Include the Summary Table in My Grant Proposal?

Due to space limitations, the summary table is not typically included in the actual grant proposal submission. Regardless, the table will still be critical in your writing process. Your acquired grasp of the prior published literature in your area—the number of studies and their trends as to methods, findings, and gaps—will readily come across as discussed in the *Significance and Innovation* section. However, as a side benefit, the table may be useful for writing a review article and submitting that for publication.

3.7 EXAMPLE LITERATURE REVIEW OUTLINE AND SUMMARY TABLE

USE OF NON-STEROIDAL ANTI-INFLAMMATORY DRUGS (NSAIDS) AND RISK OF ENDOMETRIAL CANCER IN POSTMENOPAUSAL WOMEN

LITERATURE REVIEW OUTLINE

I. Significance and Innovation
  A. Importance of endometrial cancer
    i. Public health impact of endometrial cancer
      a. Prevalence and incidence of endometrial cancer in the United States overall, in women, and in postmenopausal women
      b. Sequelae of endometrial cancer
      c. Established risk factors for endometrial cancer
      d. Prevalence of NSAIDS use
    ii. Physiology of the relationship between NSAIDS and endometrial cancer
      a. Hormone-mediated mechanism
      b. Insulin-mediated mechanism
      c. Inflammatory mechanism
    iii. Epidemiology of the relationship between NSAIDS and endometrial cancer
  B. How previous research is limited (research gap) (Table 3.5)

TABLE 3.5 Example Summary Table for a Proposal to Evaluate the Use of NSAIDS and Risk of Endometrial Cancer in Postmenopausal Women,

AUTHOR, YEAR	STUDY DESIGN	STUDY POPULATION	NSAIDS TYPE	EXPOSURE WHEN/HOW	EXPOSURE STRATIFIED BY	OUTCOME WHAT	OUTCOME HOW	EFFECT ESTIMATE	ADJUSTMENT FACTORS
Smith et al., 2021	Case-control study	400 matched pairs, age 35–50, received medical services at Georgia Hospital, 2010–2012	A: Aspirin	Self-administered questionnaire	BMI	Cases: endometrial cancer; controls: nonneoplastic conditions	Cases and controls identified from tumor registry	(1) ↔A: Regular users vs. nonusers OR: 0.96 (95% CI: 0.71–1.31) (2) ↓A: Obese users vs. normal weight users OR: 0.45 (95% CI: 0.22–0.87)	Age, education, BMI, parity, age at menarche, and menopause
Jones et al., 2021	Prospective cohort study	50,000 female teachers, age 30–55 years in the US	A: Aspirin, NA: Non-aspirin NSAIDS	Self-administered questionnaire at baseline	BMI	Self-reported cases of endometrial cancer	Cases confirmed by physicians reviewing medical records	(1) ↔A: Past vs. never users RR: 1.17 (95% CI: 0.94–1.47); (2) ↔A: Current vs. never users RR: 1.08 (95% CI: 0.88–1.32) (3) ↔A: Obese current users vs. obese never users RR: 0.61 (95% CI: 0.41–0.91)	Age, BMI, smoking, oral contraceptive use, menopausal hormone therapy age at menarche and menopause, hypertension, diabetes

(Continued)

TABLE 3.5 (CONTINUED)   Example Summary Table for a Proposal to Evaluate the Use of NSAIDS and Risk of Endometrial Cancer in Postmenopausal Women

AUTHOR, YEAR	STUDY DESIGN	STUDY POPULATION	NSAIDS TYPE	EXPOSURE		OUTCOME			EFFECT ESTIMATE	ADJUSTMENT FACTORS
				WHEN/HOW	STRATIFIED BY	WHAT	HOW			
Frances et al., 2020	Case-control study	200 cases, 205 controls, age 50–70, New York	*Any:* Any NSAIDS, *A:* Aspirin, *NA:* Non-aspirin NSAIDS	Interview	BMI	Cases of endometrial cancer diagnosis	Cases: Dept. of Health and State Cancer Registry; controls of <65 years of age by random dig. dialing; controls of >65 years by Center for Medicare & Medicaid Services (CMS) data		(1) ↓*Any:* Users vs. nonusers OR: 0.6 (95% CI: 0.4–0.98) (2) ↓*A:* users vs. nonusers OR: 0.6 (95% CI: 0.3–1.0) (3) ↓*NA:* Users vs. nonusers OR: 0.7 (95% CI: 0.4–1.3) (4) *NA:* Lower vs. higher BMI ↓OR: 0.7 (95% CI: 0.4–1.4)	Age, BMI, education race, menarche, hormone therapy, oral contraceptive use age at menopause, parity, family history of endometrial cancer
Dodge et al., 2019	Prospective cohort study	65,000 women in Taipei Diet and Health Study, age 50–71 years, 2010–2013	*Any:* Any NSAIDS, *A:* Aspirin, *NA:* Non-aspirin NSAIDS	Mailed questionnaire	BMI	Cases of endometrial cancer	North American Association of Central Cancer Registries		(1) ↔*Any:* Users vs. nonusers RR: 0.7 (95% CI: 0.5–0.97) (2) ↔*A:* Users vs. nonusers RR: 0.7 (95% CI: 0.4–1.0) (3) ↔*NA:* Users vs. nonusers; RR: 0.8 (95% CI: 0.5–1.3) (4) *A:* Obese users vs. obese nonusers RR: 0.7 (95% CI: 0.4–1.4)	Age at menarche and menopause, race, PMH use, parity, oral contraceptive use, smoking, BMI, physical activity, diabetes, hypertension, heart disease, family history of breast cancer

(Continued)

TABLE 3.5 (CONTINUED)   Example Summary Table for a Proposal to Evaluate the Use of NSAIDS and Risk of Endometrial Cancer in Postmenopausal Women

| AUTHOR, YEAR | STUDY DESIGN | STUDY POPULATION | EXPOSURE | | | OUTCOME | | EFFECT ESTIMATE | ADJUSTMENT FACTORS |
			NSAIDS TYPE	WHEN/HOW	STRATIFIED BY	WHAT	HOW		
Grainger et al., 2019	Case-control study	250 cases and 405 controls, age 50–74 years (2007–2010)	Any: Any NSAIDS, A: Aspirin	In-person interview	BMI	Cases of endometrial cancer; controls: cases of ovarian cancer	Cases: cancer surveillance system affiliated with SEER; controls: random dig. dialing	(1) ↔Any: Users vs. nonusers OR: 1.01 (95% CI: 0.8–1.5); (2) ↔A: Users vs. nonusers OR: 1.02 (95% CI: 0.6–1.77); (3) ↔Any: Obese users vs. nonusers OR: 0.91 (95% CI: 0.61–1.42)	Age, residence, calendar year, BMI, hormone therapy use
Roth et al., 2018	Prospective cohort study	12,000 females, age 55–69 years, Western Health Study 2000–2010	A: Aspirin, NA: Non-aspirin NSAIDS	Mailed questionnaire at baseline	BMI (data not shown)	Cases of endometrial cancer	Identified from State Health Registry	(1) ↔A: Users vs. nonusers HR: 0.77 (95% CI: 0.59–1.01); (2) ↔NA: Users vs. nonusers HR: 0.87 (95% CI: 0.67–1.10)	Age, BMI, age at menarche and menopause, history of oral contraceptive use, history of diabetes and hypertension

Choosing the Right Funding Source

4

This chapter will walk you through choosing the right funding source for your grant proposal. It is divided into three parts—Part I: "Developing Your Grant-Funding Plan" provides strategic advice for launching your grantsmanship career in collaboration with a mentor, Part II: "Funding Mechanisms for Early-Career Grants," and Part III "Step-by-Step Advice for Finding the Right Funding Source at NIH" go over considerations in choosing the right funding source. Navigating the NIH grant system can be overwhelming; however, NIH is the most typical funding source for epidemiology and preventive medicine, particularly for larger awards—the ultimate career goal. Indeed, the NIH Office of Extramural Research is the largest funder of biomedical research in the world, and NIH funds research in just about every area that's remotely related to human health and disease.

In November 2019, NIH published an updated Notice of Interest in Diversity (https://grants.nih.gov/grants/guide/notice-files/NOT-OD-20-031.html). This Notice explains that innovation and scientific discovery are enhanced by including individuals from diverse groups including those that are underrepresented in the biomedical, clinical, behavioral, and social sciences. NIH defines underrepresented individuals as those from underrepresented racial and ethnic groups, individuals with disabilities, individuals from disadvantaged backgrounds, and women. This chapter describes selected diversity-related funding opportunity announcements, and a complete list can be found at https://extramural-diversity.nih.gov/guidedata/data.

4.1 PART I: DEVELOPING YOUR GRANT-FUNDING PLAN

4.1.1 Steps for Success

4.1.1.1 Step #1: Locate a Mentor for Grantsmanship

As noted in Chapter 1, "Ten Top Tips for Successful Grant Proposal Writing," one of the top ten tips (Tip #1: Start Small but Have a Big Vision) was to create a vision of your ultimate large grant project with the help of a mentor. If you do not currently have a mentor, speak to your department chair and ask whether she or he can provide you with one. Consider both on-site and off-site faculty as potential mentors. For example, if the work of your departmental colleagues does not relate to your primary area of interest, then seeking external mentors is particularly important. Chapter 1 goes on to provide additional tips for locating a mentor and what constitutes an ideal mentor.

4.1.1.2 Step #2: Develop Your Overall Grantsmanship Goal

Once you have identified a mentor or mentorship team, it is best to sit down together to create your overall grantsmanship plan. Each small grant—be it a seed grant, a predoctoral fellowship, or an early-career award—should be viewed as providing preliminary data for one or two of the specific aims of your ultimate larger grant. Typically, large grants are funded by the NIH R01 mechanism.

DOI: 10.1201/9781003155140-5

Let's assume that a typical R01 contains three to five specific aims. Start with applying to small grant mechanisms in which each application is designed to support **one or two** of these ultimate aims. These small grants should not be designed to provide the definitive answer to these aims but instead to show that the aims are feasible and/or provide preliminary data in their support. These small grants will be limited by smaller sample sizes and budgets but will be able to demonstrate proof of principal—that you can *pull it off.* See Chapter 1, "Ten Top Tips for Successful Grant Proposal Writing," for an example of putting this tip into action.

4.1.2 Plan for a Steady Trajectory of Grants from Small to Large

Start out by capitalizing on funding mechanisms designed to support small projects targeted to early-career faculty or postdoctoral fellows. Below is an example schematic demonstrating the progression from a small internal seed grant to modest NIH grants (e.g., Career Awards) and then culminating in the receipt of an NIH R01 (Figure 4.1).

Note that the **order of the smaller steps is flexible**. For example, you might consider submitting an application to NIH for a Career Development Award (K award) prior to an R21 or R03 due to the limited time period of eligibility for mentored individual career awards (e.g., within six years of your postdoctoral degree). Then, you might consider applying for an R21 or R03 second.

4.1.2.1 Avoid Classic Pitfall #1: Don't Skip Straight to Large Funding Mechanisms

Early-career faculty want to be successful and, as such, are often tempted by the wish to immediately make a big impact and *land a big grant*. Others are under pressure from their institutions and department chairs to immediately apply for a large grant (e.g., an NIH R01) without a track record of smaller grant funding. In my experience as an NIH review panel member, this approach is almost certainly destined to fail.

The majority of review panels consider a large grant to be the culmination of a growing body of work. That is, a desirable grant-funding history starts from small seed grants progressing to larger and larger awards in a cumulative fashion. Reviewers like to see evidence of this stairway to success, and it's your job to demonstrate that you have been on this stairway.

Smaller grants provide critical evidence to reviewers that you can successfully:

- Write grant applications
- Manage the logistics of grant projects
- Translate these grants into publications

Several exceptions to the above pitfall are described below.

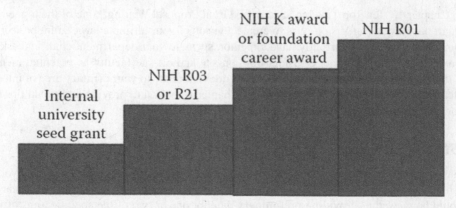

FIGURE 4.1 Example trajectory of grants from small to large.

4.1.3 Serve as a Co-Investigator on Established Teams or Consider a Multiple PI Grant

Given today's difficult grant-funding climate, another way to ensure grant success is to also serve as a **co-investigator** on a grant led by one of your more senior colleagues while launching your own **independent** research track. For example, you may be an early-career faculty member within a research team that already has a track record in your area. Joining an established research project also provides you with the opportunity to apply for supplementary funding that builds upon the established methods and successes of these ongoing grants. Research supplements are described later in this chapter.

Remember that this collaborative work only needs to serve as one of the several streams of your research track. As noted in Chapter 1, "Ten Top Tips for Successful Grant Proposal Writing," developing your own independent line of research funding is of high priority. Therefore, you may want to consider engaging a more senior investigator as a co-investigator on your grant. This will give you a head start as you gain both their expertise and the advantage of including any preliminary data they may have as *the team's* preliminary data in your application. However, as described in Chapter 20, "Review Process," one of the key criteria upon which a grant is scored is the expertise of the PI. Regardless of your investigative team, if you are the PI, the reviewers will be looking for *your* track record in managing such a large grant. It is unlikely you will be able to provide this assurance of feasibility at an early stage in your career.

Therefore, an alternative approach to consider is the multiple PI (MPI) proposal. The MPI approach requires that each PI brings substantive expertise to complementary components of the proposal. In other words, the goal is to encourage collaboration among *equals* when that is the most appropriate way to address a scientific problem. For example, you may have expertise in the content area (e.g., genetic epidemiology) while your co-PI has a track record with managing large epidemiologic grants. In other words, care should be taken with the MPI approach as these grants are not designed to be mentored grants such as Fellowship Grants or Career Development Awards (see Chapter 18, "Fellowship Grants," and Chapter 19, "Career Development Awards").

4.1.4 Plan for More Than One Potential Funding Pipeline

As noted in Chapter 1, "Ten Top Tips for Successful Grant Proposal Writing," given today's grant-funding climate, the only way to ensure grant success is to have several proposals in the pipeline and/or under review **at the same time**. All of these grants, ideally, should support the ultimate envisioned aims of a larger grant (e.g., an NIH R01). For example, you could submit a small grant proposal to support Aim #1 of your ultimate R01 to an internal seed grant opportunity at the same time that you submit a small grant proposal to support Aim #2 of your ultimate R01 to NIH as an R03. Because all these initiatives fit within your overall grantsmanship goal, in the wonderful event that all are funded, they can all serve as pilot data for your larger R01-type grant.

Consider multiple funding options for the same application Another strategic approach is to consider multiple funding options for the *same* application. In other words, submit the same (or very similar) grant application to multiple potential funders. For example, submit a small grant proposal to support Aim #1 of your ultimate R01 for (1) an internal seed grant as well as to (2) a small foundation and (3) to NIH for a smaller grant mechanism. On the highly unusual chance that you obtain funding for this grant from more than one source, you will simply be faced with the luxury of declining one of these sources. Most often, the grant submission requirements differ between these funding agencies, such that you will already have made modifications between each version of the proposal. The **key** here is that you are being efficient by taking the same small grant topic and shaping it to apply to several granting mechanisms.

4.2 PART II: FUNDING MECHANISMS FOR EARLY-CAREER GRANTS

4.2.1 Focus on Grants Targeted to Early-Career Faculty and Postdoctoral Fellows

Grant funding is challenging to obtain. However, graduate students and early-career faculty have certain advantages that they can capitalize upon. **Doctoral and postdoctoral training grants or fellowships** as well as **early-career awards** provide the highest chances for success. A primary advantage of these mechanisms is that they typically do not require significant preliminary data. Instead, funding decisions for these awards rely most heavily on your promise and potential as a candidate. This potential is indicated by three items: (1) your education to date, (2) the mentors with which you have surrounded yourself, and (3) the public health importance of your topic.

A key advantage of these funding mechanisms is that, unlike larger grant awards, you will be competing in a smaller pool of investigators, all of whom will be at a comparable stage in their career as yourself. Thus, you avoid competing against senior investigators who already have established track records. As one senior investigator once advised me, "Avoid competing against the 'big boys and girls' as long as you can!" This advantage that you now have will quickly be over after several years pass by, and you find yourself no longer eligible for these early-career investigator awards.

Therefore, if you are a **graduate student**, seek out grant mechanisms designed for graduate students; if you are an **early-career faculty** member, look for grants designed for early-career faculty members. Section 4.3.2 (Step #2: Choose a Funding Mechanism Sponsored by Your Selected NIH Institute) in this chapter goes over each of these targeted funding sources. You may also want to explore the All About Grants podcast in which the NIH Office of Extramural Research provides advice for new and early-career scientists (https://grants.nih.gov/news/virtual-learning/podcasts.htm#3).

4.2.2 Internal University Funding

Internal awards vary by institution but may include small seed grants and faculty research grants. Take advantage of these opportunities as these grants are typically designed for early-career faculty, and therefore, the institution will be motivated to award these to you as they are invested in your success. In these applications, highlight that the proposed work is critical to the ultimate submission of a larger grant to show your clarity of purpose and the key role that this smaller grant will play.

4.2.3 Foundation Grants

Many foundations have grants targeted for career development. Foundation websites are the best place to start. Examples are as follows:

- The American Diabetes Association Junior Faculty Development Award and the Minority Junior Faculty Development Award
- The Alzheimer's Association Research Grant to Promote Diversity
- The Charles A. King Trust Postdoctoral Research Fellowship Program
- The American Heart Association Career Development Award
- The March of Dimes Starter Scholar Research Award

These grants can total as much as $150,000–$200,000 in direct costs per year and provide support for anywhere from two to five years, but these specifics vary widely by foundation.

4.2.4 Resources for Selecting the Right Funding Source

Universities have resources to help you find grants relevant to your interest area and level. For both graduate students and early-career faculty, your university's office of research will help you identify **funding databases** and **funding sources** and subscribe to **funding alerts**.

Selected examples include:

The Foundation Directory Online is an extensive database of philanthropic giving. Access to this directory may be provided through your university.

Grant Forward features more than 10,000 research funding opportunities from US federal agencies and private foundations. It includes subject search capabilities, a customizable alert service, and an expertise profile service.

Grants.gov is a centralized, searchable clearinghouse for over 1000 grant programs from federal grant-making agencies. Several email alert features are available so that you can receive notifications of new grant opportunity postings.

NIH Guide for Grants and Contracts (https://grants.nih.gov/funding/searchguide/index.html#/) provides daily updates and weekly funding alert email notifications of research priorities and open solicitations from NIH to subscribers.

NIH RePORTER (http://projectreporter.nih.gov/reporter.cfm) allows you to search a repository of NIH-funded research projects and access publications resulting from NIH funding. You can limit your search to particular key terms and to particular funding mechanisms.

National Science Foundation (NSF) funds research and education in most fields of science and engineering and accounts for about one-fourth of federal support to academic institutions for basic research. The website allows you to search a repository of NSF-funded research projects and search for funding.

4.2.5 Look at Who and What They Funded before You

As noted in the Chapter 1, "Ten Top Tips for Successful Grant Proposal Writing," given today's Funding agencies will often make publicly available a list of prior grant awardees. These lists may include the grant title, recipient name, amount awarded, and institution. If the granting agency does not provide a list of past grant recipients, your own institution's office of grants and contracts may have a list of investigators on your campus who have obtained these same grants. Look over this list and see whether you or your mentors know any of these investigators.

This is useful for several reasons. First, it shows the interest of the funding agency in funding research in **epidemiology, biostatistics, and preventive medicine**. Some funding agencies simply don't have the interest or track record in funding population-based research and instead limit their funding to laboratory studies (e.g., *bench science*). Second, it is reasonable to consider asking successful fundees to share their successful applications with you, particularly if you, or your mentors, recognize any names on the fundee list or see that they are from your institution. Reassure these successfully funded investigators that you are simply seeking a model for the appropriate scope and depth of the research plan, not the actual content of their aims. When framed in this manner, people are typically willing to share.

4.2.6 Look at Who Serves as Reviewers

In addition to posting prior grant awardees on their website, funding agencies may also post a list of prior and current grant reviewers and their affiliations. Go through this list and review the expertise of these investigators. Ask yourself if their expertise overlaps with your study aims and methodology.

For example, are any of these investigators population health researchers? Are any from similar departments/divisions to yours? It would be a high-risk proposition to write a proposal for a foundation that does not include reviewers with expertise in epidemiology or preventive medicine on their review panels.

4.3 PART III: STEP-BY-STEP ADVICE FOR FINDING THE RIGHT FUNDING SOURCE AT NIH

The NIH websites are expansive and require considerable time to read and navigate, therefore this section of the chapter focuses on recommended sources of NIH funding for graduate students, postdoctoral fellows, and early-career faculty.

Below, I provide a step-by-step approach for finding the right funding mechanism at NIH (Table 4.1).

4.3.1 Step #1: Determine Which NIH Institute's Mission Encompasses Your Topic

Once you have identified a mentor, created your overall grantsmanship goal, and "bitten off" a chewable section of that larger goal into a first feasible grant proposal (as described in Chapter 1, "Ten Top Tips for Successful Grant Proposal Writing"), the next step is to view the NIH institute websites. NIH is made up of **27 institutes and centers**, each with a specific research agenda, often focusing on particular diseases or body systems (Table 4.2). Go to their websites to see which NIH institute's mission encompasses your

TABLE 4.1   Step by Step: Finding the Right Funding Mechanism at NIH

Step 1: Determine which NIH institute's mission encompasses your topic.
Step 2: Choose a funding mechanism sponsored by your selected NIH institute.
Step 3: Choose the corresponding funding opportunity announcement (FOA) (Program Announcement [PA] or Request for Application [RFA] number).

TABLE 4.2   NIH Institutes

National Cancer Institute (NCI)	National Eye Institute (NEI)
National Heart, Lung, and Blood Institute (NHLBI)	National Human Genome Research Institute (NHGRI)
National Institute on Aging (NIA)	National Institute on Alcohol Abuse and
National Institute of Allergy and Infectious Diseases (NIAID)	Alcoholism (NIAAA)
National Institute of Child Health and Human Development (NICHD)	National Institute of Arthritis and Musculoskeletal and Skin Diseases (NIAMS)
National Institute of Diabetes and Digestive and Kidney Diseases (NIDDK)	National Institute on Deafness and Other Communication Disorders (NIDCD)
National Institute of Environmental Health Sciences (NIEHS)	National Institute of Dental and Craniofacial Research (NIDCR)
National Institute on Minority Health and Health Disparities (NIMHD)	National Institute on Drug Abuse (NIDA)
	National Institute of Mental Health (NIMH)
National Institute of Nursing Research (NINR)	National Institute of Neurological Disorders and Stroke (NINDS)

topic. At the same time, search on NIH RePORTER using the keywords associated with your topic of interest. Search "hits" will provide a "details" tab which lists the NIH institute(s) supporting that grant.

4.3.2 Step #2: Choose a Funding Mechanism Sponsored by Your Selected NIH Institute

Now that you have identified a relevant NIH institute(s), go to their website and see which funding mechanisms they offer and who/what it is designed to support. For example, does the institute fund Career Development Awards (K series), and if so, which ones? Do they fund Research Awards (R Series such as R03s and R21s)? Not all NIH institutes offer every funding mechanism. In addition, even for the same funding mechanism, each institute may have different emphases and program requirements. Therefore, it is perfectly appropriate to contact the relevant institute staff member early in the process to determine whether your planned research and/or training fall within their mission for that type of award.

The funding mechanisms listed in Table 4.3 are particularly suited to early-career faculty and doctoral students.

4.3.2.1 Doctoral and Postdoctoral Fellowship Grants (F Series) "Ruth L. Kirschstein Individual National Research Service Award" (NRSA)

Doctoral and Postdoctoral Fellowships (F series) are named after Dr. Ruth L. Kirschstein, an accomplished scientist in polio vaccine development, who became the first female director of an NIH institute. She was a champion of research training and a strong advocate for the inclusion of underrepresented individuals in the scientific workforce. The goal of these fellowship awards is to ensure a diverse pool of highly trained scientists in appropriate scientific disciplines to address the Nation's biomedical, behavioral, and clinical research needs (https://researchtraining.nih.gov/programs/fellowships).

Chapter 18, "Fellowship Grants," provides tips and strategies for successful submission of a fellowship grant application. In brief, these fellowship awards require a proposed **research and training plan**, which will be conducted under the supervision of a **mentor (sponsor)**. The sponsor and any cosponsors are also expected to have a successful track record of mentoring and provide an assessment of the applicant's qualifications and potential for a research career.

TABLE 4.3 Selected Examples of Funding Mechanisms Suitable for Early Grants

	DOCTORAL STUDENTS	POSTDOCTORAL FELLOWS	EARLY-CAREER FACULTY
Mentored/training awards			
Doctoral and postdoctoral fellowships (F series)			
F30, F31	×		
F32		×	
Training grants (T series)	×	×	×
Individual mentored career development awards (K series)			
K08, K22, K99/R00		×	
K01, K07, K23, K25			×
Loan repayment program (LRP)		×	×
Research supplements	×	×	×
Independent awards			
Research awards (R series)			
R03, R15, R21		×	×

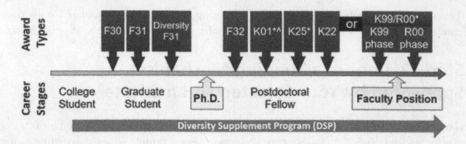

FIGURE 4.2   Training grants and fellowships for researchers. *Faculty may also be eligible for K01 and K25. ^K01 awardees may also be eligible for the Limited Competition: Small Research Grant Program for K01/K08/ and K23 Recipients (R03).

Below, I highlight selected fellowship grants (Figure 4.2). Note that fellowship recipients must be a citizen or non-citizen national of the United States or a permanent resident. Individuals on temporary or student visas are not eligible.

For Doctoral Students
F30 Individual Predoctoral MD/PhD and Other Dual Doctoral Degree Fellowships   This award provides support to doctoral candidates enrolled in a formally combined MD/PhD program to perform a research project in clinical or basic sciences. This fellowship is awarded to applicants with the potential to become productive, independent, highly trained physician-scientists, and other clinician-scientists, including patient-oriented researchers in their scientific mission areas.

F31 Individual Predoctoral Fellowships   This award provides support for promising doctoral candidates to perform dissertation research and receive training in scientific health-related fields relevant to the missions of the participating NIH institutes.

F31 Individual Predoctoral Fellowships to Promote Diversity in Health-Related Research   This award is identical to the F31 but provides support for promising doctoral candidates who are from underrepresented racial and ethnic groups, individuals with disabilities, and individuals from disadvantaged backgrounds.

For Postdoctoral Fellows
F32 Individual Postdoctoral Fellowships   This award provides support for promising postdoctoral fellows to perform a research project within the broad scope of biomedical, behavioral, or clinical research.

4.3.2.2 Training Grants (T Series) "Ruth L. Kirschstein Individual National Research Service Award"

Training Grants (T series) are also named after Dr. Ruth L. Kirschstein. Training grants are Institutional awards to support research training activities for predoctoral students and/or postdoc *trainees* selected by the institution. They are **awarded to universities** under the direction of a senior faculty member who serves as the training project director (PD)/PI. These programs require a program director and experienced faculty to serve as mentors (https://researchtraining.nih.gov/programs /training-grants).
    Therefore, you would not apply directly to NIH yourself for a training grant. Ask your chair or mentor if this type of program is available at your institution. Then, you would follow **internal university guidelines** to apply to be a fellow in this program. Note that recipients of training grant awards must be a

citizen or non-citizen national of the United States or a permanent resident. Individuals on temporary or student visas are not eligible.

For Doctoral Students and Postdoctoral Fellows
T32 Institutional Research Training Grants are awarded to support predoctoral and postdoctoral research training to help ensure that a diverse and highly trained workforce is available to assume leadership roles related to the nation's biomedical, behavioral, and clinical research agenda. The training grants tend to require a proposed **research and training plan**, which will be conducted under the supervision of a **mentor or preceptor**. Often, the next step for a T32 fellow is to apply for a K award.

4.3.2.3 Career Development Awards (K Series)

Most **individual mentored** career development awards are designed for applicants who have completed their academic or clinical training and who have accepted (or have recently started) a faculty position. The goal of these awards is to develop a diverse pool of highly trained scientists in appropriate scientific disciplines to address the Nation's biomedical, behavioral, and clinical research needs (Figure 4.2).

Chapter 19, "Career Development Awards," provides tips and strategies for successful submission of an individual mentored career award application. In brief, proposals for these K awards require a proposed **research project** and a **career development training plan** to be conducted under the supervision of a *mentor*. As with other mentored awards, the mentor, co-mentor, or mentoring team should be recognized as accomplished investigators in the proposed research area and have a track record of success in training and placing independent investigators. The mentor must be at a domestic (US) institution. The mentor and any co-mentors are also expected to provide an assessment of the applicant's qualifications and potential for a research career and a plan for mentoring and monitoring the candidate's research, publications, and progression toward independence. In addition, the proposals also require a description of the candidate's background, career goals and objectives, and training in the responsible conduct of research.

In terms of eligibility, note that some career development awards limit eligibility to those with a limited number of years of postdoctoral experience at the time of application (e.g., four to six years depending upon the type of award). It is important to note that you will not be eligible for a career development award if you have already received a large NIH R01 grant (as PI) but that you are still eligible if you have been awarded an NIH small grant (R03), exploratory/developmental grant (R21), or dissertation award (R36). Therefore, these eligibility limitations make a K award an excellent choice for an early-career faculty member. This NIH website walks you through selecting the right career award for your level: https://researchtraining.nih.gov/programs/career-development. Below, I briefly describe selected career awards.

Selected Individual Mentored Career Development Programs
For Postdoctoral Fellows
- *K08 Mentored Clinical Scientist Research Career Development Award*: To provide the opportunity for promising clinician-scientists with demonstrated aptitude to develop into independent investigators, or for faculty members to pursue research, and aid in filling the academic faculty gap in health profession's institutions.
- *K22 Career Transition Award*: To provide support to outstanding newly trained basic or clinical investigators to develop their independent research skills through a two-phase program; an initial mentored research experience, followed by a period of independent research.
- *K99/R00 Pathway to Independence Award*: To support an initial mentored research experience (K99) followed by independent research (R00) for highly qualified, postdoctoral researchers to secure an independent research position (e.g., faculty appointment). Award recipients are expected to compete successfully for independent R01 support during the R00 phase.

For Early-Career Faculty
- *K01 The Mentored Research Scientist Career Development Award*: For support of a post-doctoral or early-career research scientists committed to research, in need of both advanced research training and additional experience.
- *K07 Academic Career Development Award*: To support either a mentored or an independent investigator to develop or enhance curricula, foster academic career development of promising young teacher-investigators, and to strengthen existing teaching programs.
- *K23 Mentored Patient-Oriented Research Career Development Award*: To provide support for the career development of clinically trained professionals who have made a commitment to patient-oriented research and who have the potential to develop into productive, clinical investigators.
- *K25 Mentored Quantitative Research Career Development Award*: To support the career development of investigators with quantitative scientific and engineering backgrounds outside of biology or medicine who have made a commitment to focus their research endeavors on basic or clinical biomedical research.

4.3.2.4 Loan Repayment Programs

Loan repayment programs (LRPs) are designed to recruit and retain highly qualified health professionals into biomedical or biobehavioral research careers. The program is an excellent option for postdoctoral fellows and early-career faculty.

LRPs offer up to $50,000 per year to repay qualified educational debt (i.e., student loans) in return for a commitment to engage in NIH mission-relevant research. Note that eligibility is limited to US citizens, US nationals, or permanent residents of the United States by the LRP award start date.

LRPs require that you commit at least two years to conducting qualified research. Loan repayment benefits are in addition to your institutional salary. The application requires a description of your current or proposed **research and training** plan as well as a statement from the **mentor(s)** (if you are an early-career faculty member, your mentor can be your department chair) (https://www.lrp.nih.gov/).

There are six LRPs—each with a different focus:

1. Clinical research
2. Pediatric research
3. Health disparities research
4. Contraception and infertility research
5. Clinical research for individuals from disadvantaged backgrounds
6. Research in Emerging Areas Critical to Human Health (REACH)

4.3.2.5 Research Supplements

This program provides administrative supplements to existing, active NIH research grants for the purpose of supporting full-time or part-time research by individuals meeting the eligibility criteria described below. Therefore, if your mentor is a PI of an active research grant with 2 years or more remaining on that active grant, they may be eligible to submit an administrative supplement to the grant to support you and your research project. In this way, a research supplement could fund the collection of preliminary data for a subsequent K-award application. Indeed, there is an expectation that this type of award will be followed by a subsequent application for NIH support. Note that while the mentor will be listed as the PI on this supplement, you will be listed as the *candidate*. There are a variety of different types of supplements. Examples are as follows:

For Postdoctoral Fellows and Early-Career Faculty
Research Supplements to Promote Diversity in Health-Related Research These supplements are designed to improve the diversity of the research workforce by supporting and recruiting students, postdoctoral

fellows, and eligible investigators from groups that have been shown to be underrepresented in health-related research.

Research Supplements to Promote Reentry into Biomedical and Behavioral Research Careers   These supplements are designed to support individuals with high potential to reenter an active research career after an interruption for family responsibilities or other qualifying circumstances. The purpose of these supplements is to encourage such individuals to reenter research careers within the missions of all the program areas of NIH.

4.3.2.6 Research Awards (R Series)

The smaller Research Awards such as R21s and R03s are **not mentored** and are designed to support your **independent research**. While they typically provide smaller budgets than an R01, they are well suited to early-career faculty as they do not require preliminary data. In addition, receipt of these awards does not remove your NIH **early-stage investigator** advantage as described below. However, it is important to note that these awards are not offered by all NIH institutes.

For Postdoctoral Fellows and Early-Career Faculty
R03 NIH Small Grant Program   This award provides support for small research projects that can be carried out in a short period of time (i.e., two years) with limited resources. Preliminary data are not required to receive these awards and in contrast, such projects are actually well suited to collect such data. Therefore, excellent topics for R03 applications include pilot or feasibility studies, collection of preliminary data, secondary analysis of existing data, small research projects, or development of new research technology. Direct costs are generally quite limited (e.g., up to $50,000 per year). Note that this funding mechanism is not utilized by all the NIH institutes.

R15 NIH Academic Research Enhancement Award (AREA)   This award is designed to stimulate research in educational institutions that have not been major recipients of NIH support. They are intended to support small-scale research projects proposed by faculty members from these eligible institutions, to expose students to meritorious research projects, and to strengthen the research environment of the applicant institution. The project period is limited to three years, and preliminary data are not required. Check with your institution's office of grants and contracts regarding your eligibility for an R15. The majority of NIH institutes utilize this award.

R21 NIH Exploratory/Developmental Research Grant Award   This award is designed to encourage exploratory/developmental research by providing support for the early and conceptual stages of project development. Exploratory studies are defined as novel studies that break new ground or extend previous discoveries toward new directions or applications. High-risk/high-reward studies that may lead to a breakthrough in a particular area or result in novel techniques, agents, methodologies, models, or applications that will impact biomedical, behavioral, or clinical research are an excellent fit for R21s. Direct costs (e.g., $275,000 over two years) are typically higher than an R03. Again, no preliminary data are required. Note that this funding mechanism is not utilized by all the NIH institutes.

R01 NIH Research Project Grant   An R01 is for a mature research project that is hypothesis-driven with strong preliminary data. R01s provide up to five years of support, with a budget that reflects the costs required to complete the project. R01s can be investigator-initiated or can be solicited via a Request for Applications. The Research Project (R01) grant is an award made to support a discrete, specified, circumscribed project to be performed by the investigator in an area representing the investigator's specific interest and competencies, based on the mission of the NIH. As a general rule, R01 application budgets are not limited but need to reflect the actual needs of the proposed project. Those requesting $500,000 or more in direct costs in any year must receive permission from a scientific/research contact at NIH.

Typically, new investigators do not skip directly to this funding mechanism, and if they do, their budgets are typically well below the $500,000 cap. However, if you are a new investigator, and are trying to determine whether to submit an R01 application, ask yourself the following:

- Do you have strong preliminary data that support your hypothesis/hypotheses?
- Is there a strong rationale for the proposed study?
- Do you have a proven track record of experience in the field, including publications in scientific journals?
- Do you or your collaborators have sufficient expertise to accomplish the goals of the proposed work?

4.3.2.7 Choosing between an R03 and an R21

R03s are smaller in budget, but don't have the high impact requirement of an R21. However, given the current funding environment, one could argue that all grant proposals have to be high impact to be competitive. This doesn't mean that as an epidemiologist or preventive medicine specialist, you have to propose to create a new methodology for an R21 proposal. Instead, high impact could be defined as the early investigation of a novel hypothesis or use of better methods to evaluate an existing hypothesis for which prior findings have been conflicting. R21 grants are intended to encourage exploratory/developmental research by providing support for the early and conceptual stages of project development. However, if you propose a "small R01 style" research project for an R21 mechanism, you may find that two years is not long enough to yield enough data for publication or generates sufficient preliminary data for an R01 application.

In contrast, projects of limited cost or scope that use widely accepted approaches and methods are likely better suited for the R03 small grant mechanism. For example, as noted in Chapter 1, "Ten Top Tips for Successful Grant Proposal Writing," reproducibility and validity studies and pilot feasibility studies are excellent topics for small grants like the R03 as they have clearly defined parameters and aims and are feasible to conduct.

4.3.2.8 Early-Stage Investigator Advantages

Once you reach the step of applying for an NIH R01 award, you will have several advantages as an early-career faculty member.

NIH defines **new investigators** as PIs who have **not** received a substantial NIH independent research award such as an R01. In other words, you will remain a *new investigator* even after you receive early-stage or small research grants (e.g., an R03 or R21) or Training Grants/Fellowships (e.g., T and F series awards), infrastructure (e.g., R15 awards), or Career Development Awards (e.g., K series awards).

NIH defines **Early-Stage Investigators (ESIs)** as a subset of new investigators. In other words, if you are a new investigator and you are also within ten years of your terminal degree.

Applications from ESIs, like those from all new investigators, are given special consideration during peer review and at the time of funding. Peer reviewers are instructed to focus more on the proposed approach than on the track record and to expect less preliminary data than might be provided by an established investigator.

Check your specific NIH institute of interest for their policies for new investigators and/or ESIs. These **special considerations** may include funding priority and ensured years of support. For example, some NIH institutes have separate pay lines (e.g., more generous) for awards to ESI applicants and/or monitor their new investigator pool to make sure that a certain percent has ESI status.

4.3.3 Step #3: Choose the Corresponding Funding Opportunity Announcement Number

Once you have followed the steps above, then you will need to choose the corresponding funding opportunity (FOA). NIH advertises availability of grant support through FOAs. Search for an FOA specific to your area of interest, or apply to one of the parent announcements (https://grants.nih.gov/grants/guide/parent

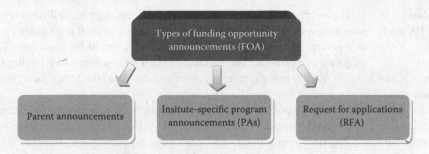

FIGURE 4.3 Types of funding opportunity announcements.

_announcements.htm). You can search for FOAs in the NIH Guide for Grants and Contracts (https://grants .nih.gov/funding/index.htm) or in Grants.gov.

There are three types of FOAs as described in Figure 4.3. The type of FOA that you list on your submission cover/face page will dictate the specific submission instructions that you will follow (as described in Chapter 17, "Submission of the Grant Proposal") and will also have implications for your probability of receiving funding as described below.

Parent announcements (PAs) refer to general investigator-initiated, unsolicited research. More simply stated, this means that if you, as the PI, propose a grant on any topic within the breadth of the NIH mission, it will likely fit under a general parent announcement. In other words, the individual grant project design reflects the ideas and creativity of the investigator. For example, R03, R21, and R01 grants described above fall under general parent announcements. In addition, all **training grants** are in the form of PAs. This is a key advantage that should not be overlooked—and if at all possible, you should see whether your grant topic relates to one of the PAs. Submission dates are standard (approximately three times per year), and the funding pay line is determined by the NIH institute of choice. **Advantages** of parent announcements are your flexibility in topic.

Institute-Specific Program Announcements are similar to parent announcements but are generated by the specific NIH institute themselves and reflect the institute's broad research interests or a reminder of a scientific need. Again, if you, as the PI, have a grant proposal on any topic within the breadth of that particular institute, it will likely fit under an institute-specific PA. You will find R03, R21, and R01 mechanisms here. Many research topics span multiple institutes and you will be able to cross list these on your application (more on this in Chapter 17, "Submission of the Grant Proposal." Submission dates are standard (approximately three times per year). **Advantages** of institute-specific PAs are that the institute may have flexibility in funding **above the pay line**.

Example Choice of FOA

The National Institute on Drug Abuse (NIDA) offers the parent R03 (PA-20-200). In addition, at one time they also offered a **specific** R03, which was focused on "Alcohol and Other Drug Interactions: Unintentional Injuries and Overdoses (R03) (PA-18-861)." If your R03 topic happened to be focused on this topic, then applying for this institute-specific PA (PA-18-861) would be preferable. Instead, if your R03 topic focused on another area relevant to NIDA, then you would apply through the parent R03 announcement (PA-20-200).

Request for Applications (RFAs) are formal statements inviting applications on a well-defined area with specific objectives. They have specific, one-time application receipt dates and plan to fund a limited prespecified number of awards. RFAs use a special review panel that is convened on a one-time basis. There are several **disadvantages** of RFAs:

- Revising and resubmitting your proposal are typically not possible as there is only one review.
- The review panel has not worked together before, which may make the review process more unpredictable.
- The topic is not investigator-initiated.

How to choose between a PA and an RFA I advise early-career investigators to prioritize their overall research/grantsmanship vision over and above RFAs with a single receipt date unless your research is a perfect fit. And, even in that situation, I would be cautious. Given that the majority of grants are not funded on their first submission, having the opportunity to resubmit is key for early-career investigators. In other words, avoid the temptation to substantively alter your research vision in response to a specific RFA with a single receipt date.

Instead, search for an institute-specific PA that fits closely with your overall research vision or that simply requires a few modest tweaks to your research vision. If you are unable to identify a relevant institute-specific PA, then apply under the more general parent PA. In other words, do not substantively alter your research in response to a specific PA or RFA. As you will see in Chapter 18, "Submission of the Grant Proposal," your application is scored by a study section at NIH which is **independent** from the NIH institutes. As long as you receive a strong scientific score from this study section, you will have a high chance of success. Response to an institute-specific PA simply gives you an extra boost, as it gives the NIH institute more flexibility in their pay line for what scores are funded.

4.3.3.1 Read the FOA Carefully!

Finally, be sure to read the FOA carefully for specific eligibility requirements as well as any special review criteria or application instructions before writing your application. **Then take a second look!**

4.4 EXAMPLES OF CHOOSING THE RIGHT FUNDING SOURCES

4.4.1 Example #1: A Postdoctoral Researcher Transitioning to Early-Career Faculty

Below is our example, provided in Chapter 1, "Ten Top Tips for Successful Grant Proposal Writing," of the overall grantsmanship goal of a postdoctoral researcher and Table 4.4 outlines the corresponding grantsmanship timeline.

Example Overall Grantsmanship Goal/Research Theme
To obtain an R01 grant to conduct a large prospective study of vitamin D intake and risk of depression.
Specific Aims of the R01
Specific Aim #1: To evaluate the association between self-reported vitamin D and risk of depression.
Specific Aim #2: To evaluate the association between a biomarker of vitamin D and risk of depression.
Specific Aim #3: To evaluate whether the impact of vitamin D on depression risk is stronger among those with gene x as compared to those without the gene.

TABLE 4.4   Grantsmanship Timeline Example for a Postdoctoral Researcher

SUBMISSION YEAR WITHIN CAREER STAGE	FUNDING MECHANISM	TOPIC
Postdoctoral Fellow		
Year 01	F32 Individual Postdoctoral Fellow through NIMH	Small Grant Proposal to Support Aims #1 and #2: A reproducibility and validity study of the proposed vitamin D questionnaire against an objective measure.
Year 02	K99/R00 Pathway to Independence Award (NIMH)	Small Grant Proposal to Support Aims #1, #2, and #3: A pilot/feasibility study of recruiting a prospective cohort study at the proposed study site.
Assistant Professor		
Year 01	Internal Faculty Research Grant	Small Grant Proposal to Support Aim #3: Evaluate the influence of gene x on the association between vitamin D and depression using an existing dataset.
Year 01	Continuation of K99/R00 through NIMH	
Year 02	American Society for Nutrition—Starter Scholar Award[a]	Small Grant Proposal to Support Aims #1 and #2: A reproducibility and validity study of the proposed depression questionnaire against a clinical diagnosis of depression.
Year 02	R03 NIH Small Research Grant Program at NIMH	Small Grant Proposal to Support Aims #1 and #2: A reproducibility and validity study of the proposed depression questionnaire against a clinical diagnosis of depression (Note in case American Society for Nutrition grant not awarded).
Year 03	Resubmission and/or conduct of above grants	
Year 04	R01 at NIMH	Proposal to conduct a large prospective study of vitamin D intake and risk of depression.

[a] Hypothetical foundation grant.

4.4.2 Example #2: An Early-Career Faculty Member

The example below provides the overall grantsmanship goal of a faculty member and Table 4.5 outlines the corresponding grantsmanship timeline.

Example Overall Grantsmanship Goal/Research Theme
To obtain an R01 grant to conduct a randomized trial of exercise in the prevention of obesity in early childhood.
Specific Aims of the R01
Specific Aim #1: To evaluate the impact of the six-month exercise intervention on BMI.
Specific Aim #2: To evaluate the impact of the six-month exercise intervention on markers of insulin resistance.
Specific Aim #3: To evaluate the impact of the six-month exercise intervention on levels of cardiovascular risk factors.
Specific Aim #4: To evaluate the efficacy of the six-month exercise intervention on measures of compliance (i.e., exercise and diet).

TABLE 4.5   Grantsmanship Timeline Example for an Early-Career Faculty Member

TIME	FUNDING MECHANISM	TOPIC
Assistant Professor		
Year 01	Internal Faculty Research Grant	Small grant Proposal to Develop the Intervention: Conduct focus groups among at-risk children.
Year 01	American Diabetes Association Junior Faculty Award	Small grant Proposal to Support Aim #4: To evaluate the efficacy of the exercise intervention on measures of compliance.
Year 02	R21 NIH Small research grant Program NIDDK[a]	Small grant Proposal to Support Aims #1, 2, 3, and 4: A pilot feasibility study of the proposed intervention among a sample of at-risk children.
Year 03	Resubmission and/or conduct of above grants	
Year 04	R01 from NIDDK	Proposal to conduct a randomized trial of exercise in the prevention of obesity in early childhood.

[a] In response to a specific PA from NIDDK for "Home and Family Based Approaches for the Prevention or Management of Overweight or Obesity in Early Childhood (R21) and (R01)."

Scientific Writing

5

Before you put pen to paper, this chapter focuses on writing style and provides tips as well as stylistic guidelines for writing with a scientific audience in mind. As with any writing, factor in time for (1) writing a first draft; (2) editing (i.e., checking the draft for completeness, cohesion, and correctness); and (3) rewriting in response to your coinvestigators' comments.

5.1 TIP #1: CONSIDER YOUR AUDIENCE

Your target audience in grant proposal writing is the general scientific community and not just experts in your field. As noted in Chapter 1, "Ten Top Tips for Successful Grant Proposal Writing," grant reviewers do not always have expertise in your proposed subject area. That is, while one reviewer may have a specific background in your area, some others are assigned based on their expertise with your proposed methodology (e.g., epidemiology), and others may be assigned to review your statistical analysis section. For example, a grant designed to identify risk factors for uterine cancer may be assigned to the following three reviewers: (1) an oncologist, (2) an epidemiologist who has conducted case-control studies among cancer patients, and (3) a statistician. It is even possible that the physician or the epidemiologist will not have direct experience with uterine cancer specifically but are instead more generalist reproductive cancer researchers.

However, it is reassuring to note that, if your proposal is well written, even a generalist reviewer will be able to assess (1) whether your goals are clearly stated, (2) whether your proposal justifies how it extends prior work in the field, (3) what is innovative about your proposal, as well as (4) the impact of your potential findings on public health and clinical practice.

5.2 TIP #2: OMIT NEEDLESS WORDS

A common aphorism is that, in most writing, every third word can be eliminated. Of course, this cannot be taken literally, but at its heart, this phrase means that all writing has a *flab* factor, particularly in early drafts. I can recall reviewing few grant proposals that would not be strengthened by some condensation.

Vigorous writing is concise. As described in the classic guide to writing by Strunk and White:

> A sentence should contain no unnecessary words, a paragraph no unnecessary sentences, for the same reason that a drawing should have no unnecessary lines and a machine no unnecessary parts. This requires not that the writer make all his sentences short, or that he avoid all detail and treat his subjects only in outline, but that every word tell.

George Orwell was an early-20th-century English novelist and journalist who had a profound impact on language and writing. His writing reflects clarity, intelligence, and wit. Orwell was unhappy with vague writing and professional jargon and felt that poor writing was an indication of sloppy thinking. He excused neither the scientist nor the novelist from his strict requirement for good, vigorous writing.

DOI: 10.1201/9781003155140-6

Orwell's Writing Rules

1. Never use a long word where a short one will do.
2. If it is possible to cut a word out, always cut it out.
3. Never use the passive where you can use the active.
4. Never use a foreign phrase, a scientific word, or a jargon word if you can think of an everyday English equivalent.
5. Break any of these rules sooner than say anything outright barbarous.

Therefore, in rereading your proposal for a second and third time, your main focus will be removing extraneous words that detract the reviewer from quickly seeing your main points (e.g., the research gap and how your proposal extends the prior literature on this topic). The strict page limitations in most grants will also provide motivation to follow this tip. On the other hand, if you do not use up the space allotted (e.g., by leaving blank lines/white space at the end of the proposal), reviewers may wonder why you did not provide more detail.

Many expressions in common use violate this principle:

- *The question as to whether* … can be written as *Whether* …
- *There is no doubt but that* can be written as *no doubt (doubtless)*.
- *This is a subject that* … can be written as *This subject* …
- *The reason why is that* … can be written as *Because* …

The use of definite, specific, concrete language is the surest way to arouse and hold the attention of the reviewer:

- *Since* actually refers to a span of time and should not be used in place of *Because*.
- *Though* can be written as *Although*.
- *In order to* … can be written as *To* ….

In this spirit, in 2005, the *American Journal of Epidemiology* (Vol 161, No 5) included an editorial titled "Please Read the Following Paper and Write this Way!" To this day, this editorial remains a valuable resource for learning how to write succinctly within the context of scientific writing. The improved example below omits needless words from a sentence found in the Significance and Innovation section of a proposal.

Example Revision of Needless Words
Original Version Needs Improvement
Using accelerometers, light-intensity physical activity *has been found to* be positively associated with kidney function.
Improved Version
Using accelerometers, light-intensity physical activity *has been* positively associated with kidney function.

5.3 TIP #3: AVOID PROFESSIONAL JARGON

In the spirit of writing clearly and concisely, it is critical to avoid the use of professional jargon. (Or, if you must include the jargon, then also add a brief explanation.) *Professional jargon* in epidemiology often occurs when describing potential study limitations. For example, terms such as *selection bias*, *information bias,* and *confounding* require a brief layperson description. Even for an audience of experts, simply using these terms without describing the bias scenario that you are concerned about puts the burden on the reviewer to imagine it. More importantly, clarifying your jargon with simple terms will show the reviewers that you have a clear grasp of the potential bias scenario. This advice follows the principle of being *kind* to the reviewer.

Example Revision of Professional Jargon
Consider that you are conducting a study of oral contraceptives and risk of diabetes.
Original Version Needs Improvement
Findings of an increased risk of diabetes among oral contraceptive users may be due to detection bias.
Improved Version
Detection bias is possible because women who take oral contraceptives are monitored more closely for diabetes than nonusers of oral contraceptives.

The improved example retains the term *detection bias* but also includes a clear explanation of what detection bias means in this scenario.

5.4 TIP #4: AVOID USING THE FIRST-PERSON SINGULAR

Use of the first-person singular voice puts you at risk of sounding subjective and expressing simply a personal opinion. In other words, the first-person singular (e.g., *I* or *myself*) is appropriate for writing an editorial but not for writing a grant proposal, with the one important exception of the candidate's sections in a Fellowship Grant (see Chapter 18) or a Career Development Award (see Chapter 19).

Example Revision of First-Person Singular
Original Version Needs Improvement
In this section on Significance and Innovation, I will establish what I believe to be a major weakness in the literature on weight loss programs. Namely, my observation is that most of the evidence on the impact of the programs on cardiovascular disease risk factors is purely descriptive and anecdotal. While reading this section, you should keep in mind …
Improved Version
The popularity of weight loss programs has resulted in numerous articles reporting claims about the impact of such programs.[1-7] The articles tend to provide: (1) purely descriptive, anecdotal accounts of the programs' impact on cardiovascular disease risk factors[1-3] and (2) descriptions of design and guidelines for developing a weight loss program.[5-7]

The *improved version* has a number of advantages:

First, the improved version avoids the use of the first-person singular by not referring to the writer(s) at all. You can also use the term *we* when referring to publications by your research team (e.g., any of your coinvestigators). "*We*" is always preferable to the term "*I*" unless you are writing a fellowship (F series) or career award grant (K series) (see Chapters 18, "Fellowship Grants," and Chapter 19, "Career Development Awards"). Note that the improved version will be viewed as more scientifically sound as it does not appear that the proposal writer is stating their own personal opinions.

Second, the *improved version* cites scientific publications to support the points raised. This further reinforces the objectivity of the assertions made.

Third, the use of a numbered list in the *improved version* provides structure and organization to the paragraph and gives the impression that the writer has conducted a thorough review and knows how to organize and present results.

Overall, the impression given by the *improved version* is one of rigor and fact as opposed to conjecture and personal conversation.

5.5 TIP #5: USE THE ACTIVE VOICE

Use the active voice (as opposed to the passive voice) as much as possible in scientific writing. A clear active voice gives a stronger impression than a passive voice and has other advantages: it avoids indirect sentence constructions that are harder to read and takes up less space—vital when writing a page-limited grant proposal.

If you read scientific journals (always recommended to improve your writing!), you will see that these journals provide further evidence that the active voice is preferable. For example, one of the highest-ranked and rigorous journals, *The New England Journal of Medicine*, uses active voice. A quick glance through a typical article in *The New England Journal* will yield such sentences as the following:

Example Revision of Passive Voice
Original Version #1 Needs Improvement
In the study by Smith et al., it was found …
Improved Version
Smith et al. found that …
Original Version #2 Needs Improvement
Patients were recruited who …
Improved Version
We recruited patients who were …

As you can see, the improved version is more concise and easier to read.

5.6 TIP #6: USE THE POSITIVE FORM

This tip is closely related to Tip #5: Use the Active Voice suggesting the use of active voice. The use of positive form is always recommended for proposals. Simply, in place of stating what you chose *not* to do, instead state what you chose to do. The one exception to this rule would be the section on study limitations and alternatives (see Chapter 15, "How to Present Limitations and Alternatives"). Only in this section, would you discuss what you chose *not to do* and why. In other words, put your best foot forward.

Example Use of Positive Form
Original Version Needs Improvement #1
We did not think that a case-control design was appropriate for our proposed study.
Improved Version #1
We thought a prospective cohort study was the appropriate design for our proposed study.
Original Version Needs Improvement #2
We chose not to recruit women who were less than age 16 years
Improved Version #2
We chose to recruit women who were aged 16 years and older.

5.7 TIP #7: AVOID USING SYNONYMS FOR RECURRING WORDS

The use of synonyms can lead to reviewer confusion and frustration. We are taught in creative writing courses to find synonyms for terms in order to keep reader interest and to avoid being repetitive. In contrast, this approach is discouraged in scientific writing. Given the complexity of the terms and methods used in proposals, the more consistent you can be in your word choices, the easier it will be for the reviewer to understand your proposal and thereby to evaluate its merits.

Example Revision of Synonym Use
(Underlining used to denote synonyms)

Original Version Needs Improvement
The <u>Athena cohort</u> was taught to correctly identify heart-healthy food groups and was brought back to be studied by three researchers twice, once after six months and again at the end of the year. The <u>other group</u> of youngsters was asked to answer the set of questions only once, after six months; but they had been taught to label the food groups by name rather than by health effects. The performance of <u>Group 1</u> was superior to the performance of <u>Group II</u>. The superior performance of the <u>experimental group</u> was attributed to ...

Improved Version
The experimental group was taught to identify heart-healthy food groups and was retested twice at six-month intervals. The control group was taught to identify the food groups by name and was retested only once after six months. The performance of the experimental group was superior to the performance of the control group. The superior performance of the experimental group was attributed to ...

You probably found yourself reading the original example several times to make sense of it. Imagine your frustration as a grant reviewer facing a stack of proposals to read with an impending deadline. Specifically, the original example used several synonyms for the same study group: *Athena cohort*, *Group 1*, and *experimental group*. It was also unclear who constituted the *other group of youngsters*. Confusion grows because we don't know if Group 1 refers to the Phoenix cohort, the *other group of youngsters*, or represents a third group that has yet to be defined. In the improved example, it is now clear that there are only two groups—the *experimental* group and the *control* group.

5.8 TIP #8: USE TRANSITIONS TO HELP TRACE YOUR ARGUMENT

This tip fits under the concept of being kind to your reviewer (as described in Chapter 1, "Ten Top Tips for Successful Grant Proposal Writing"). For example, if you want to introduce three related points, begin sentences or paragraphs that describe each point with the terms *first*, *second*, and *third*. These terms provide guideposts for your reviewer helping them to identify inter-relationships between sections of your proposal. They ensure that you are internally consistent and do not add extraneous points, or even worse, inadvertently drop one of your arguments. Other transition phrases include: *in the next example*, *in a related study*, and *a counterexample*. Use these transition phrases as much as possible—they alert the reviewer to the purpose of each paragraph and therefore are *kind* to the reviewer.

5.9 TIP #9: AVOID DIRECT QUOTATIONS BOTH AT THE BEGINNING AND WITHIN THE RESEARCH STRATEGY

While the use of direct quotations is not unusual in creative writing, they should be avoided in scientific writing. This is particularly important when summarizing the conclusions of prior published papers or the results of a review article written by leaders in the field.

First, by definition, direct quotations are presented out of context and, as such, may not convey the original author's intent. Explaining the context of the quotation uses even more space, can serve to detract from your main purpose, and may even confuse the reviewer with nonessential details.

Instead, paraphrasing prior literature in your own words is always preferable. This technique eliminates disruptions in the flow due to different writing styles and avoids extraneous details.

Example Avoidance of Direct Quotations
Consider a grant proposal to evaluate the association between socioeconomic status and overall health status that starts with the following quote:

Original Version Needs Improvement
"The place and roles that individuals take up in the socioeconomic structure of the society shapes and defines the life conditions that characterize the different social classes and are the source of the differences in the quality of life and the differential exposure to conditions (e.g., different types of behaviour and lifestyle characteristics of different social groups) that on the one hand protect and benefit health and on the other hand deteriorate and limit health, resulting in the appearance of disease and death (Smith et al. 2012)."
Improved Version
Socioeconomic status constitutes a variety of factors (e.g., lifestyle and behavioral factors) and, in turn, has been found to impact morbidity and mortality.[1-3]

The first concern is that the quote is very dense, the wording is cumbersome, and it is unlikely that the writing style and terminology used in the rest of the proposal will be consistent with this quote. Second, note the potential for differences in style and spelling conventions between the quote (i.e., the use of the British spelling *behaviour*) and what is likely to be in the body of the proposal. The quote also uses synonyms for socioeconomic status (e.g., *socioeconomic structure*, *social class*, *social groups*). (See Tip #7: Avoid Synonyms for Recurring Words). Instead, your proposal should have one voice—your own.

5.10 TIP #10: AVOID SAYING *THE AUTHORS CONCLUDED* ...

When describing the findings of prior studies, try to avoid phrases such as *the authors concluded*. Instead, it is more impressive to state your own conclusions from the authors' work. It may be surprising to learn that, instead of gaining credibility by directly quoting the authors, you will be inadvertently undermining the reviewer's confidence in your own abilities as an independent researcher.

Remember that authors are not always correct in their conclusions. Some authors might minimize the impact of potential biases on their study findings. Other authors may either incorrectly describe their study design or use a vague term when describing their study design (e.g., retrospective study vs. *case-control study*).

Example Revision of the Phrase "The Authors Concluded"

Original Version Needs Improvement
The authors concluded that their findings were unlikely to be due to selection bias.
Improved Version
Because women who participated in the study did not differ significantly from women who did not participate in the study in terms of sociodemographic factors, it is unlikely that the findings could have been due to selection bias.

Note that the improved version has the additional advantage of avoiding the use of epidemiologic jargon (Tip #3: Avoid Professional Jargon) by defining *selection bias* in layperson's terms.

5.11 TIP #11: PLACE LATIN ABBREVIATIONS IN PARENTHESES; ELSEWHERE USE ENGLISH TRANSLATIONS

The following examples list the correct usage of some standard Latin abbreviations which are almost always used *within parentheses*. Note that English translations of these terms are almost always used *outside of parentheses*. Caution should be taken with the punctuation used in the Latin abbreviations, although software spell-checkers should correct any errors you make in use of these terms:

- (i.e.,) = that is
  "We propose to evaluate diabetes risk factors (i.e., glucose, insulin, adiponectin)."
  Or, "We will evaluate diabetes risk factors, that is, glucose, insulin, adiponectin."
- (e.g.,) = for example
  "We propose to evaluate sociodemographic factors (e.g., age, income, education)."
  Or "We propose to evaluate sociodemographic factors, for example, age, income, and education."
- (vs.) = versus
- (etc.) = and so forth
- et al. = and others (note that this is the only exception where the Latin abbreviation goes outside of parentheses)

5.12 TIP #12: SPELL OUT ACRONYMS WHEN FIRST USED; KEEP THEIR USE TO A MINIMUM

Proposal writers often resort to acronyms as a way to save space. While this is acceptable for commonly accepted acronyms (e.g., MI for myocardial infarction), this practice is discouraged for acronyms that are either not commonly used or, even worse, that are created solely for the purposes of your proposal.

Consider that you are writing a proposal to evaluate the risk of high-impact physical activity and you find yourself using that term repeatedly. It is still not acceptable to create a new acronym to save space (e.g., HIPA for high-impact physical activity). Using such nontraditional or customized acronyms will make your proposal more difficult for a reviewer to follow—leading to frustration. Some proposal writers, intent on saving space, have tried to get around this tip by inserting an acronym glossary near the beginning of their proposal. However, such a glossary requires the reviewer to constantly flip back and forth to refer to the glossary, impeding the flow of their reading. Anything to make the review process easier for the reviewer, even at the expense of a slight increase in word count, will pay off in terms of a happier reviewer who can clearly see the impact of your application.

5.13 TIP #13: AVOID THE USE OF CONTRACTIONS

Another technique that proposal writers sometimes use to save space is the use of contractions. Contractions are common in casual usage (and in this textbook!) but are not appropriate for scientific writing. Common contractions include such words as *don't*, *didn't*, and *can't*. The use of contractions runs the risk of diminishing the quality of your proposal by prioritizing space-saving over scientific writing quality.

Example Revision of Contractions

Original Version Needs Improvement
Given the differences in barriers to physical activity according to ethnicity, it's critical to evaluate whether the findings differ by ethnic group.

Improved Version
Given the differences in barriers to physical activity according to ethnicity, it is critical to evaluate whether the findings differ by ethnic group.

5.14 TIP #14: SPELL OUT NUMBERS AT THE BEGINNING OF A SENTENCE

All numbers, no matter how large, must be written out when they appear at the beginning of a sentence. It is common to see numbers less than ten written out, and this is actually required by many scientific journals. However, to avoid having to write out larger numbers, try not to put them at the beginning of a sentence. It would certainly be cumbersome to start a sentence with *One thousand eight hundred seventy-six* women were enrolled. In other words, rearrange your sentence.

Example Revision of Use of Numbers in a Sentence

Original Version Needs Improvement
1876 women were enrolled in the study.
First Improved Version
A total of 1876 women were enrolled in the study.
Second Improved Version
We enrolled a total of 1876 women in the study.

The second improved version is even further improved by using active voice *and* avoiding starting the sentence with a large number.

5.15 TIP #15: PLACEMENT OF REFERENCES

In writing a grant proposal, you will cite published articles in the body of your proposal (in-text citations), and the references in full will appear at the end of your proposal in a reference list. For an NIH grant, the choice of reference style is up to you. There are several issues to consider. First, given that space is typically at a premium in a grant proposal, the choice of superscript references like this[1] is often the best choice. This style also has the second advantage of allowing the text to flow in a relatively unimpeded fashion. Other in-text citation types range from first author's name and publication date in parentheses (e.g., Smith et al. 2012) to all authors' names and publication date (Smith A, Jones B, Brown C, 2006), both of which take up more space.

If it is important to make reference to particular authors by name, you may want to select the reference style that includes author name and date. Or alternatively simply refer to the author in the body of the sentence and maintain the superscripted references like this: Smith et al.[1] This may be particularly relevant in an area where there is a small body of research. Either way, it is important to note that the reviewer will have access to the full citation in the reference list—the question is whether or not you feel it is critical that they see all the authors' names in real time as they read your study rationale.

It is also important to note that superscripted in-text citations are always placed after punctuation like this.[1] In contrast, when proposal guidelines require in-text citations to be in parentheses, they are placed before the punctuation like this (1). Or like this (Smith A, Jones B, Brown C, 2006).

5.16 STRIVE FOR A USER-FRIENDLY DRAFT

To ensure a happy reviewer, it is vital to meticulously read your draft. The avoidance of spelling and grammatical errors and consistency in style and terminology reflects well upon you as a researcher. It is certainly true that some of the brightest researchers have not been strong writers, and vice versa. However, from a reviewer's standpoint, the grant proposal writing style is the first impression that you make. It is rare that a meticulously written proposal does not represent a conscientious researcher. Therefore, your writing style not only provides evidence of your care in preparation but also avoids errors that will detract from your proposal and reflect poorly on the quality of your scholarship.

Classic errors to avoid are lack of callouts to figures and tables in the text or misnumbered figures or tables. While these mistakes seem small, they can lead to a very frustrated reviewer who is trying to hunt down the appropriate figure/table.

Other reviewer-friendly stylistic practices include the use of standard margins and avoidance of *cute* touches such as clip art or any other special touches that may distract the reviewer by calling attention to the format of your paper instead of its content. While some granting agencies, such as NIH, allow the use of color highlighting, it is important to note that many reviewers print out their assigned proposals on their own black and white printers. Therefore, take care that any point that you were trying to highlight can still be visualized in black and white (e.g., in graphs, use dotted lines vs. dashed lines as opposed to different colored lines). In the text, consider the use of bolding or underlining, being sure to follow the granting agency's guidelines at all times. You could also consider italics, but some reviewers find italics difficult to read.

5.17 TAKE ADVANTAGE OF WRITING ASSISTANCE PROGRAMS

Most universities have writing centers. Similarly, university faculty development offices often offer grant-writing workshops or other writing assistance. As noted in Chapter 1, "Ten Top Tips for Successful Grant Proposal Writing," some departments will fund early-career faculty to attend local and national grant-writing workshops and will compensate outside scientists, with expertise on the proposed topic, to review and critique your grant proposals. Lastly, many departments will support their early-career faculty by making the services of a grant writer available. This person will likely not be an expert in your field but will be well able to review your application and ensure that you are clearly and concisely conveying your aims and methods. By encouraging you to be as clear as possible, the best grant writers help you further refine your specific aims and convey the potential impact of your findings.

5.18 SOLICIT EARLY INFORMAL FEEDBACK ON YOUR PROPOSAL

As noted in Chapter 2, "Setting Up a Time Frame," it is always best to get as much feedback as possible on your draft grant proposal, as early in the process as possible, when there is still time to make changes. We call this early feedback *low stakes*. The more feedback you can receive from your colleagues and mentors—even if they are not experts on your topic—the less likely that you will hear concerns from reviewers that you have not already addressed. Even a generalist reviewer will be able to assess (1) whether your goals are clearly stated, (2) how the grant extends prior work in the field (i.e., its innovation), and (3) and the impact of your potential findings on the field. These aspects are often the most critical in the assigned score for an application.

The more rigorous the comments the better, as it is more than likely that the NIH reviewers would have the same comments. Remember, as noted in Chapter 1, "Ten Top Tips for Successful Grant Proposal Writing," some of your assigned grant reviewers will also not have expertise in your area of interest.

After writing a first draft, ask your readers to point out elements that are not clear. It's best if this process can be conducted face-to-face (in person or virtually).The process of verbally responding to their concerns and points of confusion in your proposal will be invaluable in helping you to better articulate your thoughts in writing. First, such an interchange will enable you to identify areas that you have not clearly conveyed to the reader. Second, through orally explaining any confusing concepts to the reader, you will learn how to better explain these concepts when you return to writing. This practice of peer reviewing and receiving verbal comments back in real time has been an invaluable practice that I use in my course on scientific writing.

5.18.1 Solicit Feedback on Content, Not Just Style

It is important to get feedback on the *content* early in the redrafting process. If your first draft contained stylistic and organizational errors, such as misspellings or misplaced headings, your reviewer may feel compelled to focus on these stylistic errors and defer comments on content until the manuscript is easier to read. If this occurs, be prepared to ask for comments on content. Did you cover the literature adequately? Are your conclusions about the topic justified? Are there gaps in your review? How can the proposal be improved? It is critical to get this feedback on the *content* early in the redrafting process.

5.19 WHO MUST READ YOUR PROPOSAL

All coinvestigators and consultants on your grant should be given the opportunity to review the complete proposal. As noted in Chapter 2, "Setting Up a Time Frame," ideally, provide your coinvestigators with a complete copy of the draft of your proposal at least one month before it is due. In this way, they will have two weeks to read the proposal, and then you have time to incorporate their comments and to follow-up with a revised draft or requests for clarification. It will be even better if you've already incorporated the coinvestigator feedback much earlier in the process with their review of your specific aims. There is nothing more inconsiderate of a colleague's time than to ask for their comments at the last minute—it implies either that they do not have competing responsibilities or that you will not be incorporating their comments. This is not to say that you cannot disagree with their preliminary feedback, but instead ensure that there is time to discuss these differences in opinion with your coinvestigators. In particular, it will be important to talk about any substantive suggestions that you choose not to incorporate. Then, allow plenty of time for the redrafting process and sending the draft to your coinvestigators again for another round of review.

5.20 INCORPORATING FEEDBACK

In this process of review, it is essential to remember that the reader is always right. In other words, if one person misunderstands your points, or finds them confusing, then it is highly likely that some of the reviewers will also misunderstand your points.

It will be tempting to defend the draft proposal. Instead, try to determine why the reader did not understand it: Did you provide insufficient background information? Would the addition of more explicit transition terms between sections make it clearer? These questions should guide your discussion with the reader.

Early in one's career, it is instinctive to blame the reader. *They just don't understand my points* is a common reaction. Further complicating this is the tendency of early-career faculty to mistakenly believe that they have to write using jargon in order to impress. Instead, the most impressive writing is the simplest writing. It takes much longer to write something short and concise, than to write a long thought laden with jargon, that when closely scrutinized may not really have substance. Then, allow plenty of time for the feedback and redrafting process.

One way to get an *ear* for how to write in a scientific manner is to read numerous reviews of literature, paying attention to how they are organized and how the authors make transitions from one topic to another. And, as noted above, read the *American Journal of Epidemiology* (Vol 161, No 5) editorial titled "Please Read the Following Paper and Write this Way!"

5.21 HOW TO RECONCILE CONTRADICTORY FEEDBACK

It is inevitable that you will encounter differences of opinion among those that read your draft. The likelihood for contradictory feedback increases in direct proportion to the number of people that you solicit as readers. This is not to say to limit the number simply to make the process easier but instead to choose carefully such that each investigator/committee member is playing a key role. This will ultimately be appreciated by grant review agencies and can lead to a higher review score.

Reconcile contradictory feedback by seeking clarification from the readers. Consider the scenario in which one reader asks for additional details about a prior study by, for example, Smith et al., while another suggests that you not include that study at all. First, consider the possibility that these different opinions are due to lack of clarity in the proposal. This would be the easiest misunderstanding to clear up. If not, seek further clarification from both sources and negotiate a resolution. After such a discussion, the grant proposal should be revised to clarify the relevance of that citation. For example, *while Smith et al. studied the relationship between x and y, this does not directly relate to our work which used a different technique to study the relationship between x and y.* This added text shows that you have a mastery of the literature and did not accidently leave out the study by Smith et al. It also avoids a potential reviewer concern that you were not even aware of the Smith study. Instead, it shows enough familiarity with the study to say why this work was not relevant. Remember that it is possible that Smith may be one of your proposal reviewers!

5.22 ANNOTATED EXAMPLE: NEEDS IMPROVEMENT

A PROPOSAL TO EVALUATE THE ASSOCIATION BETWEEN OBESITY AND HEAT ILLNESSES AMONG A MILITARY POPULATION.

PARAGRAPH #1

A hot topic among environmentalists today is global warming and the corresponding public health need to study risk factors for heat-related illnesses. Current findings suggest an increase in the number of heat waves resulting in the unforeseen deaths of hundreds of US children and adults alike.

Comment: In general, the tone in paragraph #1 is too casual and the paragraph sounds more like an editorial or a commentary for the lay press. Suggestions to improve include:

- Insert citations throughout.
- Specify changes in the incidence rates of heat illnesses over time.
- Add information on the impact of heat illnesses on other diseases or disabilities or work lost days.

PARAGRAPH #2

Dozens of heat illness studies have shown that the primary populations at risk are the young and the elderly. The one prior study of obesity and heat illness found no association (RR = 1.1, 95% CI 0.9–1.2) between obesity and heat illnesses (2). However, as the authors noted, possible recall and selection biases were weaknesses of the study. Therefore, this proposal will focus on the hypothesis that among soldiers, those with obesity (body mass index [BMI] >25 kg/m^2) are at higher risk of heat stroke and exhaustion than those of normal weight (BMI 18.5 to <25).

Comment: Overall, paragraph #2 is too vague. Suggestions to improve include:

- Insert citations throughout.
- Add a physiologic and epidemiologic justification for the proposed hypothesis. While it is often a strength to be conducting an early study in an area, the lack of any studies could be due to the fact that the hypothesis is not adequately grounded in either the physiologic or the epidemiologic literature.
- Cite the incidence/prevalence rates of obesity and heat illnesses in soldiers to highlight that soldiers are at particular risk of heat illnesses and, therefore, are important to study.
- Avoid professional jargon (e.g., recall bias and selection bias) without clarifying the study limitations in simple terms.
- Avoid the phrase *as the authors noted*, and instead state your own view.

PART II

The Grant Proposal
Section by Section

Scientific component of grant proposal: Outline

I. Scientific Component
  a. Title
  b. Project Summary/Abstract (30 lines of text)
  c. Project Narrative (2–3 sentences)
  d. Introduction to Application (for Resubmission and Revision applications)
  e. Specific Aims
  f. Research Strategy (6–12 pages depending on the type of grant)
    I. Significance and Innovation
    II. Approach
      A. Preliminary Studies
      B. Study Design and Methods
      C. Data Analysis Plan
      D. Power and Sample Size
      E. Alternatives and Limitations
  g. Training Information for Fellowship Grants (F series)
  h. Candidate Information for Career Development Grants (K series)
  i. PHS Human subjects and Clinical Trials Information
  j. Bibliography and References Cited

Specific Aims

6

Welcome to Part II of this textbook, "The Grant Proposal: Section by Section." In this part of the text-book, I will walk you through the scientific sections of the grant proposal step by step, with a particular focus on strategically meeting the NIH guidelines specific to each section. As noted earlier, NIH is the most typical funding source for grants in epidemiology and preventive medicine, particularly for larger awards—the ultimate career goal.

In Chapter 3, "Identifying a Topic and Conducting the Literature Search," I described a step-by-step process for ascertaining a research gap via a targeted literature search. Chapter 3 started with how to create a literature review outline, techniques and tips for conducting the search, and ending with how to assimilate those search findings into a summary table. After identifying the research gap with the help of this summary table and confirming and/or refining your topic, you are now ready for the process of actually writing the Research Strategy (i.e., Significance, Innovation, and Approach) section of the grant proposal.

6.1 PURPOSE OF THE SPECIFIC AIMS PAGE

The Specific Aims page can arguably be considered the most critical component of the entire proposal. After the Abstract (described in Chapter 16, "Project Summary/Abstract"), the Specific Aims page is the first section, and sometimes the only section, to be read by the entire review panel and therefore is of paramount importance. A well-written Specific Aims page serves not only to *grab* the reader's attention but also immediately brings to the forefront *what is new here*—along with the scientific importance and the impact of the proposal.

As noted in Chapter 1, "Ten Top Tips for Successful Grant Proposal Writing," the majority of the NIH review committee, with the exception of the three to four reviewers assigned to your application, may only ever read the Project Summary/Abstract and Specific Aims page of your proposal. Yet all reviewers will be scoring your proposal! Even, more importantly, they may be reading this page just moments before your review. Therefore, the Specific Aims page has to grab their attention, be clear and easy to read, give a quick snapshot of the study methods, as well as the overall impact of the study findings. The *so what* factor has to be quickly addressed. Give the reader a reason to read on!

As noted in Chapter 1, most funding agencies, including NIH, consider the overall impact of the proposal as one of the top criteria in funding decisions. Specifically, as discussed in Chapter 20, "Review Process," the NIH directs reviewers to "provide an **overall impact** score to reflect their assessment of the likelihood for the project to exert a sustained, powerful influence on the research field(s) involved." An application does not need to be strong in all categories (e.g., Significance, Investigators, Innovation, Approach, Environment) to be judged likely to have major scientific impact. For example, a project that by its nature is not innovative may be essential to advance a field.

6.2 A WORD OF CAUTION

If you have skipped directly to this chapter in an attempt to move more quickly through the proposal-writing process, you will actually find the opposite. A key part of your proposal's potential to have a strong overall impact is your ability to clarify how the proposed work will **extend prior research in the field**. Only after your work in reading, organizing, and identifying the research gap in the prior literature will you have set the stage appropriately for this step.

Your choice of specific aims will be designed to fill this gap and will dictate the content of the remainder of your proposal. That is, it is only after the identification of your research gap that the writing process will flow easily. Each section of a well-written grant proposal flows directly from and mirrors components of the specific aims.

6.3 OUTLINE FOR THE SPECIFIC AIMS PAGE

The NIH grant application starts with a **one-page** description of your specific aims. The goal of this page is not only to list your specific aims but also to provide a brief summary of the significance and innovation and a synopsis of the study design. You will have room to expand upon all these items in the body of your proposal, but brief summaries are key components of this page.

6.3.1 Goals of the Specific Aims Page

The first goal of the Specific Aims page is to give an overview of the problem—What is known? What is the remaining question? Your second goal is to explain—How are you going to answer the question? What is the long-term goal of this line of research?

The majority of grant proposals in epidemiology and preventive medicine aim to identify an association between an exposure of interest and an outcome of interest. According to the NIH guidelines, the Specific Aims should:

State concisely the goals of the proposed research and summarize the expected outcome(s), including the impact that the results of the proposed research will have on the research field(s) involved. List succinctly the specific objectives of the research proposed (e.g., to test a stated hypothesis, create a novel design, solve a specific problem, challenge an existing paradigm or clinical practice, address a critical barrier to progress in the field, or develop new technology).

During my time as a standing and ad hoc member of several NIH study sections, I have found the outline listed in Table 6.1 to be the most successful approach for the Specific Aims page.

TABLE 6.1 Detailed Outline for the Specific Aims Page

SPECIFIC AIMS PAGE	
I. Significance and Innovation	One to two paragraphs
A. Importance of the topic	
i. Public health impact of the outcome	
ii. Physiology of the exposure–outcome relationship(s)	
iii. Epidemiology of the exposure–outcome relationship(s)	
B. How previous research is limited (research gap)	
C. The overall goal of your proposal and how it will fill this research gap	
III. Highlights of the Approach (Methodology)	One paragraph
A. Study design	
B. Sample size	
C. Measurement tools	
D. Preliminary study findings (if applicable)	
II. Specific Aims and Hypotheses	Half page
IV. Summary of the Significance and Innovation	Two to three sentences

6.3.2 Paragraphs #1–#2: Significance and Innovation

6.3.2.1 A. Importance of the Topic

This one-to-two paragraph section should first briefly summarize the public health importance of your topic—typically your outcome of interest—using citations. Second, the paragraph should summarize the physiological or behavioral mechanisms that link your exposure to your outcome. And third, it should summarize the prior epidemiologic literature between your exposure and outcome. Recall that you gathered literature to support these sections in Chapter 3, "Identifying a Topic and Conducting the Literature Search," in the area and highlight the research gap.

Remember that a fully developed section on each of these items will be part of the full 6-to-12-page Research Strategy of your grant proposal. Instead, here in the Specific Aims page, your goal is to be **brief**. It is always more difficult to write a short explanation than a long one!

6.3.2.2 B. How Previous Research Is Limited

The importance of the research gap Failure to identify a research gap is one of the most common flaws of an application. It is critical that the Specific Aims page clarifies, through the gap, how it will extend prior research in this area. Simply proposing to repeat prior studies is typically not sufficient to receive funding. Gaps can range widely—from methodological weaknesses to limited sample sizes. Luckily, you will have already identified this research gap (Table 6.2) by creating and reviewing the summary table as described in Chapter 3.

6.3.2.3 C. The Overall Goal of Your Proposal and How It Will Fill This Research Gap

At the end of this subsection, you can state your long-term goal and the goal of the current proposal.

A pitfall to avoid There is an old adage among reviewers that there is an inverse association between the amount of time spent on the background in an abstract and the odds of funding! Excess time spent defining well-known terms or providing background takes space away from identifying a research gap and describing the approach (methodology). The research gap should be readily apparent to the reviewer by the end of the first paragraph at the latest. Lastly, the final sentence of this paragraph can present your overall study goal.

TABLE 6.2 Example Research Gaps

Prior Literature Is …
Limited to particular study designs
Limited to particular methodology
Limited sample size
Conflicting findings
Limited control for confounding factors
Limited to particular study populations
Limited number of prior studies

Example Paragraph #1 with Research Gap Bolded

Women diagnosed with gestational diabetes mellitus (GDM) are at substantially increased risk of developing type 2 diabetes and obesity, currently at epidemic rates in the United States.[1,2] **GDM, therefore, identifies a population of women at high risk of developing type 2 diabetes and thus provides an excellent opportunity to intervene years before the development of this disorder**. Rates of both GDM and type 2 diabetes are higher among. Hispanic women as compared to non-Hispanic white women.

It is well recognized that acute as well as chronic physical activity reduce fasting plasma glucose as well as improve glucose tolerance in type 2 diabetes.[3] Similarly, increased physical activity improves insulin sensitivity and glucose control in pregnant patients with GDM.[4] Recent epidemiologic studies have suggested that women with higher levels of physical activity have reduced risk of GDM.[5–10] Prior exercise interventions among women at risk of GDM were limited by reliance solely on self-reported physical activity and were conducted primarily among non-Hispanic white women.[11–15] **Therefore, we propose to test the hypothesis that an exercise intervention is an effective tool for preventing GDM among Hispanic women with a history of GDM.**

6.3.3 Paragraph #3: Highlights of the Approach (Methodology)

This third paragraph of your Specific Aims page should provide a brief summary of your study methods. It is critical in this paragraph to provide the:

- Study design
- Sample size
- Name/source of the dataset to be used (if relevant)
- Measurement tools that will be used (e.g., food frequency questionnaires, activity monitors, and biomarkers)

Leaving these key pieces of information of an abstract out of an abstract is a common pitfall even among experienced investigators. Their omission will leave the reviewer wondering how you will be conducting the study.

It may be helpful here to know that your primary assigned NIH reviewer is tasked with describing your proposed approach to the rest of the review panel—who have not yet read your proposal. A well-written synopsis of the proposed study methods can serve as the reviewer's script in presenting your proposal. By having written this *script* for them, not only are you being kind to the reviewer but also you are ensuring that their *pitch* to the committee will be accurate and cover all the key points. If there is space, this paragraph can reappear later in the proposal in your Research Strategy section at the beginning of the Approach subsection as a synopsis of your protocol (see Chapter 11, "Study Design and Methods").

Lastly, if you have any prior grant funding or publications relevant to the proposed topic and/or methods to be used, this is a key place to mention them. Citing the specific grant number is even more impressive as it makes it apparent that this funding was externally obtained. You can do this concisely by stating the grant number, funding source, and your role in parentheses (e.g., ADA #xxxx; Dr. Smith PI).

Example Synopsis of the Study Methods

A total of 320 multiparous women who had GDM in a prior pregnancy (58% will be from minority groups) will be recruited in early pregnancy (10 weeks gestation) and randomized to either an exercise intervention (n = 160) or a comparison health and wellness intervention (n = 160). The overall goal of the intervention is to encourage pregnant women to achieve the American College of Obstetricians and Gynecologists Guidelines for physical activity during pregnancy. The intervention consists of a 12-week program ending at routine GDM screen (24–28 weeks gestation) with approximately 14 weeks of follow-up (ending at birth). The intervention draws from the theory of stages of motivational readiness for change and social cognitive theory constructs for physical activity behavior and will take into account the specific challenges faced by women of diverse socioeconomic and ethnic backgrounds. GDM will be assessed via American Diabetes Association criteria, and biochemical factors associated with insulin resistance will be collected at baseline and 24–28 weeks gestation. Physical activity will be assessed via seven days of accelerometer monitoring at baseline, at 22–24 weeks gestation, and at 32–34 weeks gestation. **The intervention protocol builds upon findings from our pilot work[1] (American Diabetes Association Career Award #1234; PI: Yourself)** and can readily be translated into clinical practice in underserved and minority populations.

6.3.4 Paragraph #4: Specific Aims and Corresponding Hypotheses

This paragraph will be a numbered list of your specific aims and hypotheses using the techniques described in the next chapter (Chapter 7, "How to Develop and Write Hypotheses").

A typical small grant proposal to NIH typically has three related aims, while a larger NIH proposal (e.g., the R01 mechanism) often has as many as five related aims. The trick is to avoid being too ambitious while at the same time not being too narrow. Mentors, outside readers, and coinvestigators can help you identify the appropriateness of your aims. Feedback from this group should very quickly be obtained from them before proceeding further. NIH RePORTER (https://reporter.nih.gov/) is also invaluable in providing a sense of what would be considered appropriate and not too ambitious.

Take care to use measurable terms in your aims. For example, reviewers may be concerned that terms such as "healthcare utilization," "quality of care," and "disparities" are too general in this section and need to be operationalized. For more details, see Chapter 7, "How to Develop and Write Hypotheses."

Example Specific Aims

Specific Aim #1: To evaluate the impact of a 12-week individually targeted exercise intervention on risk of recurrent GDM among prenatal care patients with a history of GDM.

Hypothesis #1: Compared to subjects in the comparison health and wellness intervention, women in the individually targeted exercise intervention will have a lower risk of recurrent GDM.

Specific Aim #2: To evaluate the impact of a 12-week individually targeted exercise intervention on biochemical factors associated with insulin resistance among prenatal care patients with a history of GDM.

Hypothesis #2: Compared to subjects in the comparison health and wellness intervention, women in the individually targeted exercise intervention will have lower fasting concentrations of glucose, insulin, leptin, TNF-α, CRP, and higher concentrations of adiponectin.

Specific Aim #3: To evaluate the impact of a 12-week individually targeted exercise intervention on the adoption and maintenance of physical activity during pregnancy among prenatal care patients with a history of GDM.

Hypothesis #3: Compared to subjects in the comparison health and wellness intervention, women in the individually targeted exercise intervention will participate in more physical activity in mid- and late pregnancy.

6.3.5 Paragraph #5: Summary of Significance and Innovation

The final paragraph of the Specific Aims page should summarize the significance and innovation of your proposal. The specific words, *significance* and *innovation* should be highlighted in bold. Remember that these factors are essential in obtaining funding, and reviewers are instructed to summarize these aspects of your proposal as part of their critique forms. A good reviewer will search for these key terms in your Specific Aims page.

6.3.5.1 Significance

Describe the expected contribution of your project by clarifying how the results of the proposed study (or the achievement of your long-term goals described in paragraph #1 above) will change public health and/or clinical practice. In other words, how disseminating the findings of your research will benefit the field. Note if the proposal is relevant to an NIH Institute's priority, quote this priority area. You can find a list of NIH Institutes' research priorities on their websites.

The NIH defines **significance** as addressing the following questions:

- Does the project address an important problem or a critical barrier to progress in the field?
- If the aims of the project are achieved, how will scientific knowledge, technical capability, and/or clinical practice be improved?
- How will successful completion of the aims change the concepts, methods, technologies, treatments, services, or preventive interventions that drive this field?

As you can see from these questions, *significance* in this context does not **only** mean that you plan to study a very important public health issue. *Significance* is also assessed by reviewers in terms of how data from your study will **inform the field**. Be clear as to how currently available data need to be refined and extended. For example, obesity is a significant public health problem in the United States. But how will your study drive the field forward: Will it identify susceptibility genes or maybe point the way to better preventive interventions?

A perfectly designed study about an unimportant question is not considered significant. Vice versa, a study that considers a topic of extremely high public health significance but has flaws in the study design that can affect validity of the findings is not significant either.

6.3.5.2 Innovation

Examples of innovation in epidemiology, biostatistics, and preventive medicine could include applying established techniques to a new area, or the use of stronger/more advanced techniques or theoretical constructs to address questions which have already been examined (e.g., the application of a more advanced statistical technique to an area in which it hasn't been used before). Innovation could also involve the use of objective measurement tools to address an exposure that had previously relied upon self-reported assessment.

Remember that you don't necessarily have to be the very first to do anything, but that using newer/stronger techniques in an area of sparse research can be considered innovative.

Most importantly, don't rely upon the reviewers to figure out how your research plan is innovative; tell them how it is innovative!

The NIH defines **innovation** as addressing the following questions:

- Does the application challenge and seek to shift current research or clinical practice paradigms by utilizing novel theoretical concepts, approaches or methodologies, instrumentation, or interventions?

- Are the concepts, approaches or methodologies, instrumentation, or interventions novel to one field of research or novel in a broad sense?
- Is a refinement, improvement, or new application of theoretical concepts, approaches or methodologies, instrumentation, or interventions proposed?

6.3.5.3 An Important Caveat

Don't feel that you have to propose the development of a new methodology to achieve the *innovation* guidelines. Often in epidemiology and preventive medicine, you will be proposing to use standard population-based methods to achieve your specific aims. In this case, while your methods will not be innovative, your aims may be innovative through addressing **novel hypotheses**. In other words, a project that employs standard methodologies can nevertheless result in essential information that will advance the field.

Example Summary of Significance and Innovation
This proposal is **innovative** in being the first, to our knowledge, to test a physical activity intervention designed to prevent gestational diabetes mellitus (GDM) among high-risk women. We focus on the previous understudied Hispanic population and use multidimensional (subjective and objective) measures of physical activity, and multiple and fasting measures of biochemical factors associated with insulin resistance. The **significance** of the study lies in the fact that changes in modifiable risk factors may reduce the morbidity associated with GDM and risk of subsequent type 2 diabetes, obesity, and cardiovascular disease in women. The 2020–2025 NIDDK Strategic Directions for Research calls for more research on how "multiple factors, such as exercise and diet contribute to GDM" (Goal 1.1).

6.4 WHEN TO CONSIDER DISCARDING YOUR ORIGINAL AIMS AND HYPOTHESES

If, after reading the above guidelines, you find you cannot clearly articulate the significance and innovation of your specific aims, it may be reasonable to consider substantially revising or discarding your original aims and starting over.

A pep talk It is common to become discouraged if you find that a study has already been published evaluating your exposure–outcome relationship of interest. As mentioned earlier in this text, many studies of varying designs and methodologies are required before causality can be determined. In addition, often these previously published studies may have conflicting findings. That is, some studies may have observed associations that were not statistically significant, while others observed an increased or decreased risk of your health outcome of interest among those who were exposed. In this situation, the Specific Aims page should state this research gap (e.g., *few studies have evaluated the relationship between x and y, and among these studies, findings have been conflicting*). The Aims page can then go on to briefly state potential reasons for these conflicts—such as different measurement tools and limitations in methodology. In other words, even in the situation of previously published studies on your exposure–outcome relationship, you should be able to clearly identify a worthy research gap. One doesn't have to be proposing the first study in an area in order for the proposal to be of high scientific importance. As discussed in Chapter 20, "Review Process," the overall impact of your specific aims is the driver of the final score of an NIH grant.

Reasons to consider discarding or revising your original aims are as follows:

- If you cannot identify the public health or clinical significance of your potential findings.
- If you cannot identify a means by which your aims will extend the prior published literature (i.e., the research gap). Think broadly on this topic and remember to consider the list of possible research gaps from Chapter 3, "Identifying a Topic and Conducting the Literature Search" (e.g., via a new study population, study design, or measurement tool, etc.).
- When, after conducting power calculations, you discover that you have insufficient statistical power even after considering such techniques described in Chapter 13, "Power and Sample Size."

6.5 SHOULD YOU AIM TO CONDUCT ANALYTIC OR DESCRIPTIVE STUDIES?

Specific aims in epidemiology and preventive medicine typically propose to assess measures of association between an exposure of interest and an outcome of interest. These types of aims are termed *analytic*. However, for pilot or feasibility studies, it is reasonable to propose specific aims designed simply to measure the distribution of an exposure or an outcome, independent of their association with each other. These types of aims are termed *descriptive* or univariate. The main point to keep in mind is that these descriptive-type analyses are typically only appropriate for feasibility or pilot studies or as a Specific Aim #1 in a proposal which also contains analytic aims as Specific Aims #2, #3, and/or #4.

Example Descriptive vs. Analytic Aims

Descriptive Aim
Specific Aim #1: To estimate seasonal trends in the prevalence of tick-borne diseases in the Northeastern United States.
Analytic Aim
Specific Aim #1: To evaluate the association between seasonal trends in the prevalence of tick-borne diseases and corresponding trends in Lyme disease incidence.

In the example above, the descriptive aim simply describes the prevalence of an exposure (i.e., tick-borne diseases). In contrast, the analytic aim evaluates the association between tick-borne diseases (the exposure) with Lyme disease incidence (an outcome).

6.6 AIMS INVOLVING THE USE OF AN EXISTING DATASET—PROS AND CONS

As many diseases are relatively rare, epidemiologic studies typically require large numbers of participants and many years of follow-up. In addition, if you aim to recruit participants yourself, the Institutional Review Board (IRB) approval process for human subjects' protection can be quite lengthy. In contrast, proposing to evaluate your specific aims within the context of an existing dataset capitalizes on work already conducted and is an excellent first step in your proposal-writing career. This approach can also be viewed by funding agencies as a cost-efficient way to answer an important research question. Such existing datasets could be local (e.g., collected by a mentor or colleague) or national (e.g., collected as part of a national surveillance system). It is important to note that this approach would still require that your aims and hypotheses address important research questions. In addition, you would want to ensure that your proposed aims are not already included as part of the aims of the original grant that funded the existing dataset.

In summary, there are several **advantages** to utilizing an existing dataset:

- In a climate of low NIH funding pay lines, this approach can be seen as a cost-efficient way to *mine* existing data for other important questions.
- By nature of the fact that you would be working on an existing project, you will have the accompanying benefit of an established research team. These investigators can be an invaluable resource for you, and listing them on your proposal as part of your research team will be seen as a strength.
- You will not be subject to the risk of not meeting your stated recruitment and follow-up rates. Your power calculations will be based on real numbers and the reviewers can be assured that you already have the data in hand. Therefore, they are more likely to have confidence that you will be able to achieve the stated aims of the application.

There are also several **disadvantages** to utilizing an existing dataset:

- Because the overall study was not designed with your research topic in mind, you may be missing data on important covariates.
- Exclusions may have been made to the original sample that are not relevant to your research question.
- Detailed data on your exposure and outcome variables of interest may not be available.

However, these disadvantages are usually somewhat addressable as indicated in the below example.

Example Method to Minimize a Disadvantage to Utilizing an Existing Dataset
Consider that you are proposing to examine the association between smoking and risk of preterm birth within the context of a colleague's existing larger dataset designed to examine the association between physical activity and gestational diabetes.
As part of the original grant, your colleague had already collected information on smoking as well as preterm birth as covariates, however, they did not collect information on history of preterm birth—a key potential confounding factor in your proposed association of interest. To minimize this concern, you propose to conduct a sensitivity analysis, repeating your primary analysis among women who are nulliparous. In other words, by proposing to repeat the analysis within a stratum of women that had no history of preterm birth, you can assure the reviewers that you will able to evaluate the extent of potential confounding by this variable.

6.7 HOW TO DECIDE WHETHER TO INCLUDE EXPLORATORY OR SECONDARY AIMS

It is common practice for proposal writers to include exploratory or secondary aims when they lack the statistical power to achieve these aims. The advantage of including such aims is that you can show off the potential of your project to achieve numerous other goals—thereby increasing its potential value.

By labeling these aims as *exploratory* or *secondary*, you may reduce the risk of being held accountable for such a lack of power. However, it is important to keep in mind that each aim, regardless of whether it is *primary, secondary, or exploratory*, should be supported in the Significance and Innovation section and will require corresponding methods in the Approach section. By including these extra aims, you run the risk of exceeding your page requirements or short-shifting your primary aims. One compromise is, instead, to simply add a sentence about the future potential uses of your collected data.

Example Future Aims
The collection and storage of cord blood as part of this proposal will also facilitate future applications designed to evaluate the association between the *in utero* environment and the risk of childhood diseases.

6.8 TIP #1: HOW TO DEAL WITH THE ONE-PAGE LIMITATION FOR THE SPECIFIC AIMS PAGE

Specific Aims are designed to be concise and to the point. How, therefore, does one decide what merits mentioning in the aims and hypotheses aside from the independent and dependent variables and the proposed direction of effect? One of the key determinants is whether the additional details will make a critical difference to reviewers in determining whether to fund your study—again with the thought in mind that some reviewers will only read your abstract and aims. Therefore, prioritize study attributes that reflect key advances in the field. In other words, if a reviewer were **only** to read your aims and hypotheses, what key attributes (i.e., advances) of your proposal would you want them to know?

6.9 TIP #2: DO NOT PROPOSE OVERLY AMBITIOUS SPECIFIC AIMS

An *ambitious* grant proposal submitted by a new investigator is one of the most common reasons for an application to receive a poor score or to be streamlined. (For a definition of the term *streamline*, often known as *triage*, see Chapter 20, "Review Process.") Overly ambitious aims for a large R01 could include aims that are interdependent (see Tip #3: Avoid Interdependent Aims), the inclusion of too many aims (see Tip #4: Avoid Including Too Many Specific Aims), or aims without supporting preliminary data. Instead, it is much more impressive to exercise restraint and have focused and cohesive aims in your early grant proposals.

6.9.1 Recommendation for a Feasible Topic for a First Grant

As described in detail in Chapter 10, "Pilot Grants: Reproducibility and Validity Studies," make excellent choices for early-career grant proposals. Due to their fairly small size and delineated methods, they are quite feasible for early-stage investigators. Furthermore, their critical role in the development of a larger project makes them particularly appealing for reviewers—as it is clear that they are a critical first step toward answering a larger question in your next grant proposal submission.

It is perfectly appropriate for a proposal for a small pilot study to state that its ultimate objective is to support the submission of a larger award. The specific aims can conclude by saying, *Findings from this study will yield critical evidence to support the subsequent submission of an R01 application*. Reviewers like to see evidence of a carefully thought out plan for the future. It demonstrates that the findings from the proposal will have future utility.

The other advantage of starting small in this fashion (see Chapter 1, "Tip #1: Start Small but Have a Big Vision") is that it is easier to grow in a stepwise fashion from smaller to larger grants. First, such smaller grants like an NIH Career Development award or a Fellowship grant will be more likely to be funded due to their critical role in supporting your subsequent career plans—this is often the main funding criteria used by reviewers of these grant mechanisms. Second, having successfully applied for, received, and conducted any type of smaller grant will demonstrate to the reviewers that you have the ability to successfully carry out larger projects. Third, publications from these smaller grants will indicate that you can translate findings into publications—another key factor in reviewers' eyes.

6.10 TIP #3: AVOID INTERDEPENDENT AIMS

Years ago, when NIH funding pay lines were higher, it was often considered acceptable to include a pilot feasibility or a validation study as the first specific aim of a large R01-type grant application. For example, Specific Aim #1 would be to develop the tools/intervention/methods that would then be used in Specific Aims #2–#5.

In the current economic climate, reviewers do not look favorably upon this practice. They naturally ask, "What if the pilot/validation study finds that the methods are not successful? How would the investigator accomplish the subsequent aims of the project?" If Specific Aim #1 subsequently fails to find that the questionnaire is valid, then how can the remainder of the specific aims succeed? These are termed **interdependent aims**, and reviewers often consider such aims to be a fatal flaw of a proposal.

Therefore, such pilot feasibility and validity aims need to be achieved prior to applying for an R01—for example, as part of a smaller Research Award (e.g., R21 or R03), Career Development Award, Fellowship grant, or a foundation grant.

6.11 TIP #4: AVOID INCLUDING TOO MANY SPECIFIC AIMS

As a general rule of thumb, for a large NIH grant, avoid having more than four to five aims. For a smaller grant, three aims are likely sufficient, and it is particularly dangerous to include more without being viewed as overly ambitious. Because this is a common pitfall of new investigators, review panels are particularly wary of multiple aims in small grant proposals. However, there are several alternative approaches to consider.

Consider that you are writing a large R01-type NIH grant and you find yourself with eight aims; consider the following options:

Ask yourself if the aims form natural groupings. For example, is there a natural split where four aims fit under one overall goal, while the other four fit under another overall goal? If so, consider two separate grant proposals if you already have preliminary studies to support each set of aims. If you have more preliminary data for one set of aims than another, then consider limiting the proposal to focus on the set that has the most preliminary data. After submitting that application, gather more preliminary data for the second grouping of aims and consider submitting that for a separate grant submission. Remember Tip #2: Focus on Small Grants Targeted to Early-Career Investigators in Chapter 1, "Ten Top Tips for Successful Proposal Writing," that it is always preferable to have several "pots simmering on the stove" (i.e., several applications under review) at any one time.

If you truly find you cannot delete any aims, consider listing some as *exploratory aims*. Exploratory aims should be limited in number, and while they may require a data analysis plan, they do not typically require power calculations. However, caution should be taken with this approach. Reviewers will carefully examine your application to detect whether you are labeling a key aim as *exploratory* as a way to hide poor power.

Alternatively, ask yourself whether your aims are too specific. Consider how broadly or narrowly you will be writing your aims.

Example Specific Aims That Are Too Narrow
Original Version Needs Improvement
Specific Aim #1: We propose to evaluate the association between light-intensity physical activity and risk of gestational diabetes.
Specific Aim #2: We propose to evaluate the association between moderate-intensity physical activity and risk of gestational diabetes.
Specific Aim #3: We propose to evaluate the association between vigorous-intensity physical activity and risk of gestational diabetes.
Improved Version
Specific Aim #1: We propose to evaluate the association between light-, moderate-, and vigorous-intensity physical activity and risk of gestational diabetes.

The improved example recognizes the fact that the three subtypes of physical activity all fall within one overall domain of physical activity and therefore can be combined into one aim. Note, however, that the improved example still mentions these three subtypes by name to demonstrate the breadth of data available and to make clear that the findings will shed light on these aspects of physical activity.

6.12 TIP #5: IF YOU PLAN TO EVALUATE EFFECT MODIFICATION IN YOUR METHODS, INCLUDE IT AS A HYPOTHESIS

If you plan on evaluating the presence of interaction or effect modification in your data analysis, include this *a priori* as a study aim(s) and hypothesis. This will help to assure your reviewers that you will not be *data dredging* for statistically significant findings if you fail to observe an overall association between your exposure and outcome of interest. In other words, when writing the proposal, carefully consider which factors might be possible effect modifiers of the relationship between your exposure and disease, based upon feasible physiological mechanisms and/or findings from the prior literature. For a definition of effect modification (i.e., interaction) and how it differs from confounding, see Chapter 14, "Study Limitations to Consider."

It is often difficult to avoid the use of epidemiologic jargon in writing this type of aim, but it is essential to try to do so. This will ensure that the aim is clear to all reviewers. A general template for an effect modification aim could be:

Specific Aim: To evaluate whether the association between [exposure] and [outcome] differs according to [effect modifier] (Figure 6.1).

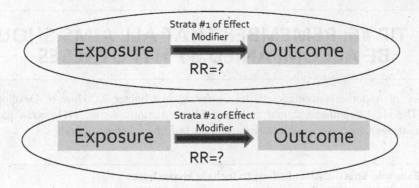

FIGURE 6.1   Effect modification by a two-level effect modifier.

Example Specific Aims for Effect Modification
Original Version Needs Improvement
Specific Aim #1: To explore the role of obesity as a potential effect modifier of the association between menopausal hormone therapy and Alzheimer's disease.
Improved Version
Specific Aim #1: To evaluate whether the association between menopausal hormone therapy and Alzheimer's disease differs according to obesity status.
  Hypothesis #1a: The impact of menopausal hormone therapy on Alzheimer's disease will be stronger among women with obesity than among women without obesity (Figure 6.2).

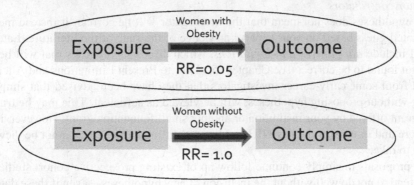

FIGURE 6.2   Effect modification by obesity.

A common pitfall is to write this aim as if the effect modifier is the exposure. Instead, this aim is designed to evaluate whether association between menopausal hormone therapy and Alzheimer's disease differs among strata of obesity. The corresponding data analysis plan could involve conducting your analysis among women with obesity only and then repeating this analysis among women without obesity. Then compare your findings—does the observed association between menopausal hormone therapy and Alzheimer's differ between these groups? Additional and/or alternative approaches to evaluate effect modification would be to include an interaction term (e.g., menopausal hormone therapy × obesity status) in your multivariable models.

6.13 TIP #6: REMEMBER THAT ALL AIMS SHOULD BE ACCOMPANIED BY HYPOTHESES

The importance of hypothesis writing will be described in Chapter 7, "How to Develop and Write Hypotheses." The ideal hypothesis should make testable predictions. As an NIH review panel member, I've seen grants triaged, or considered fatally flawed, for failing to include hypotheses.

Example Specific Aims Failing to Include Hypotheses
Specific Aim #1: To identify activities in each trimester that are major contributors to total energy expenditure.
Specific Aim #2: To directly measure the metabolic cost (intensity) of physical activity.

The example above is a simple to-do list, informally termed a *laundry list*. The act of writing hypotheses requires the investigator to assimilate the prior literature and state of evidence in a particular area and to take the next step of proposing what direction of effect they expect to see in their proposed study. The need for hypotheses is vital **even** if your aims are simply designed to be *hypothesis generating*.

Hypotheses are also critical regardless of your study methods—that is, they are necessary for both qualitative and quantitative studies. For example, Specific Aim #1 above could be an aim for a qualitative study using focus groups to generate hypotheses for major contributors to total energy expenditure. Alternatively, Specific Aim #1 could be an aim for a quantitative analysis of an existing dataset. Regardless, it requires a hypothesis. For example, **Hypothesis #1a** could be as follows: *Sports and exercise will be the major contributors to total energy expenditure, while occupational and household activities will be minor contributors.*

Including hypotheses does not mean that the investigator will be correct. It instead means that it is your best educated guess based on your expert knowledge of the state of the literature. Later in the proposal, you will include *alternatives and limitations*, which discuss approaches that will be taken if the hypothesis is not found to be correct (see Chapter 15, "How to Present Limitations and Alternatives"),

I've heard from some early-career investigators that they have been advised that simply proposing to collect data, without proposing hypotheses, will be viewed as sufficient. This may be true for a small internal seed grant offered by your institution or another small foundation grant. However, in the current economic culture and in view of the low NIH pay lines, omitting hypotheses cannot be viewed as a strategic approach to take.

Similarly, proposals to simply continue follow-up of existing prospective cohort studies or existing data registries tend to not do well without the inclusion of new hypotheses—even if these data sources are unique. This has become even more apparent with decreasing NIH pay lines. Instead, you need to include hypotheses that justify the continued follow-up of this cohort.

6.14 TIP #7: CONSIDER INCLUDING A FIGURE IN YOUR SPECIFIC AIMS PAGE

Space is limited on the one-page Specific Aims page, but if you find there is adequate space, a figure of your specific aims is highly recommended and can be viewed as a kindness to your reviewers. Note that figures may no longer be allowed in the Abstract page as per a future NIH policy aimed to avoid copyright infringement, but this policy does not, at this time, relate to the Specific Aims page. If space is not

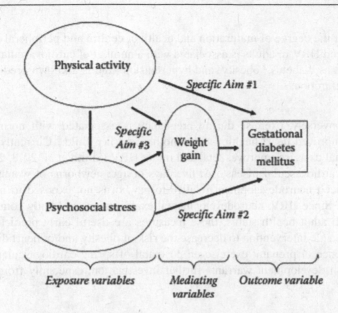

FIGURE 6.3 **Example s**pecific aims figure from a proposal to evaluate the association between physical activity, stress, and risk of GDM.

adequate, this figure can be placed in the Research Strategy section (see Chapter 8, "Significance and Innovation").

Figure 6.3 shows a proposal to conduct an observational cohort study to evaluate how physical activity (exposure #1) and stress (exposure #2) impact risk of GDM (outcome) via certain physiological and behavioral mediating variables. This one figure clearly displays the proposed relationships between the exposure variables, mediating variables, and outcome variables and the corresponding aims.

6.15 ANNOTATED EXAMPLES

6.15.1 Example #1: Needs Improvement

R03 PROPOSAL

THE IMPACT OF MATERNAL EXERCISE ON NEONATAL CARDIOVASCULAR HEALTH

Specific Aims Page

Paragraph #1: Sedentary behaviors during pregnancy are associated with weight gain, increased risk of disease, and poor pregnancy outcomes. For example, excessive weight gain in pregnancy increases the risk of hypertension, gestational diabetes, post-partum weight retention, childhood obesity of offspring. Lack of physical activity is associated with cardiovascular disease and obesity, which are two leading causes of mortality in the United States.[1] Furthermore, obesity and cardiovascular disease in adults and children has dramatically increased in the US leading to generational cycles of disease. In order to detect these conditions, heart rate variability (HRV) is used as a noninvasive physiological indicator of health and disease. Heart rate variability is the beat-to-beat variation in the duration of the R-R interval recorded via an electrocardiogram. Furthermore, metrics of HRV in the developing fetus, infant, child, and adult is a measure of cardiac autonomic balance and serve as a proxy for the degree of maturation and health of central and peripheral nervous systems. For instance, reduced HRV in adults is associated with a number of cardiovascular risk factors and disease states, such as diabetes,[2] obesity[3] and hypertension[4] and is a known predictor of mortality after myocardial infarction. [2,3]

Paragraph #2: Conversely, exercise during pregnancy is associated with normalized maternal weight gain and improved heart health for the mother and her child.[5] Currently, research shows that regular maternal exercise improves fetal and infant HRV (Smith et al. 2018, 2020), suggesting decreased risk of cardiovascular disease. At five days of age, newborns of women who exercised demonstrate advanced neurodevelopment relative to newborns not exposed to maternal exercise (Jones et al. 2015). Since HRV, neurodevelopmental examination, and body composition analysis are associated with adult health status, these measures are useful early predictors of long-term health outcomes. A safe intervention to decrease the risk of obesity and/or heart disease is physical activity. The influence of prenatal exercise on postnatal offspring cardiovascular health, obesity, and nervous system development warrants further investigation, especially from a public health perspective.

Comment

- Too much time is spent on background and brings up that old reviewer adage that the more time spent on background, the less likely the project is to be funded!
- Most importantly, by the end of the paragraphs the reader is still not clear on the research gap.
- The previous prior prenatal exercise interventions are not described—how many studies have been conducted? How would this proposed intervention extend this body of research?
- Bolding or otherwise highlighting key sentences would make the most important points in each paragraph clearer to the reviewers.
- There is excessive reliance upon one citation (Jones et al. 2015).
- The choice of citation style should be consistent. In general, superscripted references should be used to save space.
- Avoid citing unpublished literature in the specific aims page.

Paragraph #3: Our pilot research suggests that regular maternal exercise benefits the cardiovascular system of the developing fetus. Additional data show that children exposed to maternal exercise in utero are leaner and have improved heart efficiency into childhood as well. Further we have demonstrated a relationship between the level of maternal exercise activity and the amount of fetal heart change. The feasibility of this work is demonstrated by the ongoing study, and by preliminary data suggesting differences between exercisers relative to controls in fetal heart rate, birth weight, and length.

Comments

- As written, this paragraph may lead the reviewer to become concerned that this preliminary data may have already filled the research gap. Instead, any preliminary findings presented should be clearly tied to the need to address the proposed specific aims.

- Pilot data should be accompanied by parenthetical details on the funding agency, grant number, and PI name (e.g., ADA1234; PI: Smith).
- Most importantly, the reader has not been provided with the proposed study design, sample size, study population, and methodology? How many study arms will participants be randomized to?

Paragraph #4

Primary Aims

Specific Aim #1: To determine if regular maternal exercise is cardioprotective in offspring.

  Hypothesis #1a: We will test the hypothesis that maternal exercise is associated with lower heart rate (HR), increased heart rate variability (HRV), and improved cardiac efficiency (i.e., increased stroke volume and ejection fraction) at 36 weeks gestational age and one-month postnatal compared to offspring of non-exercisers (controls).

Secondary Aims

Specific Aim 2: To determine if regular maternal exercise improves neuromuscular maturation in neonates.

  Hypothesis #2a: We will test the hypothesis that exercise throughout pregnancy is associated with improved one-month infant neurological examination scores compared to controls.

Specific Aim #3: To determine if regular maternal exercise protects offspring from obesity, specifically decreased fetal and infant body fat measures, but normal growth measures.

Comments

- There should be more primary aims than secondary aims (e.g., three primary aims and one secondary aim would be preferable).
- As written, reviewers may immediately become concerned that there is inadequate statistical power to achieve Specific Aims #2 and #3 and that is why they are listed as *secondary*.
- Secondary Specific Aim #3 is not accompanied by a hypothesis.
- Italicized font can be difficult for reviewers to read and historically has been used to mark revisions in a resubmission. They should be avoided here.

Paragraph #5 (Final Paragraph): This study will determine if the offspring (fetus/neonate) of pregnant women have improved heart health, improved neuromuscular maturation, and decreased adiposity in response to chronic exercise throughout gestation relative to offspring of women who do not exercise during pregnancy. The data from this study will be the beginning of a longitudinal study to follow children exposed and not exposed to maternal exercise in utero to determine long-term health benefits. Additionally, these data will help determine if HRV can be utilized as a noninvasive means to detect these conditions in utero. This proposal is suited for this program since it aligns with the mission of promoting wellness and improving the quality of life of women and children.

Comments

- The terms *significance* and *innovation* do not appear in this paragraph. These terms are key factors in funding decisions.

6.15.2 Example #2: Does Not Need Improvement

EXERCISE INTERVENTION TO REDUCE GESTATIONAL DIABETES

SPECIFIC AIMS PAGE

Women diagnosed with gestational diabetes mellitus (GDM) are at substantially increased risk of developing type 2 diabetes and obesity, currently at epidemic rates in the United States.[1,2] **GDM, therefore, identifies a population of women at high risk of developing type 2 diabetes and thus provides an excellent opportunity to intervene years before the development of this disorder**. Rates of both GDM and type 2 diabetes are higher among Hispanic women as compared to non-Hispanic white women.

It is well recognized that acute as well as chronic physical activity reduce fasting plasma glucose as well as improve glucose tolerance in type 2 diabetes.[3] Similarly, increased physical activity improves insulin sensitivity and glucose control in pregnant patients with GDM.[4] Recent epidemiologic studies have suggested that women with higher levels of physical activity have reduced risk of GDM.[5–10] Prior exercise interventions among women at risk of GDM were limited by reliance solely on self-reported physical activity and were conducted primarily among non-Hispanic white women.[11–15] **Therefore, we propose to test the hypothesis that an exercise intervention is an effective tool for preventing GDM among Hispanic women with a history of GDM**.

A total of 320 multiparous women who had GDM in a prior pregnancy (58% will be from minority groups) will be recruited in early pregnancy (ten weeks gestation) and randomized to either an exercise intervention (n = 160) or a comparison health and wellness intervention (n = 160). The overall goal of the intervention is to encourage pregnant women to achieve the American College of Obstetricians and Gynecologists Guidelines for physical activity during pregnancy. The intervention consists of a 12-week program ending at routine GDM screen (24–28 weeks gestation) with approximately 14 weeks of follow-up (ending at birth). The intervention draws from the theory of stages of motivational readiness for change and social cognitive theory constructs for physical activity behavior and will take into account the specific challenges faced by women of diverse socioeconomic and ethnic backgrounds. GDM will be assessed via American Diabetes Association criteria, and biochemical factors associated with insulin resistance will be collected at baseline and 24–28 weeks gestation. Physical activity will be assessed via 7 days of accelerometer monitoring at baseline, at 22–24 weeks gestation, and at 32–34 weeks gestation. The intervention protocol builds upon findings from our pilot work[1] (American Diabetes Association Career Award #1234; PI: Yourself) and can readily be translated into clinical practice in underserved and minority populations.

Specific Aim #1: To evaluate the impact of a 12-week individually targeted exercise intervention on risk of recurrent GDM among prenatal care patients with a history of GDM.

  Hypothesis #1: Compared to subjects in the comparison health and wellness intervention, women in the individually targeted exercise intervention will have a lower risk of recurrent GDM.

Specific Aim #2: To evaluate the impact of a 12-week individually targeted exercise intervention on biochemical factors associated with insulin resistance among prenatal care patients with a history of GDM.

> **Hypothesis #2**: Compared to subjects in the comparison health and wellness intervention, women in the individually targeted exercise intervention will have lower fasting concentrations of glucose, insulin, leptin, TNF-α, CRP, and higher concentrations of adiponectin.

Specific Aim #3: To evaluate the impact of a 12-week individually targeted exercise intervention on the adoption and maintenance of physical activity during pregnancy among prenatal care patients with a history of GDM.

> **Hypothesis #3**: Compared to subjects in the comparison health and wellness intervention, women in the individually targeted exercise intervention will participate in more physical activity in mid- and late pregnancy.

This proposal is **innovative** in being the first, to our knowledge, to test a physical activity intervention designed to prevent gestational diabetes mellitus (GDM) among high-risk women. We focus on the previous understudied Hispanic population and use multidimensional (subjective and objective) measures of physical activity, and multiple and fasting measures of biochemical factors associated with insulin resistance. The **significance** of the study lies in the fact that changes in modifiable risk factors may reduce the morbidity associated with GDM and risk of subsequent type 2 diabetes, obesity, and cardiovascular disease in women. The 2020–2025 NIDDK Strategic Directions for Research calls for more research on how "multiple factors, such as exercise and diet contribute to GDM" (Goal 1.1).

How to Develop and Write Hypotheses

7

The importance of writing hypotheses cannot be underestimated. A well-written research hypothesis describes the results that a researcher expects to find. In effect, it is a testable prediction. Therefore, the act of creating hypotheses will require you to assimilate the prior literature and state of evidence in a particular area and to take the next step of proposing what direction of effect you expect to see in your proposed study. Thus, the process of crafting hypotheses shapes your strategy for the remainder of the proposal.

The guidelines and stylistic tips described in this chapter will walk you through the hypothesis writing process. At first, these guidelines and tips might appear deceptively simple. But, almost without exception, once you try your hand at writing your own hypotheses, you will find that they are more challenging than they seem!

7.1 NEED FOR HYPOTHESES

With few exceptions, all proposals considered compelling and fundable by granting agencies must include hypotheses. The need for hypotheses is vital **even** if your aims are simply designed to be hypothesis generating. Hypotheses are also critical regardless of your study methods—that is, they are necessary for both qualitative and quantitative studies. While most early-career faculty know that they need to include specific aims in their proposals, they often omit or have trouble articulating hypotheses. This omission is even true at the senior faculty level. As an NIH review panel member, I've seen grants triaged, or considered fatally flawed, for failing to include hypotheses.

As shown in the accompanying Figure 7.1, hypotheses should be nested within specific aims. In a grant application, the Specific Aims section is one of the first sections of your proposal to be read by reviewers. The maxim that *first impressions matter* is particularly true in this case.

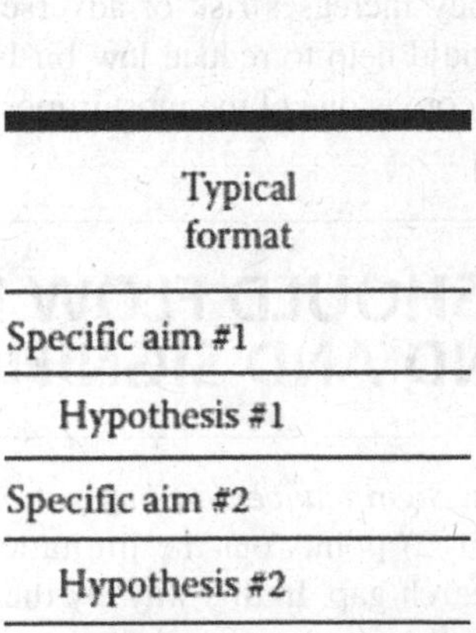

Typical
format

Specific aim #1

Hypothesis #1

Specific aim #2

Hypothesis #2

FIGURE 7.1 Typical format for specific aims and corresponding hypotheses.

DOI: 10.1201/9781003155140-9

7.2 MORE ABOUT THE DISTINCTION BETWEEN HYPOTHESES AND SPECIFIC AIMS

Specific aims are a list of tasks that you, as an investigator, propose to accomplish. Essentially, specific aims outline what you propose to *do* in the project; they are a *to-do list* of tasks. In contrast, hypotheses state the relationship that you expect to *observe*, that is, your anticipated findings. This may sound difficult, and indeed it is. The formulation of hypotheses can only occur after a comprehensive review of the prior literature on your proposed topic (see Chapter 3, "Identifying a Topic and Conducting the Literature Search"). Hypotheses must extend logically from this prior research and be a reasonable expectation by anyone who has read this prior work. Thus, including hypotheses indicates that you have a clear grasp of the literature.

As you can see in the example below, if one views the specific aims without the hypotheses, the proposal is simply listing tasks to be accomplished. In contrast, with the addition of hypotheses, it becomes clear that the investigator has assimilated the prior literature and, more importantly, has an educated hunch as to what they will find.

Example Specific Aims Missing Hypotheses
Original Version Needs Improvement
Specific Aim #1: To evaluate the association between pregnancy stress and risk of adverse birth outcomes in African American women.
Specific Aim #2: To evaluate the association between pregnancy stress and risk of hypertensive disorders of pregnancy in African American women.
Improved Version
Specific Aim #1: To evaluate the association between pregnancy stress and risk of adverse birth outcomes in African American women.
　Hypothesis #1: There will be a positive association between pregnancy stress and risk of preterm birth and low birth weight.
Specific Aim #2: To evaluate the association between pregnancy stress and risk of hypertensive disorders of pregnancy in African American women.
　Hypothesis #2: There will be a positive association between pregnancy stress and risk of preeclampsia and gestational hypertension.

Hypotheses indicate your *overall impact* — A key advantage to including hypotheses is that they indirectly show off the *overall impact* of your proposal. In other words, by articulating what you anticipate to be the potential results of your study, the reviewer can begin to envision how your findings might influence public health and clinical practice. In the example above, discovering that stress during pregnancy increases risk of adverse birth outcomes might inform future prenatal intervention programs that would help to reduce low birth weight. As discussed in Chapter 20, "Review Process," the *overall impact* score is one of the most important factors in NIH funding decisions.

7.3 HYPOTHESES SHOULD FLOW LOGICALLY FROM THE BACKGROUND AND SIGNIFICANCE SECTION

Hypotheses are the climax of your proposal — A well-written *Significance and Innovation section* in your Specific Aims page (paragraphs #1–2) points out the limitations of the current research and highlights the research gap. In this way, by the time the reviewer gets to the specific aims and hypotheses, they should be craving for someone to fill this research gap. The hypotheses serve to fulfill this desire. In this manner, the hypotheses can be viewed as the *climax* of the Specific Aims page.

Example Hypotheses Flowing Logically from Paragraphs #1–2 of the Specific Aims Page

Imagine a proposal to evaluate the long-term impact of a vitamin D supplementation program. In Paragraph #1 of your Specific Aims page, you described the prior studies of vitamin D supplementation. In particular, you highlighted the point that the prior literature was limited to evaluating the short-term impact (e.g., 3 months) of these programs and that no investigators had evaluated the long-term impact of such programs. This was your "research gap."

End of Paragraph #1 of the Specific Aims Page

These findings suggest that vitamin D supplementation programs for reproductive aged women are likely to yield short-term improvements in depression. It is not clear, however, whether such improvements can be maintained over time. Therefore, our overall goal is to evaluate the long-term impact of vitamin D on depression in women.

Specific Aims and Hypotheses

Specific Aim #1: We propose to conduct a randomized controlled trial of a vitamin D supplementation program for reproductive aged women.

Hypothesis #1: We hypothesize that after one year, women randomized to a vitamin D supplementation program will report fewer depressive symptoms as compared to women randomized to the placebo group.

7.4 HOW TO WRITE HYPOTHESES IF THE PRIOR LITERATURE IS CONFLICTING

Often, prior studies are contradictory. In terms of the above example, what if some prior vitamin D supplementation programs found no impact on depression, while others observed some improvement? Or, even more extreme, what if some studies found an adverse impact? In these situations you, as a proposal writer, will be faced with choosing a hypothesized direction of effect. This task can be daunting at first. However, it may be a relief to know that the most persuasive approach is for you to be as transparent as possible regarding your decision-making process. That is, *include* the thought process behind this choice in your proposal. This process is described in detail in Chapter 8, "Significance and Innovation."

In brief, the first step is to acknowledge that you are aware that the prior literature is conflicting. This reassures the reviewer that you are knowledgeable about the state of the research in this field. Then to determine which "side" you will take, review the summary table that you created in Chapter 3, "Identifying a Topic and Conducting the Literature Search." Look at the quality of these prior studies. Consider whether studies that were methodologically stronger were more likely to observe a certain direction of effect. Ideally, the methods used in these studies should be similar to the methods that you are proposing. More heavily weigh the direction of effect observed by prior studies that used a validated measurement tool or were conducted in a study population similar to your own. Other criteria to consider are strength of study design (e.g., case-control vs. prospective study) and sample size and power to observe an effect.

If available, also read the recommendations of review articles in this area.

Use this evidence to clarify your rationale for proposing a direction of effect in your hypotheses. State why you feel that the evidence is more persuasive in one direction (e.g., a protective effect) as opposed to another direction (e.g., an adverse effect or a null effect). Be sure to cite those key studies from your summary table as well as any relevant review articles.

Key pitfalls to avoid   With the above approach, you avoid the pitfall of appearing unaware of prior work—which would not be viewed favorably by reviewers. Indeed, some of the reviewers may have been the authors of studies that reported alternative findings. Reviewers would rather have you acknowledge the complexity of the situation, and then clarify your thought process, rather than gloss over contradictory findings.

7.5 HOW TO WRITE HYPOTHESES IF THE PRIOR LITERATURE IS NULL

In the situation where prior studies have been null, and did not indicate an effect in either one direction or another, formulating a hypothesis can be even more challenging. Highlight for the reviewer why your study will be more likely to observe an effect (e.g., by nature of your larger sample size and therefore enhanced power) as compared to those prior null studies. Other reasons for why you might be more likely to observe an effect than prior studies could include your use of improved measurement tools, a stronger study design, or your focus on a high-risk population.

7.6 HOW TO WRITE HYPOTHESES IF THE PRIOR LITERATURE IS SPARSE OR NONEXISTENT

As noted in Chapter 3, "Identifying a Topic and Conducting the Literature Search," if you determine that there is no literature with a direct bearing on one or more aspects of your topic, this should be cautiously viewed as good news. That is, you may have identified a research gap, given that no one has evaluated your proposed association of interest. However, it is still essential that you assure the reviewers that your proposed hypotheses are reasonable. This can be achieved in several ways.

First, you can justify your hypothesized direction of effect based upon the proposed physiologic association between your exposure and your outcome in formulating your hypotheses.

In addition, as noted in Chapter 3, you can summarize the findings of studies with the same exposure as yours, but a different, albeit physiologically related, outcome. The concept is to choose an outcome similar to your own, so that a reviewer would consider it reasonable that a similar mechanism might link your exposure to your outcome.

Similarly, you can summarize the findings of studies with a different exposure but the same outcome as yours. Again, the idea is to select an exposure similar in nature to your exposure. The argument that you will use in your proposal is that if these other similar exposures impact risk of your outcome, then it might be reasonable to assume that your exposure also impacts your outcome in the same manner.

The plus side of this challenging situation is that, with no prior studies, the need for your study should be even clearer. Highlight this dearth of research and the novelty of your hypotheses to the reviewer.

The following are a set of guidelines to help you formulate the strongest hypotheses possible while avoiding common pitfalls.

7.7 GUIDELINE #1: A RESEARCH HYPOTHESIS SHOULD NAME THE INDEPENDENT AND DEPENDENT VARIABLES AND INDICATE THE TYPE OF RELATIONSHIP EXPECTED BETWEEN THEM

In epidemiology and preventive medicine, the independent variable is termed the *exposure variable*. This term is used broadly to encompass both risk factors and protective factors for some type of outcome (typically a disease). A common misperception is to view *exposures* as referring to adverse factors (e.g., cigarette smoking, drug use), but the definition is actually more broad. Specifically, the independent variable is any factor that may lead to a health outcome. In a similar fashion, dependent variables or *outcomes* in epidemiology and preventive medicine are often diseases but can also be positive outcomes such as psychological well-being.

Below is a simple example of a hypothesis that contains an independent and dependent variable and describes their relationship.

Example Hypothesis Naming the Independent and Dependent Variable and the Relationship between Them
Hypothesis: There will be a positive relationship between level of coffee intake and risk of Parkinson's disease.

In this example, the level of coffee intake is the independent variable (i.e., the exposure variable) and Parkinson's disease is the dependent variable (i.e., the outcome variable). Note that this example also clarifies the direction of effect. In other words, that coffee increases risk of Parkinson's disease.

Example Hypothesis Lacking Clarity in Relationship
Original Version Needs Improvement
Elderly adults will differ in their acid blocker use and they also will differ in their vitamin B12 levels.
Improved Version
Among elderly adults, there will be an inverse relationship between their acid blocker use and their vitamin B12 levels.

The improved version clarifies the direction of effect between the exposure (acid blocker use) and the outcome (vitamin B12 levels).

7.8 GUIDELINE #2: A HYPOTHESIS SHOULD NAME THE EXPOSURE PRIOR TO THE OUTCOME

This guideline may appear intuitive but is not often followed in practice. Remember that reviewers are reading your proposal for the first time. While you are thoroughly familiar with which variable is your exposure variable and which variable is your outcome variable, the reviewer is just learning this. Therefore, consistently stating the exposure variable prior to the outcome variable will result in a proposal that is easier to read and understand. This is a kindness to the reviewer that can save them precious time, and its importance should not be underestimated. In contrast, a hypothesis that lists the outcome variable first can often lead to reviewer confusion as to which is the exposure and which is the outcome variable. This is of particular concern when there may be *bidirectional* relationships between your exposure and outcome.

Consider the following example in which a diagnosis of diabetes is the exposure of interest and depression is the outcome of interest.

Example Misordered Hypothesis
Original Version Needs Improvement
There will be a positive relationship between depression and diagnosis of diabetes.
Improved Version
There will be a positive relationship between diagnosis of diabetes and depression

This improved version lists the exposure (diabetes) before the outcome (depression). In the original version, the reviewer could have mistakenly assumed that depression was the exposure and that the proposal was hypothesizing that depression may physiologically lead to an increased risk of diabetes. Indeed, there is a body of research that has proposed such an association. However, the proposal was hypothesizing the reverse: that those diagnosed with diabetes are more likely to become depressed. It is only by a consistent ordering of exposure prior to disease that such confusion can be avoided.

Example Hypothesis Listing the Outcome before the Exposure
Original Version Needs Improvement
More physical activity will be observed among children who watch less television.
Improved Version
Children who watch less television will participate in more physical activity than those who watch more television.

This improved version lists the exposure (television) before the outcome (physical activity) and also states the comparison group (see Guideline #3).

7.9 GUIDELINE #3: THE COMPARISON GROUP SHOULD BE STATED IF YOU HAVE A CATEGORICAL EXPOSURE

Hypotheses for study designs in epidemiology and preventive medicine usually involve the comparison of two or more groups, typically termed the *exposed* and *unexposed*. The general structure of a hypothesis therefore tends to follow the format "Do exposed people have a greater risk of disease than unexposed people?" In the following original version, you will see that the comparison group is not stated.

Example Hypothesis Lacking a Comparison Group
Original Version Needs Improvement
Adults who are overweight will have an increased risk of hypertension.
Improved Version
Adults who are overweight will have an increased risk of hypertension as compared to adults who are normal weight.

In the original example, failure to state the comparison group could lead the reviewer to believe that the comparison group might be adults who are *underweight* or perhaps adults who are *obese*. In other words, failure to specify the comparison group gives the reviewer more work to do (i.e., spending time trying to determine who is your comparison group) and may result in a misidentification of your comparison group.

Example Hypothesis Lacking a Comparison Group
Original Version Needs Improvement
Among endometrial cancer patients, there will be a high level of talc use.
Improved Version
Talc users will have an increased risk of endometrial cancer as compared to those who do not use talc.

The improved version not only specifies the comparison group (*those who do not use talc*) but also lists the exposure before the outcome.

A caveat   You may be interested in evaluating the impact of your exposure as a continuous variable or as a categorical variable (e.g., exposed vs. unexposed), or as both a continuous and a categorical variable. Several hypotheses can be included—as shown in the example below—one for the categorical variable and one for the continuous exposure variable.

Example Hypotheses Corresponding to Categorical vs. Continuous Exposure Variables
Hypothesis for a Categorical Exposure
Hypothesis #1a. Children exposed to formaldehyde will have an increased risk of asthma as compared to those not exposed to formaldehyde.
Hypothesis for a Continuous Exposure
Hypothesis #1b. Dose of formaldehyde exposure will be positively associated with asthma risk.

Note that the hypothesis for the continuous version of the exposure variable (hypothesis #1b) does not specify a comparison *unexposed* group because the idea is that risk of the outcome increases with increasing level of the exposure. Your hypothesis would specify the shape of the dose–response relationship that you expect to observe (e.g., positive, J-shaped, U-shaped, etc.)

7.10 GUIDELINE #4: WHEN YOUR STUDY IS LIMITED TO A PARTICULAR POPULATION, REFERENCE TO THE POPULATION IN YOUR SPECIFIC AIMS AND/OR HYPOTHESES

This guideline is particularly critical to follow when one of the key aspects of your proposal is your particular study population. For example, if you will be the first investigator to examine an association within a high-risk group, highlight this key feature in the specific aims and/or the hypotheses—it will certainly increase your chances of having the proposal funded. Another reason to highlight your study population is when that population is a relatively understudied group. In other words, refer to your population in your specific aims if your proposal fills a *research gap* by focusing on this particular population.

Third, if your study will be very large and/or use national data, highlight the study population in Specific Aims. For example, proposing to use data from a national surveillance study (e.g., the Behavioral Risk Factor Surveillance System [BRFSS]) improves your ability to observe an effect (via the large sample size) and the representative nature of the sample greatly enhances the generalizability of your potential findings.

In terms of readability, it is preferable to highlight the study population in an introductory parenthetical phrase followed by a comma, as is done in the improved example below.

Example Hypothesis Highlighting the Study Population
(Underlining for emphasis)
Original Version Needs Improvement
Specific Aim #1: To evaluate the association between mobility and quality of life among elderly adults.
   Hypothesis #1: Elderly adults differ in their levels of mobility and they differ in their self-reported quality of life.
Improved Version
Specific Aim #1: To evaluate the association between mobility and quality of life in a population-based sample of US elderly adults.
   Hypothesis #1: Among elderly adults in the US, there will be a positive relationship between level of mobility and self-reported quality-of-life scores.

This improved example, aside from now highlighting the population of interest, is also improved because it shows the hypothesized direction of effect between the exposure and the outcome (guideline #1). Also, note, however, that this approach would be less useful, for example, if your study population is a convenience sample and/or is not significantly different from the population used by prior studies in the area. In this case, highlighting the study population could actually reduce the impact of your hypotheses and add unnecessary wordiness. At worst, it could detract from the real novelty of your proposal, which, for example, might be a new assessment methodology. It is important to remember that, regardless of whether you mention your study population in your hypotheses, you will still have plenty of time to describe your study population in the *Approach* section of the Research Strategy.

In making these decisions, the key question to ask yourself is, if a reviewer only read this Specific Aims page, would they learn everything novel and innovative about your study?

7.11 GUIDELINE #5: HYPOTHESES SHOULD BE AS CONCISE AS POSSIBLE AND USE MEASUREABLE TERMS

Ultimately, hypothesis writing is a balancing act in which you weigh the benefits of being more specific with the risk of exceeding the one-page limitation for the Specific Aims page. Always keep in mind that you will be able to provide more details in the *Approach* section of the Research Strategy.

The key here is to use measurable terms. In other words, a general term for the exposure or outcome variable will not be useful if the reviewer cannot envision how this variable will be measured.

Example Hypotheses Lacking Measurable Terms
Original Version: Too Vague
There will be a positive relationship between patients' social class and their health literacy.
Revised Version: Too Detailed
Among patients, there will be a positive relationship between gross annual income in 2012 and their performance on the Smith five-level Likert cardiovascular risk factor awareness scale.
Improved Version
Among patients, there will be a positive relationship between income level and performance on a cardiovascular risk factor awareness test.

The improved version could have been written in a variety of ways. But, regardless the improved version uses of *measurable terms* in place of *social class* and *health literacy*. Specifically, it indicates that *social class* will be measured in terms of income level and that *health literacy* will be measured as performance on a cardiovascular risk factor awareness test.

As with any advice, however, it is possible to take this too far. For example, it is an ineffective use of space, to become too detailed in the hypotheses. Mentioning the title of the assessment tool is only necessary if, for example, the tool is an advance in the field, use of the tool is a strength of the study (i.e., if you are the first to use this scale), or if the majority of prior studies were based on self-report and you will be using an objective measure instead.

Again, in making these decisions, the question to ask yourself is, if a reviewer only reads this Specific Aims page, would they learn everything novel and innovative about your study?

7.12 GUIDELINE #6: AVOID MAKING PRECISE STATISTICAL PREDICTIONS IN A HYPOTHESIS

Precise statistical predictions can rarely be justified by the prior literature. For example, consider that you are proposing to conduct a study of antidepressant use on attempted suicide risk. You specifically hypothesize that risk would be reduced by exactly 50% but instead you find that risk is reduced by 52%. In this case, your hypothesis would not be supported. Indeed, findings for any other percentile other than 50% would result in the rejection of your hypothesis. Even providing a range of predictions (e.g., a 10%–20% reduction) is generally not acceptable in a hypothesis.

Example Hypothesis Needing Improvement
Original Version Needs Improvement
Cigarette smokers will have a 35% higher risk of influenza as compared to nonsmokers.
Improved Version
Cigarette smokers will have a higher risk of influenza as compared to nonsmokers.

The improved version of the example gives the direction of effect but does not give a precise amount.

7.13 GUIDELINE #7: A HYPOTHESIS SHOULD INDICATE WHAT WILL ACTUALLY BE STUDIED— NOT THE POSSIBLE IMPLICATIONS OF THE STUDY NOR VALUE JUDGMENTS OF THE AUTHOR

Traditionally, the specific aims and hypotheses themselves do not include phrases that justify the importance of your proposed research nor its possible implications. Instead, you will make these points in the section on Significance and Innovation.

Example Hypothesis Needing Improvement
Original Version Needs Improvement
Good diets will have a dramatic benefit among older adults.
Improved Version
Among older adults, those who have a Mediterranean-style dietary pattern will have a lower risk of heart disease as compared to those who eat a diet high in carbohydrates.

The improved example removes the term *dramatic* which could be viewed as reflecting the value judgments of the writer. The second advantage of the improved example is that it follows Guideline #5 by removing vague terms, such as *good diets* and *benefit,* and instead clarifies how the exposure (dietary pattern) and the outcome (heart disease risk) will be measured. The improved example also follows Guideline #3 by specifying the comparison group (e.g., diet high in carbohydrates).

7.14 GUIDELINE #8: WRITING HYPOTHESES FOR AN EFFECT MODIFICATION/INTERACTION AIM

If you plan on evaluating the presence of interaction or effect modification in your data analysis, include this a priori as a study aim(s) and hypothesis. This will help to assure your reviewers that you will not be data dredging for statistically significant findings if you fail to observe an overall association between your exposure and outcome of interest. In other words, when writing the proposal, you will want to carefully consider which factors might be possible effect modifiers of the relationship between your exposure and disease, based upon feasible physiological mechanisms and/or findings from the prior literature. For a definition of effect modification (i.e., interaction) and how it differs from confounding, see Chapter 14, "Study Limitations to Consider."

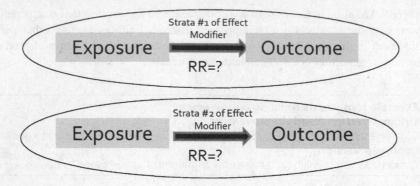

FIGURE 7.2   Effect modification by a two-level effect modifier.

As reviewed in Chapter 6, "Specific Aims," it will be key to avoid epidemiologic jargon when writing an effect modification hypothesis. This will ensure that the proposed associations are clear to all reviewers some of whom will not be epidemiologists or biostatisticians.

A general template for an effect modification hypothesis could be:

Specific Aim: To evaluate whether the association between [exposure] and [outcome] differs according to [effect modifier] (Figure 7.2).

Hypothesis: There will be a stronger positive association between [exposure] and [outcome] among [stratum 1 of the effect modifier] as compared to [stratum 2 of the effect modifier].

Or

Hypothesis: There will be a stronger inverse association between [exposure] and [outcome] among [stratum 1 of the effect modifier] as compared to [stratum 2 of the effect modifier].

Using the example from Chapter 6, "Specific Aims," we can insert an effect modification hypothesis below the corresponding aim.

Example Specific Aims for Effect Modification with Corresponding Hypotheses
Specific Aim: To evaluate whether association between menopausal hormone therapy and Alzheimer's disease differs according to obesity status (Figure 7.3).
Hypothesis #1a Original Version Needs Improvement
We hypothesize that obesity will be an effect modifier of the association between menopausal hormone therapy and Alzheimer's disease.
Hypothesis #1a Revised Version
The impact of menopausal hormone therapy on Alzheimer's disease will be stronger among women with obesity than among women without obesity.

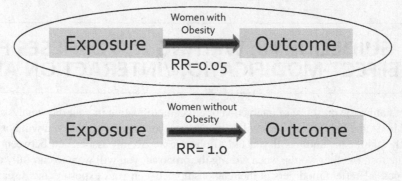

FIGURE 7.3   Effect modification by obesity.

7.15 STYLISTIC TIP #1: WHEN A NUMBER OF RELATED HYPOTHESES ARE TO BE STATED, CONSIDER PRESENTING THEM IN A NUMBERED OR LETTERED LIST

Closely related hypotheses may be arranged in a list. This approach is most useful when you have one exposure variable and several outcome variables, or vice versa.

Example Hypotheses in a List Format
Hypothesis: Females taking the alcohol awareness course will
1. be less likely to engage in binge drinking
2. be more committed to alcohol abstinence
3. obtain a higher grade point average
   as compared to those not taking the course.

In this example, the investigator plans to measure the impact of one exposure (taking the alcohol awareness course) on three possible outcomes. Note that this example above is only feasible when the comparison (non-exposed) group is identical for all three hypotheses (i.e., those not taking the course).

When to use a single hypothesis for multiple factors

In contrast, it is also permissible to include more than one hypothesis in a single sentence as long as the sentence is reasonably concise and its meaning is clear. The more connected the hypotheses are, the more desirable this approach is.

Example Hypothesis for Multiple Related Outcome Variables
Hypothesis: Premenopausal women who take oral contraceptives will experience higher rates of *cardiovascular risk factors* (i.e., HDL, LDL, triglycerides) as compared to those who do not take oral contraceptives.

In this example, the use of one sentence encompassing several sub hypotheses (i.e., outcome variables) is preferable due to the fact that there is a standardly accepted umbrella term that encompasses all these outcome variables (i.e., cardiovascular risk factors).

7.16 STYLISTIC TIP #2: BECAUSE MOST HYPOTHESES DEAL WITH THE BEHAVIOR OF GROUPS, PLURAL FORMS SHOULD USUALLY BE USED

Example Hypothesis Needing Improvement:
Original Version Needs Improvement
There will be a positive association between a midwife's years in practice and her rate of episiotomy use.
First Improved Version
There will be a positive association between midwives' years in practice and their rate of episiotomy use.
Second Improved Version
Among midwives, there will be a positive association between years in practice and rate of episiotomy use.

The first improved example replaces the term *her* with *their*. The assumption that all midwives are women is not acceptable. The second improved example has the additional benefit of removing the possessive apostrophe.

7.17 STYLISTIC TIP #3: AVOID USING THE WORDS *SIGNIFICANT* OR *SIGNIFICANCE* IN A HYPOTHESIS

The terms *significant* and *significance* most commonly refer to tests of statistical significance used by most empirical studies but can also refer to *clinical* significance. Just as we avoid making precise statistical predictions in hypotheses (see Tip #6: Remove Any Unnecessary Words), we also avoid the use of the terms *significant* or *significance* in hypotheses. Instead, you will describe the techniques that you will use to assess statistical significance, clinical significance, as well as the role of bias and confounding in the methods section of the proposal. Statistical significance refers to the probability of observing your study's results, or results even further from the null hypothesis, if the null hypothesis was true and is typically set at $p < 0.05$. Statistical significance is impacted by a number of factors including the sample size of your study (i.e., the larger the sample, the more likely that the findings will be statistically significant). In addition, even if you observe statistically significant results (i.e., $p < 0.05$), this does not rule out that your results might be due to bias (e.g., confounding, selection bias).

Clinical significance is a more subjective term and is based on the expert opinion of key leaders in the field and/or upon the prior literature. For example, consider that you conducted a study of the impact of prenatal exercise on birth weight. Let's assume that you found a 50 g difference in birth weight between exercisers (exposed group) and non-exercisers (unexposed group), which was **statistically significant** at $p = 0.01$. However, obstetricians may not consider a 50 g difference in birth weight to be **clinically significant**; that is, such a small difference in birth weight may not impact the current or future health of the baby. On the flip side, let's assume that you found a 200 g difference in birth weight that was not statistically significant (e.g., $p = 0.25$). Such a difference may be viewed as clinically significant but, due to your small sample size, was not statistically significant.

Example Hypothesis Needing Improvement:
Original Version Needs Improvement
Women with obesity will have a significantly greater risk of premenstrual syndrome as compared to women with normal weight.
Improved Version
Women with obesity will have a greater risk of premenstrual syndrome as compared to women with normal weight.

7.18 STYLISTIC TIP #4: AVOID USING THE WORD *PROVE* IN A HYPOTHESIS

Epidemiologic and biostatistical research is almost always conducted among study samples drawn from larger populations. The corresponding statistical techniques are designed to take into account this sampling variability and yield findings with observed probabilities and confidence intervals. Thus, it is critical to remember that we, as investigators, gather data that offer varying degrees of confidence regarding various conclusions. In addition, our observed findings not only may be due to chance, but they may also be due to biases such as confounding, selection bias, information bias, and misclassification. We are therefore not able to *prove* a hypothesis in our proposed study.

Consider the Bradford Hill criteria, otherwise known as Hill's Criteria for Causation, which are a group of minimal conditions necessary to provide adequate evidence of a causal relationship between an exposure and a disease in epidemiology and preventive medicine. These criteria include the *strength of association*, *biologic plausibility*, and *consistency*. Consistency refers to repeated observations of a similar association across different study populations using different study designs. Clearly, your one proposed study is not going to be sufficient to meet the condition of *consistency*.

Example Hypothesis Needing Improvement:
Original Version Needs Improvement
Our hypothesis is to prove that birth weight will be positively associated with bone density among children.
Improved Version
Birth weight will be positively associated with bone density among children.

7.19 STYLISTIC TIP #5: AVOID USING TWO DIFFERENT TERMS TO REFER TO THE SAME VARIABLE IN A HYPOTHESIS

This guideline fits under the general theme of being kind to the reviewer. Many recall their college English classes where they were told to avoid using the same term repeatedly and instead to make their writing interesting by using synonyms. While this may be appropriate for creative writing, this practice is discouraged for scientific writing. Instead, be as clear as possible by consistently using the same terms for your exposure and outcome variables throughout the proposal. While you as the proposal writer may be very familiar with your topic of interest, your reviewer may not be. Synonyms will make it difficult for a first-time reviewer of your proposal to become familiar with your key variables.

Example Hypothesis Needing Improvement:
Original Version Needs Improvement
Students who receive courses in stress reduction plus training in healthy dietary behaviors will have better attitudes toward their school work than those who receive only the new approach to stress reduction.
Improved Version
Students who receive courses in stress reduction plus training in healthy dietary behaviors will have better attitudes toward their school work than those who receive only courses in stress reduction.

In the original example, it is unclear whether *the new approach to stress reduction* refers to the *courses in stress reduction* alone or to some new approach which the writer mistakenly forgot to mention. At worst, the reviewer may decide that you inadvertently failed to describe the new approach.

Example Hypothesis Needing Improvement:
Original Version Needs Improvement
Students who take the AIDS awareness course will report fewer risk-taking behaviors than those who do not take the introductory health course.
Improved Version
Students who take the AIDS awareness course will report fewer risk-taking behaviors than those who do not take the AIDS awareness course

7.20 STYLISTIC TIP #6: REMOVE ANY UNNECESSARY WORDS

A hypothesis should be free of terms and phrases that do not add to its meaning. This guideline fits under the goal of being kind to your reviewer. Removing unnecessary words helps you to clearly and efficiently make your point and to save space. Reread your hypotheses several times to make sure that every word counts. You will find that it actually takes much longer to write a short hypothesis than a longer hypothesis. Avoid the pitfall of believing that longer hypotheses make your work appear more sophisticated; a targeted, precise hypothesis is always more impactful.

Example Hypothesis Needing Improvement:
Original Version Needs Improvement
Among naval shipyard workers, those who are working on seasonal schedules will report having more occupational injuries than those who are working in naval shipyards that follow a more traditional year-round schedule.
Improved Version
Naval shipyard workers who work on seasonal schedules will have higher injury rates than those who work on year-round schedules.

The improved version of the example is shorter, yet its meaning is clearer. Words such as *will report* and *more traditional* as well as the second repetition of *naval shipyards* are removed.

7.21 STYLISTIC TIP #7: HYPOTHESES MAY BE WRITTEN AS RESEARCH QUESTIONS—BUT USE CAUTION

Stating a hypothesis in the form of a question may, at first glance, make the hypothesis sound more compelling and potentially interesting. The question form also has the advantage of clearly pointing out to the reviewer the research gap (i.e., the question) that the hypothesis will address. However, wording a hypothesis as a question can be cumbersome. The other disadvantage of this approach could be a perceived lack of scientific rigor and the use of a style more typical of a newspaper or magazine article.

Example Hypothesis Needing Improvement:
Original Version
Do older men with high dietary glycemic load have higher levels of high-sensitivity CRP as compared to older men with low dietary glycemic load?
Improved Version
Among older men, those with high dietary glycemic load will have higher levels of high-sensitivity CRP as compared to those with low dietary glycemic load.

7.22 HYPOTHESIS WRITING CHECKLIST

- A research hypothesis should name the independent and dependent variables and indicate the type of relationship expected between them.
- A hypothesis should name the exposure prior to the outcome.

- The comparison group should be stated if you have a categorical exposure.
- When your study is limited to a particular population, reference to the population should be made in the specific aims or hypotheses.
- A hypothesis should be as concise as possible and use measurable terms.
- Avoid making precise statistical predictions in a hypothesis.
- A hypothesis should indicate what will actually be studied—not the possible implications of the study or value judgments of the author.
- When a number of related hypotheses are to be stated, consider presenting them in a numbered or lettered list.
- Because most hypotheses deal with the behavior of groups, plural forms should usually be used.
- Avoid using the words *significant* or *significance* in a hypothesis.
- Avoid using the word *prove* in a hypothesis.
- Avoid using two different terms to refer to the same variable in a hypothesis.
- Remove any unnecessary words.
- Hypotheses may be written as research questions—but use caution.

Significance and Innovation

8

The *Significance and Innovation* section falls within the Research Strategy (i.e., Significance, Innovation, and Approach) section which is limited to 6–12 pages depending upon the grant mechanism.

In Chapter 6, "Specific Aims," I provided tips for summarizing your significance and innovation at the end of the Specific Aims page. This full *Significance and Innovation* section within the Research Strategy allows you the opportunity to **expand upon** that summary. The goal of the *Significance and Innovation* section is to convince your reviewer that you have a solid command of the current research in the field and that you can be objective and thoughtful in your evaluation of this prior literature. In fact, a well-written *Significance and Innovation* section will lead the reviewer to crave to fill the same research gaps that you are addressing in your specific aims.

In this section, the NIH asks you to clarify the Significance and Innovation in the following manner.

1. **Significance**
   - Explain the importance of the problem or critical barrier to progress that the proposed project addresses.
   - Describe the strengths and weaknesses in the rigor of the prior research (both published and unpublished) that serves as the key support for the proposed project.
   - Explain how the proposed project will improve scientific knowledge, technical capability, and/or clinical practice in one or more broad fields.
   - Describe how the concepts, methods, technologies, treatments, services, or preventive interventions that drive this field will be changed if the proposed aims are achieved.

2. **Innovation**
   - Explain how the application challenges and seeks to shift current research or clinical practice paradigms.
   - Describe any novel theoretical concepts, approaches or methodologies, instrumentation or interventions to be developed or used, and any advantage over existing methodologies, instrumentation, or interventions.
   - Explain any refinements, improvements, or new applications of theoretical concepts, approaches or methodologies, instrumentation, or interventions.

As you can see from the questions above, *significance* in this context does not **only** mean that you plan to study a very important public health issue. *Significance* also relates to how your findings will **inform the field**. For example, obesity is a significant public health problem in the United States. But, how will your study drive the field forward: Will it identify susceptibility genes or maybe point the way to better preventive interventions? In other words, a perfectly designed study about an unimportant question will not be considered significant. But a study that considers a topic of extremely high public health significance but has flaws in the study design that can affect the validity of the findings is not significant either.

8.1 REFER BACK TO YOUR LITERATURE REVIEW OUTLINE

Your *Significance and Innovation* section will draw directly from your literature review outline that you developed in Chapter 3, "Identifying a Topic and Conducting the Literature Search." Table 8.1 shows a reminder of the outline for the literature review. Note that you've already collected literature that corresponds to each of the subsections.

DOI: 10.1201/9781003155140-10

TABLE 8.1 Example Significance and Innovation Outline

I. Significance and Innovation
   A. Importance of the topic
      i. Public health impact of the outcome
         a. Prevalence and incidence of the outcome
         b. Sequelae of the outcome
         c. Established risk factors for the outcome
         d. Prevalence and incidence of the exposure (optional)
      ii. Physiology of the exposure–outcome relationship(s)
      iii. Epidemiology of the exposure–outcome relationship(s)
   B. How previous research is limited (Research Gap)
   C. The overall goal of your proposal and how it will fill this research gap

Let's use the same example used in Chapter 3.

Example Specific Aims and Hypotheses

Specific Aim #1: We propose to assess the relationship between menopausal hormone therapy and Alzheimer's disease in the Phoenix Health Study.

Hypothesis #1a: Menopausal hormone therapy will be inversely associated with Alzheimer's disease.

Specific Aim #2: We propose to assess the relationship between antioxidants and Alzheimer's disease in the Phoenix Health Study.

Hypothesis #2a: Antioxidant use will be inversely associated with Alzheimer's disease.

Corresponding Outline for Significance and Innovation Section

A. Importance of the topic
   i. Public health impact of the outcome
      a. Prevalence and incidence of Alzheimer's disease
      b. Sequelae of Alzheimer's disease
      c. Established risk factors for Alzheimer's disease
      d. Prevalence of menopausal hormone therapy and antioxidant use
   ii. Physiology of the exposure–outcome relationships
      a. The physiologic relationship between menopausal hormone therapy and Alzheimer's disease (Hypothesis #1a)
      b. The physiologic relationship between antioxidants and Alzheimer's disease (Hypothesis #1b)
   iii. Epidemiology of the exposure–outcome relationships
      a. The prior epidemiologic studies on the relationship between menopausal hormone therapy and Alzheimer's disease (Hypothesis #1a)
      b. The prior epidemiologic studies on the relationship between antioxidants and Alzheimer's disease (Hypothesis #1b)
B. How previous research is limited (research gap)
C. The overall goal of your proposal and how it will fill this research gap

8.2 THE SIGNIFICANCE AND INNOVATION SECTION SHOULD BE MADE UP OF SUBSECTIONS CORRESPONDING TO EACH HYPOTHESIS

The *Significance and Innovation* section follows the above outline. In creating and titling your subsections, use the terms that appear in your hypotheses to make it clear to your reviewers that you have summarized the state of the research in *each area* of your hypotheses. This technique of cross-checking these two sections (i.e., the Specific Aims/Hypotheses with the subsections of the *Significance and Innovation* section) will ensure that there are no omissions. In other words, you want to avoid having hypotheses that you failed to support via Significance and Innovation subsections and vice versa: extra Significance and Innovation subsections that do not correspond to a hypothesis. The latter is of particular concern in grant proposals, given the strict space limitations.

8.2.1 Consider Inserting a Figure at the Beginning of the *Significance and Innovation* Section

Note that as noted in Chapter 6, "Specific Aims," if space is not adequate to insert a figure of your specific aims, this figure can instead be placed in the *Significance and Innovation* section. Such a figure is highly recommended and can be viewed as a kindness to your reviewers.

   Figure 8.1 is from a proposal to conduct an observational cohort study to evaluate how physical activity (exposure #1) and stress (exposure #2) impact risk of gestational diabetes (outcome). This one figure clearly displays the proposed Specific Aims and the relationships between the exposure variables, mediating variables, and outcome variables.

8.3 SECTION A: IMPORTANCE OF THE TOPIC

Following the above outline, the next three subsections describe tips and strategies for writing each of the following subsections of "A. Importance of the Topic." These include the following: (i) public health impact of the outcome, (ii) physiology of the exposure–outcome relationship, and (iii) epidemiology of the exposure–outcome relationship.

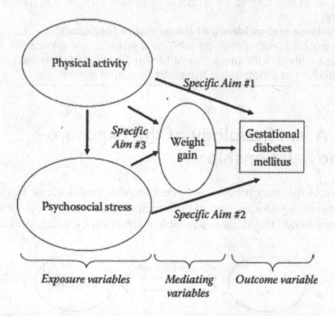

FIGURE 8.1   Example figure from a proposal to evaluate the association between physical activity, stress, and risk of gestational diabetes.

8.3.1 Section A.i.: Public Health Impact of the Outcome

The goal of this section of the grant proposal is to describe the public health significance of your outcome of interest. Start by specifying the current **prevalence and incidence rates** of your outcome (e.g., Alzheimer's disease), changes in incidence rates over time, and how many people are affected by this disorder. If your grant will be conducted among a particular subpopulation, also provide specific rates in your subpopulation (e.g., postmenopausal women) or the geographic region where the study will be conducted, if these rates are available. The goal is to start broad and then drill down as closely as possible to rates in your proposed study population.

The second important way to support the public health importance of your outcome of interest is to describe the **sequelae of your outcome/disease** (e.g., increased mortality and cardiovascular disease). For example, does your outcome (e.g., Alzheimer's disease) lead to significant future morbidity and/or mortality?

Thirdly, describe the **established risk factors** for your outcome of interest.

Finally, the public health impact of your proposal can be further enhanced by describing the prevalence and incidence of your exposure. In terms of our example above, describing the prevalence of menopausal hormone therapy would be relevant. In other words, the more the people exposed, the greater the potential public health impact of your proposal.

---

example

Example Section A. Importance of the Topic
i. **Public health impact of the outcome**
   a. **Prevalence and incidence of the outcome (Alzheimer's disease)**
      Epidemiological evidence suggests that an estimated 6.2 million Americans of all ages have Alzheimer's disease.[1] More women than men have Alzheimer's disease; almost two thirds of Americans with Alzheimer's are women.[2]
   b. **Sequelae of the outcome**
      Alzheimer's disease leads to increased rates of infection, organ failure, and eventually disability and mortality.[3]
   c. **Established risk factors for the outcome**
      Established risk factors for Alzheimer's disease include age, family history, and genetic factors.[4]
   d. **Prevalence and incidence of the exposure (optional)**
      Menopausal hormone therapy (MHT) is a relatively unexplored risk factor for Alzheimer's disease. Although the prevalence of MHT use has recently declined in the US, current rates remain high at almost one in five postmenopausal women.[5]

8.3.2 Section A.ii.: Physiology of the Exposure–
   Outcome Relationship

The goal of this section of the grant proposal is to describe the physiologic or behavioral rationale for a potential relationship between your exposure and your outcome (see Figure 8.2). In other words, your job in this section is to demonstrate that there is a feasible mechanism by which your exposure may impact

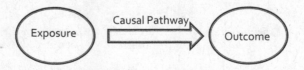

FIGURE 8.2 The causal pathway between an exposure and an outcome.

your disease. In terms of our example, describe the physiologic mechanisms by which menopausal hormone therapy could impact Alzheimer's disease.

A pitfall to avoid   As noted in the literature review outline instructions (see Chapter 3, "Identifying a Topic and Conducting the Literature Search"), it is easy to go astray when writing this section and use too much of your limited space describing the physiology of your outcome in isolation. In doing so, you'll inadvertently fail to describe the potential mechanism by which your exposure may influence your outcome. Using our example above, one can assume that the scientific reviewer is familiar, for example, with the basic etiology of Alzheimer's disease. Instead, one wants to focus on the mechanism for how your exposure, antioxidants, could *impact* Alzheimer's disease.

A similar pitfall to avoid is dedicating this section to a description of the physiology of the exposure in isolation. Using our example above, simply describing the general impact of menopausal hormone therapy on the body would not be sufficient. Instead, after a brief description of how hormones function, describe how menopausal hormone therapy could influence the occurrence of Alzheimer's disease.

Remember that reviewers are expected to have a general scientific knowledge. So, in the light of your page limitations, focus on the causal mechanisms between your exposure and your disease (see Figure 3.1).

Example Physiology of the Exposure–Outcome Relationship
Numerous animal and laboratory studies have shown that antioxidant nutrients can protect the brain from oxidative and inflammatory damage, but there are limited data available from human studies.[14-17]

Consider Inserting a Figure in the Physiology Section   A figure demonstrating the proposed physiologic pathways between your exposure and your outcome variables is highly recommended and can be viewed as a kindness to the reviewer. This is even more important when there are several potential physiological pathways. Each one should be carefully described. Figure 8.3 is an expansion of Figure 8.1 describing the physiologic and behavioral mechanisms (mediating variables) by which physical activity (exposure #1) and stress (exposure #2) may impact risk of gestational diabetes (outcome).

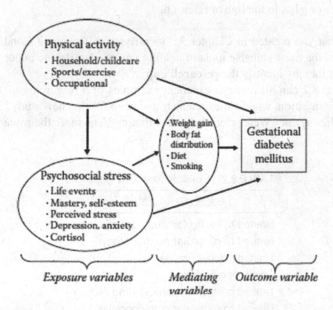

FIGURE 8.3 Mechanisms from a proposal to evaluate the association between physical activity, stress, and risk of gestational diabetes.

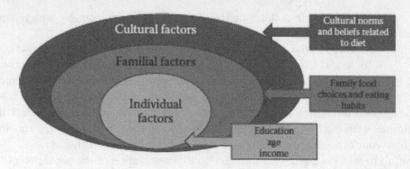

FIGURE 8.4   The underlying theoretical model behind a dietary intervention.

Figures displaying your *theoretical model*, for example, for an intervention study can also be helpful. Figure 8.4 shows the underlying theoretical model behind a dietary intervention.

8.3.3 Section A.iii.: Epidemiology of the Exposure–Outcome Relationship

8.3.3.1 Summarize the Prior Epidemiologic Literature

The goal of this section of the grant proposal is to summarize the findings of prior epidemiologic studies that evaluated the association between your exposure and your outcome. The **key strategy** is to leverage this section to make your research gap readily apparent. Highlighting the research gap is one of the most important components in a grant application and directly addresses the NIH call for applications to address the **rigor of the prior research**. Specifically, NIH Grant application instructions (and the criteria by which reviewers are asked to evaluate the scientific merit of the application) include a description of:

> The **rigor of the prior research** that serves as the key support for a proposed project to help identify weaknesses or **gaps** in the line of research.

The summary table that you created in Chapter 3, "Identifying a Topic and Conducting the Literature Search," will be one of the most valuable tools in helping you to identify the major trends or patterns in the prior literature and thereby identify the **research gap**.

The items in Table 8.2 can all serve as excellent examples of a research gap. In other words, they can serve to answer the question, what is the demonstrated need for this new study? Is this a well-studied area? Or are prior studies sparse? Were prior studies conflicting? The more the research gaps that you can

TABLE 8.2   Example Research Gaps

PRIOR LITERATURE IS...
Limited to particular study designs
Limited to particular methodology
Limited sample size
Conflicting findings
Limited control for confounding factors
Limited to particular study populations
Limited number of prior studies

TABLE 8.3   Outline for Section A.iii. Epidemiology of the Exposure–Outcome Relationship

iii. Epidemiology of Exposure–Outcome Relationship
1. Sentence #1: The total number of studies in your summary table with citations
2. Sentence #2: The number of studies in each study design
3. Sentences #3, 4, 5 etc.: Choose items that highlight your research gap. For example, the number of studies according to each category of:
   a) Study population
   b) Exposure measure
   c) Outcome measure
4. Sentence #x: The number of studies with positive, negative, and null findings, respectively
5. Sentence #x: Note relationships between study methods and study findings
6. Optional: Highlight a study (see checklist in Section 8.3.3.5)
7. Summarize study limitations (that your study will not face).

---

identify that you will be filling with your proposal, the better. In other words, at least one is necessary but more are value-added.

Therefore, in contrast to a simple listing (e.g., laundry list) of all the prior studies, the epidemiology section of the grant proposal should describe them in categories—carefully selected to highlight the research gap that your proposal will be filling. Remember that the goal is to quickly give the reviewer a synopsis of the state of the research in this area.

Table 8.3 describes a step-by-step approach for writing this section. Begin this section by noting the number and designs of the prior epidemiologic studies which have evaluated your exposure–outcome association of interest then follow along the sentences outlined in the table.

See Example #1 at the end of this chapter for how to **put this technique into action** for our example of the association between antioxidant use and Alzheimer's disease.

8.3.3.2 Choosing Categories That Highlight the Research Gap

The above outline asks you to discuss the studies in categories according to items that highlight your research gap. Your choice of categories should be dictated by the research gap that you want to highlight. For example, if one of your study strengths is your prospective cohort design, and few prior studies used this design, you will want to discuss the studies in categories by study design. In this way, you make clear to the reviewer that the number of prior prospective studies is sparse and, therefore, efficiently demonstrate that your study will be extending this prior literature by adding to the small body of prior studies of this design. You could also choose other categories by which to discuss the prior epidemiologic studies (e.g., by study population, exposure measure, outcome measure, or direction of findings; see example below).

Example Categorizing the Epidemiologic Studies by: (1) Type of Exposure and (2) Direction of Findings

A total of 15 epidemiologic studies have evaluated the relationship between antioxidant use and Alzheimer's disease.[1-15] These studies, however, have assessed women's dietary supplement use only[1-5] or dietary (non-supplement) sources only.[6-13] Only two studies have measured both supplement and dietary sources of antioxidant use.[14,15] Findings have been contradictory. Nine of the 15 published studies observed decreased risk of Alzheimer's disease for women who regularly used antioxidants compared with nonusers.[1-9] No overall association between antioxidant use and Alzheimer's disease was found in four studies.[10-13] Higher levels of antioxidant use were associated with an increased risk of Alzheimer's disease in the Framingham cohort study[14] and the Turkish case-control study.[15]

In the above example, the writer chose to group the studies according to their type of exposure assessment (i.e., dietary supplement use vs. nondietary sources) and then according to their findings (i.e., decreased risk, null, and increased risk). This laid the groundwork for the need to extend prior research by measuring *both* dietary supplement and dietary sources of antioxidants. In other words, grouping the prior studies according to their type of exposure assessment primed the reviewer to see the need for future studies to improve exposure assessment, a need that was subsequently satisfied when they reached the Approach section of your proposal.

8.3.3.3 Note the Relationships between Study Methods and Their Corresponding Findings

Use your summary table to identify possible explanations for any differences in study findings across the prior literature such as different methodologies or different populations.

Example Noting Relationships Between Study Methods and Findings
While the two studies that used mailed questionnaires support the finding that inhalant use among adolescents increased the risk of autism, the three studies that used face-to-face interviews did not observe an increased risk.

This example identifies differences in study methods (i.e., questionnaires vs. face-to-face interviews) as a possible explanation for the differences in study findings. Again, this is a useful approach to take if you are proposing to use a method that, in the past, was associated with statistically significant findings.

8.3.3.4 What Should You Do if the Prior Literature Is Conflicting?

The first and foremost approach to dealing with controversies or conflicting findings in the prior literature is not to hide them. Instead, objectively present each opposing finding or theory. Indeed, remember that your reviewers may have published in the same field and may be the authors of the very works that you are discussing. Imagine their perception of your scholarship if your proposal leaves out their findings. In other words, **let reviewers know that you are aware of controversies.**

The worst-case scenario (always healthy to imagine) is that you have left out the reviewer's study because it is not consistent with your hypothesis. In other words, you decide to only present studies that found a positive association between your exposure and outcome (and omit the reviewer's study that found an inverse association) to further justify your hypothesis of a positive association. The reviewer would conclude that not only do you not have an adequate grasp of the literature but also you are purposefully spinning prior findings. In fact, it is always a useful exercise to envision that one of the reviewers is indeed an author of one of the prior studies in the field.

Give clear reasons for taking a side In the context of prior conflicting findings, describe the decision process by which you determined your proposed hypothesis. You will want to (1) present the conflicting findings, then (2) describe the strengths and limitations of these prior studies, and finally (3) describe how you weighted these strengths and limitations to come up with your final hypothesis. In this section, do not be shy in presenting prior study limitations. Remember that you are simply proposing to test a particular hypothesis. You are not proposing to determine causality. Therefore, your goal is to convince the reviewer that you are open-minded enough to reject your hypothesis if your experimental results indicate.

8.3.3.5 Highlight Key Studies

After describing the prior epidemiologic studies, if space allows, you can highlight one or more of the key studies that were included in your groupings. As a reminder, these would be studies that appeared in your summary table of the epidemiologic association between your exposure and your outcome.

Which studies to highlight? In choosing which prior epidemiologic studies to highlight, you have several options. For example, you may choose to highlight one of the most recent studies to give a sense of the current state of the field. Or consider highlighting what you believe is the strongest prior study in the area. Details on these studies will give your reviewer a sense of the state of the art in the field and will also provide further support for your methods—if they are similar to those in these highlighted studies. You may also consider highlighting a prior study most similar to your own—to provide support for your hypotheses and/or proposed methods. Caution should be taken, however, to be sure to clarify how your study will *improve or differ from* these highlighted studies. That is, you don't want to obviate the need for your study.

Make explicit the reasons for highlighting noncurrent articles. Such reasons could include the fact that the study is a landmark study or perhaps the study is the only evidence available on a given topic; or perhaps by including this older study, it helps the reviewer to understand the evolution of a research technique that you are proposing.

How to highlight a particular study? When highlighting studies, first state why you think the highlighted study is important, for example, *In the most recent study to date, Smith et al. enrolled…* or *In the first prospective study of risk factors for Alzheimer's disease, Smith et al. enrolled…* Then, be sure to concisely delineate the following **key attributes** about the highlighted study—ideally within several sentences.

Checklist of items to note when highlighting a particular study:

- Why the highlighted study merits highlighting
- Author name
- Study design
- Size
- Brief methods
- Measure of association and variability
- Brief limitations (that your study will improve upon)

Below is an example of a highlighted study from the same proposal designed to assess the association between antioxidants and Alzheimer's disease.

Example of a Highlighted Study

In the only prospective study to assess frequency and dose of lifetime supplement use, Jones et al. administered the Antioxidant Questionnaire to 2000 women at the onset of menopause.[39] Alzheimer's disease was measured at follow-up using an interviewer-administered cognitive battery evaluating global cognition, episodic memory, and executive function. Heavy antioxidant users had a decreased risk of Alzheimer's disease (OR = 0.78, 95% CI 0.56–0.94) as compared to light users. These findings, however, may be due to self-selection; women who regularly take antioxidants could be healthier in some overall way that improves cognitive function.

Note that, as demonstrated in the example above, when describing the measure of association, the key is to provide the absolute magnitude of the results, not just whether the results are statistically significant. It is important to remember that statistical significance only indicates whether the observed findings might be due to chance. Statistical significance does *not* mean that the findings are clinically significant nor that the difference is not due to bias or confounding. In other words, the highlighted study may have found statistically significant findings, but these may have been small, clinically insignificant, or due to bias. Therefore, it is always preferable to state the actual magnitude of findings (as well as the corresponding measure of variation) that the study observed. Examples include relative risks (RRs) and corresponding confidence intervals (CIs) or mean differences (and corresponding standard errors).

Also, note that in the above example, you are not expected to dissect and discuss every flaw of each highlighted study. Instead, in a grant proposal, you are expected to only comment on the most important/ major limitations of the prior epidemiologic studies with a focus on those limitations that your proposal will improve upon.

The other strength of the example is that the authors avoided using professional jargon when briefly summarizing the study limitations. By clearly defining what they meant by *self-selection*, they demonstrated their understanding of this limitation and made it easier on the reviewer who would have been left with the task of trying to deduce their point.

8.4 SECTION B: HOW PREVIOUS RESEARCH IS LIMITED (RESEARCH GAP)

As noted in Chapter 3, "Identifying a Topic and Conducting the Literature Search," the research gap does not need to be large—but it needs to be clearly elucidated and be of scientific importance in direct proportion to the size of the grant. This is a point that I can't emphasize enough. I've found that graduate students and early-career faculty are sometimes dissuaded by the presence of even one prior study in the literature that evaluated their exposure–outcome relationship. They fear that the presence of this study removes the need for their study. However, in epidemiology and preventive medicine, it is important to remember that causality can only be determined by a multiplicity of studies of varying designs in varying study populations.

As you can see by the example above of the proposal to study antioxidants and Alzheimer's disease, a total of 15 prior epidemiologic studies in your area can be considered insufficient if, for example, their findings have been conflicting, or if few of them used your proposed study methods, or even if few of these studies utilized your study design or study population.

8.4.1 Highlight the Limitations of Prior Studies That Your Proposal Will Be Able to Address

The goal of the Significance and Innovation section is to show how you will **extend prior research**, and this can only be done by filling gaps. Below is an example of simply and directly summing up the limitations of the prior literature in the area of antioxidant use and risk of Alzheimer's disease. Note that all the limitations mentioned are those limitations that the proposal writer felt that they will be improving upon in their own proposal. (Later in the Approach section, you will discuss your own study limitations, see Chapter 15, "How to Present Limitations and Alternatives").

Example Highlighting Prior Studies' Limitations
In summary, the prior epidemiologic studies of antioxidant use and Alzheimer's disease have several limitations: (1) the majority involved small numbers of nonminority women and men limiting the generalizability of results, (2) failure to assess both supplement and dietary sources of antioxidant use, and (3) measures of Alzheimer's disease that were not validated.

In other words, if your proposal will also be using measures of Alzheimer's disease that are not validated, it will not be useful to include this phrase in your summary of the prior studies' limitations, because this is a limitation that your proposed study shares with the prior literature. Instead, you will want to highlight a research gap that your study will be filling. It is not that you will hide the problems that you share with the prior literature, but only that you will discuss them later in the Approach section.

Sometimes early-career faculty are hesitant to point out the limitations of prior studies for fear of offending the authors of these works, whom, they fear, might be serving as potential reviewers of their proposal. However, remember that all authors are aware of the limitations of their studies and even have presented these openly in the Discussion sections of their published work. It is fine to point out these concerns simply and directly. In addition, if, in your opinion, these authors have not identified all their limitations, it is also fine to factually state what you view are additional study limitations. For example, an author of a previous cross-sectional study will know that their study design has limitations, by definition, as compared to a prospective cohort study.

8.4.2 Express Your Own Opinions about a Prior Study's Limitations

It is important to show evidence of independence in your summary of the prior literature when writing a grant proposal. In other words, be sure to summarize the study limitations in your own words. Avoid quoting directly from the author's description of their own study limitations (e.g., from the Discussion section of their published article). For example, avoid sentences such as, *The authors stated that their findings might be due to confounding.* This approach is problematic for several reasons. First, the authors may be incorrect. Second, the authors are certainly not as unbiased as you theoretically are. Third, your opinion of the primary limitation of their study (which you selected to highlight the need for your own study) may differ from their opinion.

8.4.3 You May Refer to Comments from a Review Article

A review article can provide useful authority on the research gap—and be cited to support your proposed topic. In this situation, citing a review article is like calling in the *big guns*. For example, many review articles will comment upon the limitations of prior studies and point out the need for and type of future studies that should be conducted in the area. If these conclusions are consistent with the thrust of your proposed study, then it would be helpful to cite the review article.

Example Reference to a Review Article
Example #1
Prior studies were limited by lack of control for key confounding factors. In fact, in a recent review article of risk factors for bladder cancer, Taylor et al. concluded that prior studies faced uncontrolled confounding.
Example #2
In a review of risk factors for preterm delivery, Berkowitz et al.[29] concluded that there is insufficient data to assess the effect of recreational activity on prematurity.

8.5 SECTION C: SUMMARY OF SIGNIFICANCE AND INNOVATION

The goal of this section is to clarify the overall goal of your proposal and how it will fill the research gap that you identified in Section B: How Previous Research Is Limited (Research Gap). That is, why it is significant and innovative. This is your *big bang*, the culmination of all the prior sections. The below example follows directly on from Section B's description of how previous research was limited (the research gap). The specific words, *significance* and *innovation* should be highlighted in bold. Remember that these factors are essential in obtaining funding and reviewers are instructed to summarize these aspects of your proposal as part of their critique forms. A good reviewer will search for these key terms in your *Significance and Innovation* section.

Example Highlighting Prior Studies' Limitations and How You Will Fill That Gap
In summary, the prior epidemiologic studies of antioxidant use and Alzheimer's disease have several limitations: (1) the majority involved small numbers of nonminority women and men limiting the generalizability of results, (2) failure to assess both supplement and dietary sources of antioxidant use, and (3) measures of Alzheimer's disease that were not validated. **Therefore, the overall goal of this proposal is to prospectively evaluate the association between antioxidant use and risk of Alzheimer's disease.** This proposal is **innovative** in examining these associations in a racially/ethnically diverse population-based sample, using a comprehensive measure of antioxidant use (encompassing both supplements and dietary sources), as well as a validated measure of Alzheimer's disease. The **significance** of the study lies in the fact that changes in modifiable risk factors may reduce the morbidity associated with Alzheimer's disease and be instrumental in preventing or delaying decline in cognitive function.

8.6 STYLISTIC TIPS FOR WRITING THE SIGNIFICANCE AND INNOVATION SECTION

8.6.1 Tip #1: Summarize Key Sentences in Bold

Consider bolding or otherwise highlighting one key sentence in each paragraph of the *Significance and Innovation* section. This tip fits under the concept of being kind to your reviewer. That is, this bolding does the work for the reviewer of locating the key sentence in each paragraph and identifying it for them. Indeed, the act of searching for this key sentence provides you with the added benefit of ensuring that each paragraph has a key point. With space at a premium in grant proposals, each sentence needs to count. This point is particularly relevant for the *Significance and Innovation* section, as this section is usually densely packed with text, and reviewers may have difficulty picking out the key points.

Key example sentences to bold include sentences stating: (1) the research gap, (2) the long-term goal of your proposal, and (3) the overall goal of the proposal.

8.6.2 Tip #2: Avoid Broad and Global Statements

Broad and global statements are typically already well-understood by the reviewers and are not a good use of space in a grant proposal. Remember that there is an informal adage among reviewers that the longer your Significance and Innovation section, the less likely your application will receive a good score. You want to quickly pivot from what is known—to the research gap—to how your proposal will fill this gap.

Example Broad Statement to Avoid
Original Version Needs Improvement
Obesity reduction is important to both the economy of the United States and to the rest of the world. Without obesity prevention, we will face a catastrophic public health crisis in the next millennium...
Improved Version
Tailored exercise and dietary interventions have been credited as the most effective form of weight-reduction programs.[12] Over the past five years, randomized trials of such interventions have been limited due to....

The improved example clarifies the specific topic that will be evaluated, and it is now clear what will be measured and studied. Other improvements include the addition of citations and specification of the time frame of interest.

8.6.3 Tip #3: Be Comprehensive and Complete in Citations

Check that your citations are internally consistent and complete. For example, the opening sentence of a paragraph describing the prior literature should cite all the studies highlighted in this section.

Example Comprehensive Use of Citations
A total of 15 epidemiologic studies have evaluated the relationship between physical activity and birth weight.[1-15] These studies, however, have assessed women's occupational activities only,[1-5] recreational activities only,[6-11] or a combination of occupational and household activities.[12,13] Only two studies have measured total activity (recreational, occupational, and household).[14,15]

Note that in this example above, the first sentence cites references 1–15, and the subsequent sentences divide this total into subcategories (i.e., 1–5, 6–11, 12, 13, 14, 15) corresponding to the total number of 15 cited at the beginning of the sentence. In this way, the reviewer can easily see the specific number of studies in each subcategory and what percent they are of the whole body of literature on your topic.

Lastly, if you later choose to highlight particular studies, they should also have been included in the citations from this opening sentence. In other words, in the example above, any subsequent highlighted study would have a citation between 1 and 15 inclusive.

8.6.4 Tip #4: Citations Should Directly Follow the Studies That They Relate To

Avoid grouping citations at the end of the sentence when the sentence describes disparate findings derived from independent citations.

Example Revision of Citation Placement
Original Version Needs Improvement
Previous studies have found that 35%–50% of college students report participating in an online alcohol abuse prevention program.[1-3]
Improved Version
Previous studies have found that 35%[1,2] of college students to 50%[3] of college students report participating in an online alcohol abuse prevention program.

In the original example, the reviewer will not know which of the three cited studies reported which percentage. If the reviewer is questioning one of your presented rates, the burden will be upon them to look through each of your three citations. This is an example of not being kind to the reviewer. In the improved example, the citations immediately follow the corresponding percentages.

8.6.5 Tip #5: If You Are Commenting on a Time Frame, Be Specific

Example Clarification of Time Frame
Original Version Needs Improvement
In recent years, there has been an increase in child abuse.
Improved Version
Child abuse incident reports increased by 50% between 2010 and 2020, totaling almost 6 million reports in 2013.[1]

The improved version provides a time frame for the increase, making the statement less general and more specific, which is always preferable.

8.7 ANNOTATED EXAMPLES OF THE SIGNIFICANCE AND INNOVATION SECTION

8.7.1 Example #1: Section A. iii.: Epidemiology of Exposure–Outcome Relationship

Specific Aim #2: We propose to assess the relationship between antioxidants and Alzheimer's disease in the Phoenix Health Study.

This example follows Table 8.3, "Outline for Section A.iii. Epidemiology of the Exposure–Outcome Relationship." Note that selected categories used to organize the prior epidemiologic literature, and therefore highlight the research gap, are listed in [brackets].

Section A.iii. Epidemiology of the Exposure–Outcome Relationship

[*Total # of studies*]: "A total of 21 epidemiologic studies have evaluated the relationship between antioxidant use and Alzheimer's disease."[1–21]

[*Study design*]: "Of these, 16 were prospective cohort studies,[1–16] 3 were cross-sectional studies,[17–19] and 2 were case-control studies."[20,21]

[*Study population*]: "These studies, however, have been conducted in predominantly non-Hispanic white populations,[1–15] with only 3 studies conducted among African Americans, [16–19] and 2 studies conducted among Hispanics."[20,21]

[*Exposure measures*]: The majority assessed women's dietary supplement use only[1–15] or dietary (non-supplement) sources only. [16–19] Only 2 studies have measured both supplement and dietary sources of antioxidant use.[20,21]

[*Outcome measures*]: More than half of the studies relied upon assessments of Alzheimer's disease that were not validated." [1–11]

[*Findings*]: Findings have been contradictory.[1–21] Fifteen of the 21 published studies observed decreased risk of Alzheimer's disease for women who regularly used antioxidants compared with nonusers.[1–15] No overall association between antioxidant use and Alzheimer's disease was found in four studies.[16–19] Higher levels of antioxidant use were associated with an increased risk of Alzheimer's disease in the Framingham cohort study[20] and the Turkish case–control study.[21]"

[*Relationships between methods and findings*]: "While the two studies that used both supplement and dietary sources of antioxidant use support the finding that antioxidant use decreased the risk of increased risk of Alzheimer's disease,[20,21] the 15 studies that assessed women's dietary supplement use only[1–15] did not observe a decreased risk."

Optional [*Highlight a study*]: "In the only prospective study to assess frequency and dose of lifetime supplement use, Jones et al. administered the Antioxidant Questionnaire to 2000 women at the onset of menopause.[39] Alzheimer's disease was measured at follow-up using an interviewer-administered cognitive battery evaluating global cognition, episodic memory, and executive function. Heavy antioxidant users had a decreased risk of Alzheimer's disease (OR = 0.78, 95% CI 0.56–0.94) as compared to light users. These findings, however, may be due to self-selection; women who regularly take antioxidants could be healthier in some overall way that improves cognitive function."

[*Summarize study limitations*]: In summary, the prior epidemiologic studies of antioxidant use and Alzheimer's disease have several limitations: (1) the majority involved small numbers of nonminority women and men limiting the generalizability of results, (2) failure to assess both supplement and dietary sources of antioxidant use, and (3) measures of Alzheimer's disease were not validated.

Note that this format would be repeated for each specific aim/hypothesis.

8.7.2 Example #2: Section I.: Significance and Innovation

Specific Aim #1: To evaluate the association between antipsychotic drug use and risk of breast cancer.

Specific Aim #2: To evaluation whether the association between antipsychotic drug use and risk of breast cancer differs according to menopausal hormone use (MHT) [effect modification aim]

Section A.i.: Public health impact of the outcome

A. **Importance of the topic**
   i. **Public health impact of the outcome (breast cancer)**
      a. **Prevalence and incidence of the outcome**
         Among women in the United States, breast cancer is the most prevalent form of cancer and the second leading cause of mortality affecting 1 in 9 women.[1-3]
      b. **Sequelae of the outcome**
         According to the American Cancer Society, approximately 266,120 new cases of invasive breast cancer will be diagnosed in women in 2018, of which 40,920 will lead to mortality.[4] The American Cancer Society also reported that incidence rates for breast cancer among postmenopausal women in 2017 was approximately 69%.[5]
      c. **Established risk factors for the outcome**
         There are both modifiable and non-modifiable risk factors associated with breast cancer. Women who have inherited mutations to certain genes, such as BRCA1 and BRCA2, are at higher risk of developing breast cancer.[6] In addition, women with early onset of menses or menopause after the age of 55 are at an increased risk. Having a family history of breast cancer also increases the risk of breast cancer, especially when it involves a first-degree relative.[6] Modifiable risk factors include being physically active as well as moderate consumption of alcohol.[6] Certain forms of menopausal hormone therapy (MHT) as well as oral contraceptives have been found to increase breast cancer risk.[6]
      d. **Prevalence and incidence of the exposure (optional)**
         Another potential modifiable factor is medication use, particularly antipsychotic drug use. In the United States, psychiatric medication sales are among the five top drug sales in the country.[7] Based on data extracted from the Total Patient Tracker Database, approximately 7 million adults aged 45 and above use antipsychotics.[8] While these statistics do not differentiate between men and women, data have shown that nearly twice as many women compared to men reported taking psychiatric drugs.[9] Therefore, we propose to investigate the relationship between antipsychotic drug use and breast cancer risk among postmenopausal women using data from all eligible participants enrolled in the population-based Back-to-Health Women's Study between 2015 and 2020.
   ii. **Physiology of the relationship between antipsychotic drug use and risk of breast cancer**

A potential physiological relationship between antipsychotic drug use and risk of breast cancer may be explained via prolactin (PRL). Antipsychotics serve as dopamine antagonizers that block post-synaptic D2 receptors located in the pituitary gland.[7] Once dopamine binds to dopamine D_2 receptors on the membrane of the lactotroph cells, this stimulation impacts PRL gene transcription. PRL causes breast enlargement in pregnancy and is responsible for milk production during lactation.[10] Activation of the prolactin receptor (PRLR) has induced mammary carcinomas in transgenic mice[15] and human breast cancer cells have a higher expression of PRLR levels as compared to normal breast tissue.[16] PRL has been also found to stimulate the growth of malignant neighboring cells in the breast in the presence of a carcinoma.[18]

In terms of the impact of MHT on the association between antipsychotic drugs and breast cancer, MHT use has been shown to increase PRL levels.[19] Therefore, the association between antipsychotic drugs and breast cancer might be stronger in women using MHT via a synergistic effect.

iii. **Epidemiology of the relationship between antipsychotic drug use and risk of breast cancer**

Comment: After listing the total number of studies, this section categorizes the studies by (a) study design, (b) study population, (c) exposure assessment, (d) covariate assessment, and (e) assessment of effect modification. In this way, the authors are able to highlight the research gap that prior studies have not been conducted in their study population, confounding was not well controlled for, and effect modification was not well examined.

A total of seven epidemiologic studies have evaluated the relationship between antipsychotic drug use and breast cancer risk.[20-27] Of these, three were prospective cohort studies,[21,22,23] two were retrospective cohort studies[24,25] and two were case-control studies.[6,27]

The majority of these studies evaluated their findings among combined populations of pre- and postmenopausal women and men and women.[22-25] In addition, only one study compared typical antipsychotics (first-generation drugs) to atypical antipsychotics (second-generation drugs).[20] Only two of these studies accounted for important covariates such as reproductive history.[23,24] While all seven studies looked at the relationship between antipsychotic drug use and breast cancer risk, only one study in particular stratified their findings by MHT use.[20]

Findings from these prior studies have been contradictory. Three of the seven published studies found no overall association between antipsychotic drug use and risk of breast cancer.[22,23,25] An inverse association between antipsychotic drug use and risk of breast cancer was found in one study.[20] Antipsychotic drug use was associated with an increased risk of breast cancer in three studies.[21,24,26]

In the only study to stratify their findings by MHT use,[20] Smith et al. conducted a retrospective cohort study using a nested case-control analysis that involved 100,000 women in the UK. This cohort consisted of all female patients who received at least one prescription for any antipsychotic drug between January 1, 2010, and December 31, 2020. Antipsychotic drug use, breast cancer diagnosis, and MHT were all abstracted from a linked health record database. Typical antipsychotic drug users had an approximately 20% decreased risk of breast cancer (aRR = 0.81, 95% CI 0.63–1.05) as compared to atypical antipsychotic users, however this finding was not statistically significant.

B. **How previous research is limited (research gap)**

In summary, the prior studies of the association between antipsychotic drug use and risk of breast cancer faced several limitations: (1) they did not evaluate their findings among postmenopausal women only but instead combined populations of both men and women as well as pre- and postmenopausal women, (2) only one compared typical antipsychotics (first-generation drugs) to atypical antipsychotics (second-generation drugs), (3) the majority did not account for important covariates such as reproductive history, and (4) only one evaluated the potential for effect modification by MHT use.

C. Summary of Significance and Innovation

This proposal is **innovative** in being the first, to our knowledge, to study the relationship between antipsychotic drug use and risk of breast cancer among postmenopausal women. It is also **innovative** in its power to control for covariates due to its large sample size which also enables the evaluation of the role of MHT as an effect modifier. The **significance** of the study lies in the fact that antipsychotic drug use as well as breast cancer rates are growing. Established risk factors cannot account fully for these increased rates highlighting the role of potentially modifiable risk factors such as antipsychotic drug use.

8.7.3 Example #3: Section I.: Significance and Innovation

Specific Aim #1: To evaluate the association between sleep duration and risk of gestational diabetes.

Section A.i.: Public health impact of the outcome

A. **Importance of the topic**

   i. **Public health impact of the outcome (gestational diabetes)**

     a. **Prevalence and incidence of the outcome**

Gestational diabetes is a form of diabetes mellitus that develops in pregnant women and has been found in approximately 10% of all pregnancies.[4] Hispanic women are two to four times more likely to develop gestational diabetes than their non-Hispanic counterparts.[4]

     b. **Sequelae of the outcome**

Gestational diabetes leads to an increased likelihood of developing diabetes later in life.[5] It can also lead to several other negative postpartum outcomes that may subsequently affect the mother or the child.[3] Gestational diabetes can lead to low blood glucose in the child at birth, which can contribute to breathing problems as well as a higher risk of infant morbidity and obesity. Gestational diabetes can also lead to diabetes mellitus type II later in life for both the mother and the child.

     c. **Established risk factors for the outcome**

Established risk factors for gestational diabetes include family history of hyperglycemia, lifestyle and eating habits, and obesity.[6] Socioeconomic status and racial or ethnic identity are other important risk factors in the development of gestational diabetes.[5] Recently, there has been interest in the role of sleep in the incidence of gestational diabetes. Only 65.2% of all women in the United States and 65.5% of Hispanic women in the United States report adequate sleep.[6] Therefore, it is important to understand how sleep duration may affect the risk of gestational diabetes.

   ii. **Physiology of relationship between sleep duration and gestational diabetes**

Humans spend approximately one third of their lives sleeping, when their bodies are able to complete many of the "rest and digest" tasks that allow them to maintain homeostasis or a balanced physiological state.[7] As such, when humans do not obtain the optimal duration of sleep on a regular basis, there are negative consequences on a variety of bodily functions, including glucose metabolism. This relationship between sleep duration and insufficient glucose metabolism has been shown in people with type II diabetes,[7] where short sleep duration leads to insulin resistance.

The exact physiological mechanism of the relationship between sleep duration and gestational diabetes is unknown, and evidence for potential theories is limited. However, several mechanisms have been proposed, which include (1) an endocrine mechanism and (2) a behavioral (e.g., appetite) mechanism.

In terms of the endocrine mechanism, fragmented sleep leads to an increase in sympathetic activity and cortisol levels, potentially leading to morning insulin resistance and, thereby, gestational diabetes.[6] In terms of the behavioral mechanism, when people do not regularly obtain sufficient sleep duration, appetite is not suppressed properly. This then leads to greater caloric intake and ultimately promotes obesity. Obesity can in turn lead to diabetes by increasing insulin resistance and causing β-cell dysfunction, which diminishes the amount of insulin released into the bloodstream.[8]

iii.   **Epidemiology of relationship between sleep duration and gestational diabetes**

Comment: After listing the total number of studies, this section categorizes the studies by (a) study design, (b) study population, (c) exposure assessment, (d) covariate assessment, and (e) assessment of effect modification. In this way, the authors are able to highlight the research gap that prior studies have not been conducted in their study population, confounding was not well controlled for, and effect modification was not well examined.

A total of four studies have addressed the relationship between sleep duration and gestational diabetes.[11-14] Two of them were prospective cohort studies, one was a cross-sectional study, and one was a case–control study.

Three of these studies measured sleep via self-reported questionnaires[11,13,14] that were not validated. One study used a more quantitative measurement technique, specifically an Actigraph wrist watch to measure sleep duration.[11] None of the studies were conducted in Hispanic women, and most of the studies only used blood samples to establish gestational diabetes,[12-14] without confirming cases through medical record abstraction. In all the studies, short sleep duration was associated with a higher risk of gestational diabetes.[11-14]

In the most recent prospective cohort study to date, Smith et al. enrolled 500 pregnant women with obesity and 3000 pregnant women without obesity between the ages of 18 and 40 (10% Hispanic).[11] The authors used structured questionnaires to establish sleep duration in each group, with questions asking about typical sleep duration, with possible responses including: ≤ 5, 6, 7, 8, 9, or ≥ 10 hours. The authors found that women who slept less than seven hours per night had a significantly higher risk of gestational diabetes compared to women who slept eight to nine hours, even after adjusting for other major risk factors of gestational diabetes (aRR = 2.48; 95% CI = 1.20–5.13).[11] This study was limited, however, by not using a validated tool to measure sleep duration.

B. **How previous research is limited (research gap)**

In summary, no studies to date have addressed the relationship between sleep duration and gestational diabetes in Hispanic women. In addition, prior studies did not use a validated measure of sleep duration and did not confirm the diagnosis of gestational diabetes via medical record abstraction.

C. **Summary of Significance and Innovation**

Because obstetrical outcomes can differ by maternal race/ethnicity,[17] with minorities generally facing more negative health outcomes, it is important to study this topic in diverse populations. This study will be **significant** because Hispanic women have a higher rate of gestational diabetes than non-Hispanic populations. Therefore, we propose to evaluate the relationship between duration of sleep and gestational diabetes in Hispanic women. This study will be **innovative** because it will be the first, to our knowledge, to evaluate this association in Hispanic women using a validated measure of sleep duration.

Preliminary Studies

9

The Preliminary Studies section of a grant proposal broadly encompasses the Principal Investigator's (PI's) preliminary studies, data, or experience pertinent to the application. When available, preliminary studies are critical to a grant application as they provide evidence supporting your ability to achieve your proposed specific aims and hypotheses.

Preliminary data can provide support for two key factors:

- That your proposed **approach** is promising
- That your ability to carry out your proposed research is **feasible**

Ideally, preliminary studies can motivate the rationale for your proposed study—in terms of its aims, hypotheses, and approach.

Therefore, this chapter provides you with strategies for selecting which preliminary data might be relevant and strategies for how to find or collect preliminary data. Just as importantly, this chapter provides you with tips for describing and summarizing preliminary data in a manner that best positions your proposal for a successful review.

9.1 WHAT ARE PRELIMINARY STUDIES?

Preliminary studies can take two forms:

Pilot studies are small-scale preliminary studies conducted to evaluate feasibility, duration, cost, adverse events, or improve upon the study design prior to performance of a full-scale research project.

Feasibility studies are pieces of research done before a main study to answer the question "Can this study be done?" They are used to estimate important parameters that are needed to design the main study.

Most typically, **pilot studies** address the same aims, or very similar aims, to those that you are proposing in your current proposal but have with several key differences. First, pilot studies are typically conducted **with a smaller sample** than your proposed study. This small sample does not typically have adequate power to decisively answer your proposed hypotheses but ideally suggests an association. Therefore, preliminary findings from this pilot will ideally motivate the rationale for your larger proposed study. Second, pilot studies may have been conducted in a dataset or study population that differs from your proposed study in important ways—via characteristics of the study population (e.g., age and race/ethnicity), via study design (e.g., cross sectional), or via study methods (e.g., less precise measurement tools). Regardless of the type of pilot study, the goal of the pilot is to provide findings that in some way support your proposed aims and hypotheses and justify the need for your proposed study (e.g., via an improved measurement device, stronger study design, different study population).

DOI: 10.1201/9781003155140-11

Pilot Study Examples
- Testing the intervention with a small sample of participants
- Asking a small sample of participants from the target population to complete your questionnaire and then revising the questions based on their responses
- Enrolling a small sample of participants into your planned study design and following them to study completion

Feasibility studies of your proposed methods demonstrate to reviewers that you can logistically pull off your proposed study. Feasibility studies can provide key data on a number of factors. They can provide evidence that you, as a PI, are able to recruit subjects and logistically collect data within the proposed study population. Such preliminary data may have the added benefit of providing key figures necessary for calculating power and sample size calculations for your current proposal. Participant satisfaction surveys administered in a feasibility study can also provide data on the acceptability of your methods. Validation studies of your proposed methods (as described in Chapter 10, "Pilot Grants: Reproducibility and Validity Studies") can provide assurance that a study based on your proposed methods will work. Overall, the goal of a feasibility study is to show proof of principle and demonstrate to the reviewers that you can *pull it off*.

Feasibility Study Examples
- Going to a potential study site to see whether the research is possible
- Pre-testing the informed consent process with volunteers to ensure that the information is comprehensible
- Testing the reproducibility and validity of your study instruments

It is important to note that even if you are in the middle of conducting your pilot or feasibility study, but final results are not yet ready, they still may generate useful preliminary data as listed below.
Data generated from preliminary studies include:

- Eligibility rates
- Recruitment rates
- Retention rates
- Participant satisfaction survey results
- Reproducibility and validity of your proposed methods
- Descriptive statistics on your proposed exposure and outcome variables (e.g., mean and standard deviation)
- Measures of association between your variables (e.g., mean differences, correlation coefficients, relative risks)

Include preliminary studies by your co-investigators It is also important to note that preliminary studies not only are limited to your own prior work but also encompass the work of all of your co-investigators. Your co-investigators on the application are part of your *research team*, and their preliminary data are eligible to be included. Indeed, the fact that they have relevant preliminary data may be one of the reasons that you have invited them to serve as co-investigators!

9.2 WHERE TO PLACE PRELIMINARY STUDIES IN AN NIH GRANT PROPOSAL

A typical location for preliminary studies is immediately after the *Significance and Innovation* section of the proposal, at the beginning of the *Approach* section(s). Remember that the entire Research

Strategy, including the preliminary studies, must fit within the 6–12-page limit depending upon the grant mechanism.

9.3 START BY DESCRIBING YOUR RESEARCH TEAM

As noted earlier, the NIH definition of Preliminary Studies includes the PI's experience pertinent to this application. Therefore, start the Preliminary Studies section by pointing out the **expertise of your research team** in all aspects of the proposal.

Example Preliminary Study Section Describing the Investigative Team
Substantial preliminary work demonstrates the experience of the research team in all aspects of the proposed study: physical activity measurement (Drs. Jones, Thompson, and Levine), physical activity interventions (Drs. McGovern and Smith), racial/ethnic issues surrounding physical activity (Drs. Jones and Smith), gestational diabetes (Drs. Branson and Smith), obstetrics (Dr. Goldman), and statistical analysis of physical activity data (Dr. Francis).

Then, demonstrate **established relationships** among the co-investigators on your proposal. A track record of prior collaborations among you and your investigative team will reassure your reviewers that these co-investigators do not appear in name only. Relationships with more senior colleagues are critical if you are an early-career faculty. Their involvement on your proposal will be a key factor supporting your ability to logistically conduct the project—particularly if these senior investigators have a track record of conducting similar projects in similar populations.

There are several ways in which you can prove established working relationships:

- Co-authored publications
- Submitted publications under review
- Co-presentations
- An established mentoring relationship (e.g., as part of a training grant)
- Co-investigators on an already funded grant

Of course, much of this information will appear in your biosketch and that of your co-investigators. But you cannot rely on the reviewers to connect the dots between you and your co-investigators. Instead, you want to make it easy for the reviewers by clearly delineating this prior collaboration in your Preliminary Studies section.

9.4 HOW TO DESCRIBE PRELIMINARY DATA

Your description of preliminary data should be concise and include the following key items:

1. The pilot grant name, number, and Principal Investigator (PI) (if your preliminary data were supported by funded research)
2. Citations for pilot study results (if published)
3. A table/figure or narrative of the findings relevant to the current proposal
4. The relationship of the preliminary data to current proposed aims and hypotheses

If your preliminary data were based on a grant-funded pilot study, then state the grant number and PI's name early in the paragraph. If you were not the PI, then clarify in parentheses the role of that PI on your proposal (e.g., "S1234 ASPH/CDC PI: Jones, coinvestigator on the proposed study"). The body of the paragraph should contain a brief description of the methods and findings. Findings ideally should be shown via a table/figure with a brief description of the take-home message. If published, be sure to cite the publication that includes these preliminary data. Remember that publications authored by yourself or by your co-investigators are all eligible to include here.

eg
example

Example Description of Preliminary Data
Behaviors Affecting Adolescents (BAA) Study (ASPH/CDC 1234, PI: yourself): This pilot study was conducted at the proposed study site in conjunction with Drs. Taylor, Smith, and Jones (co-investigators). The primary goals were to investigate the effect of an individually tailored 12-week exercise intervention on serum biomarkers associated with insulin resistance. Adolescents (n = 25) were predominantly overweight/obese (98%), young (48% <24 years), and low income (43% <$15,000/year). After the 12-week intervention, during a time when exercise typically decreases, the exercise arm experienced a higher increase in sports/exercise (0.9 MET-hours/week) versus the control arm (−0.01 MET-hours/week; p = 0.02) (Figure 9.1).[1] Intervention participants reported being satisfied with the amount of information received (95%), and 86% reported finding the study materials interesting and useful. **These data support the feasibility and efficacy of the exercise component of the proposed lifestyle intervention in Aim #1 of the proposal.**

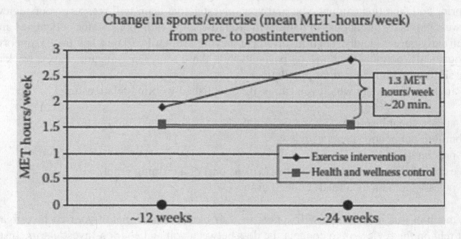

FIGURE 9.1 Preliminary data from a pilot exercise intervention.

9.5 LINK EACH OF YOUR PRELIMINARY STUDIES TO YOUR PROPOSED SPECIFIC AIMS/HYPOTHESES

A key pitfall in grant proposals is to fail to link preliminary data to one or more of your proposed specific aims or hypotheses. It is your job to clarify how each of your preliminary studies relates to or supports your proposed aims and hypotheses. You cannot rely on the reviewer to do this for you. This is often done in the first or final sentence of each preliminary study paragraph. Specify the rationale for why these preliminary data are relevant to the current proposal. Indeed, the act of creating these sentences serves the dual purpose of ensuring that you are not including extraneous preliminary findings not directly relevant to your aims, or vice versa. In other words, if you can't make the connection, then the reviewer will certainly not be able to.

Example Last Sentences of Preliminary Study Descriptions
- This study adds further evidence of our experience conducting randomized trials among at-risk Hispanic women and therefore provides **support for Aim #1**: *To conduct a randomized trial of a dietary intervention among Hispanic women.*
- This study supports our ability to recruit, retain, and intervene on weight loss, physical activity, and diet with the postpartum population and therefore provides **support for Aim #2**: *To conduct a randomized trial of a lifestyle intervention among postpartum women.*
- These data support the feasibility, acceptability, and efficacy of a high-reach, low-cost, individually tailored mailed intervention among high-risk adolescents and therefore provides **support for Aim #3**: *To conduct a randomized trial of a behavioral intervention among high risk adolescents.*

It is not considered appropriate to *pad* the preliminary studies section with preliminary studies that do not relate to one or more of your specific aims or hypotheses simply to assure the reviewers that you have research experience. They will see your experience from your biosketch. Instead, as noted above, you will want to show that each preliminary study presented relates specifically to one or more of your proposed hypotheses or, at the least, to a subcomponent of a hypothesis.

After you describe findings that are relevant to your hypotheses, then you may go on and mention other unexpected or unusual significant findings (if space permits), but the hypotheses of the proposal need to be supported first.

Example Linking Preliminary Data to Hypotheses
Hypothesis #1a: Television viewing time will be negatively associated with the school readiness of preschoolers.
Preliminary studies section
[Address hypothesis #1a first] In our pilot study, we found that television time was negatively related to school readiness ($r = -0.70$, $p = 0.02$).
[Include other findings second] We also found that children's television viewing time was significantly and negatively related to parental instruction ($r^2 = -0.35$, $p = 0.01$).

9.6 PRELIMINARY STUDIES SHOULD NOT FULLY ANSWER YOUR PROPOSED RESEARCH QUESTIONS

While your preliminary studies should directly relate to one or more of your specific aims, ideally they should not fully answer your research questions (i.e., your hypotheses). If they did, then you will have reduced reviewer enthusiasm for that aim in your current proposal. Therefore, it is critical to justify the advantage of the proposed study over and above the preliminary study, to the reviewer in the last line of each preliminary study paragraph.

For example, often your preliminary data will be based on a smaller sample than the proposed study. This small size may lead to findings that are suggestive but not statistically significant. This therefore motivates the need for a larger study (i.e., the proposed study) with adequate statistical power to follow up on the promising result that you observed in your preliminary studies.

Or your preliminary data could have derived from a lower quality measurement device, a different study population than your proposed grant, or used a more limited study design. This motivates the need for your proposed study to improve in a substantive way on these preliminary data—for example, via an improved measurement device, stronger study design, and focus on the target study population.

9.7 SHOULD I INCLUDE PRELIMINARY STUDIES EVEN IF THE GRANT DOES NOT REQUIRE THEM?

Some foundation grants and certain NIH grants do not require the inclusion of preliminary studies. These include exploratory/developmental research grants (R21/R33), small research grants (R03), and academic research enhancement award (AREA) grants (R15). For R01 applications, reviewers are instructed to place less emphasis on the preliminary data from early-stage investigators (ESIs) than from more established investigators. However, almost without exception, including the results from preliminary studies will serve to increase your chances of a favorable review. As noted above, even if you have conducted a pilot study that has not yet yielded results, preliminary recruitment rates can help to establish the feasibility and therefore the likelihood of the success of the proposed project.

9.8 DO PRELIMINARY DATA NEED TO BE PREVIOUSLY PUBLISHED?

Preliminary data can be published or unpublished. If they are published, including the citation in the proposal will further increase your chances of success. A track record of relevant publications will first provide evidence that peer reviewers considered your findings of scientific merit. Secondly, published preliminary data can provide evidence that you, as an investigator, have the ability to translate your findings into publications. This latter ability is an important concern among reviewers who want assurance that the findings of your current proposal will have an overall impact on the field. Thirdly, as noted above, any co-authored publications of preliminary findings with your co-investigators will show evidence of your track record of collaboration. Therefore, citing your preliminary study findings, when possible, is important.

9.9 PRELIMINARY STUDIES BASED ON EXISTING DATASETS

It is fairly common for grant proposals, particularly by early-career faculty, to propose to use data from an existing dataset. Such grants propose to conduct a secondary data analysis using data from a study that has already been conducted. Such a dataset may have been created by your mentor or colleagues, or it could be a national dataset to which you have access such as the Women's Health Initiative (WHI), the Behavioral Risk Factor Surveillance System (BRFSS), the National Health Interview Survey (NHIS), and/or the National Health and Nutrition Examination Survey (NHANES).

Indeed, the practice of using preexisting data is **efficient and economical**, aspects that are particularly attractive, given the current funding environment. In recognition of this, some NIH requests for proposals and program announcements are specifically limited to secondary analyses of existing datasets—as in the example below.

Example Funding Opportunity for Secondary Data Analysis
Secondary Analysis and Integration of Existing Data to Elucidate the Genetic Architecture of Cancer Risk and Related Outcomes (R01):
Through this funding opportunity announcement (FOA), the National Cancer Institute (NCI), along with the National Human Genome Research Institute (NHGRI) and National Institute of Dental and Craniofacial Research (NIDCR), encourages submission of applications proposing to conduct secondary data analysis and integration of existing datasets and database resources, with the ultimate aim to elucidate the genetic architecture of cancer risk and related outcomes (e.g., risk prediction or reduction, survival, or response to treatment, etc.).

In these situations, your preliminary studies section should include:

- A complete description of this existing dataset
  - Characteristics of the study population
  - Recruitment, eligibility, and follow-up rates
  - The final sample available for your analysis
- Your prior experience, or that of your co-investigators, with this dataset
- Your access to this dataset (refer to a letter of support included in the grant)
- Any relevant preliminary findings

Basing a proposal on an existing dataset can be a two-edged sword in that reviewers may expect you to show more preliminary data than if you were proposing a study de novo. In this situation, try to include descriptive univariate statistics on your proposed exposure and outcome variables. A table may be an efficient way to present these data and will reassure the reviewers that your study population has sufficient variability in exposure distribution such that it will be feasible to observe an association with your outcome of interest (see Chapter 13, "Power and Sample Size"). For example, if you propose to use an existing dataset to study alcohol consumption and risk of bladder cancer, but almost all your participants are nondrinkers or light drinkers, this will raise a concern among reviewers. Because reviewers know you have these data, they may think that you are hiding something by not showing it.

9.10 WHAT IF YOUR PRELIMINARY DATA CONTRADICT YOUR PROPOSED HYPOTHESES?

If your preliminary data contradict your proposed hypotheses (e.g., show the opposite direction of effect from your proposed hypotheses), this is often considered a *fatal flaw* by reviewers. First, step back and consider the statistical significance of your pilot data. Preliminary studies, by definition, are not fully powered to answer your research questions. Therefore, any pilot findings are often accompanied by a high degree of variability (e.g., a wide confidence interval) and are usually not statistically significant.

Mention alternative reasons for any contradictory findings and clarify why they will be less of a threat in the proposed study. For example, you can say that the influence of bias and confounding will be addressed in the proposed study through improvements in study design and/or the availability of data on important covariates. Indeed, a large part of the rationale for your current proposal may come from the questions raised by your preliminary work.

Avoid trying to explain away your contradictory findings by saying that they are not supported by the prior literature. If the reviewers see such opposite results from your own lab, this will call into question not only the rationale for your proposed hypothesis but also the validity of your methods.

However, if after considering these alternative explanations, you do indeed determine that your pilot findings contradict your hypotheses, then unless you have an excellent reason to explain this opposite finding and also a clear rationale for why you expect to see the opposite in your proposal—do not proceed with your hypotheses as written. Instead, consider rewriting your hypotheses or reframing the topic of the entire grant proposal.

9.11 WHAT IF YOU DO NOT HAVE PRELIMINARY DATA?

There are several approaches that you can take if you do not have preliminary data as defined above:

Does your <u>research team</u> have preliminary data? As noted earlier in the chapter, remember that your co-investigators and/or mentors in the case of a Fellowship grant or a Career Development award become your research team. If they have preliminary data, then your team, by definition, has preliminary data. The preliminary studies paragraph can state *"Our research team has also conducted …"* and then include a brief description of their preliminary studies as described above.

Consider a different funding mechanism. Certain funding mechanisms are themselves designed to generate pilot data (e.g., preliminary data) such as R21s, or R03s, or seed grants and do not require preliminary data. In contrast, an R01 requires substantial preliminary data—ideally led by the PI themselves but at a minimum by the research team. Remember that if you yourself have not been the PI of significant grant-funded research, then applying for an R01 as a sole principal investigator may be premature. Even if your *research team* has significant grant-funded research, the reviewers will still want assurance that you, as a PI, can logistically pull off a large R01 from a feasibility point of view. Choosing a co-principal investigator (co-PI) with a strong prior publication and grant record, as well as project management experience, can alleviate these concerns. The multiple PI (MPI) model is described in more detail in Chapter 17, "Submission of the Grant Proposal". Note that the co-PI role should not be confused with a co-investigator (co-I) role.

Alternatively consider taking one of your ultimate R01 aims and applying for a seed grant/R21 to support this aim. Ideally, you have already met with your mentor and mapped out your grant trajectory progression from small seed grants to small NIH grant mechanisms and/or foundation grants to the next larger sized grant, with each subsequent step providing preliminary data for the ultimate R01. This technique is described in more detail in Chapter 1, "Ten Top Tips for Successful Proposal Writing," and Chapter 4, "Choosing the Right Funding Source."

Cast a wide net and consider tangential preliminary studies. For example, if you are proposing to recruit a sample of participants, any previous experience with recruitment—even in a different setting and with different methods—may still be helpful in terms of demonstrating your experience in recruiting and retaining a study population. In this case, including a table of characteristics of your previous study population will show concrete evidence of how many participants you recruited and that you know how to collect and present data. Similarly, any prior grant management experience can also be helpful.

Again, be sure to end every preliminary studies paragraph with a sentence clarifying how these preliminary data are relevant to the current proposal.

Example Strategy to Handle Lack of Preliminary Data
Consider a proposal to conduct a randomized trial of a lifestyle intervention (which consists of diet and exercise advice) to treat diabetes in older African American men.
The following preliminary studies are relevant to include:
1. Your prior studies which only included dietary interventions or only exercise interventions even though your proposed intervention is broader.
2. Your prior studies of lifestyle interventions in non-Hispanic white populations can support your logistical experience in conducting such an intervention study.
3. Your research team's prior validation studies of the exercise and diet compliance measures that you propose to use.

9.12 TIP #1: INCLUDE TABLES AND FIGURES IN THE PRELIMINARY STUDIES SECTION

As mentioned in Chapter 1, "Ten Top Tips for Successful Proposal Writing," the more figures and tables in a grant application, the better. Not only does the process of creating these figures and tables help you to crystallize your preliminary findings, but they are also kinder to the reviewers. As compared to dense text, tables and figures are easier for the reviewer to digest and help them grasp your findings more quickly. They save space—reducing the text—critical for the page limitations of most proposals.

The example below demonstrates the advantages of a figure or a table over text alone when presenting preliminary findings.

Example Description of Preliminary Data using Text Only
A Proposal to Evaluate Coffee Drinking and Melanoma Risk
Option #1: Text Version
We investigated the association between coffee drinking (cups/day) and risk of melanoma in our pilot study. There was no increase in risk with increasing coffee consumption ($p_{trend} = 0.20$). As compared to those with no coffee consumption, the relative risk (RR) for melanoma among those with 1 cup/day of consumption was 0.79 (95% confidence interval [CI] = 0.18–1.30); for 2 cups/day of consumption, the RR was 1.47 (95% CI = 0.55–1.56); for 3 cups/day of consumption, the RR was 3.03 (95% CI = 0.95–8.55); and for 4 or more cups/day, the RR was 1.30 (95% CI = 0.54–1.35). Lack of statistically significant findings may have been due, in part, to the small sample size, particularly among those with the highest level of coffee consumption.

Example Description of Preliminary Data Using a Table
Option #2: Table version (Table 9.1)

TABLE 9.1   Preliminary Data for a Proposal to Evaluate Coffee Drinking and Melanoma Risk

COFFEE CONSUMPTION	CASES	RR	95% CI
None	15	1.0	Referent
1 Cup/day	10	7.9	0.18–1.30
2 Cups/day	9	1.47	0.55–1.56
3 Cups/day	2	3.03	0.95–8.55
4+ Cups/day	2	1.30	0.54–1.35

Example Description of Preliminary Data Using a Figure
Option #3: Figure version (Figure 9.2)

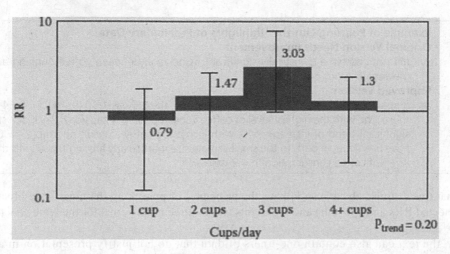

FIGURE 9.2   Preliminary data for a proposal to evaluate coffee drinking and melanoma risk.

As you can see from the example above, the figure is the clearest way to display the preliminary findings to the reviewers. It saves the reviewer the work of interpreting dense text or numerical findings. With one glance at the figure, the reviewer can see the potential trend in the findings of an increased risk of melanoma with increasing dose of coffee. At the same time, they can quickly see the statistical significance of the findings via noting if the vertical confidence interval bars cross the null value of 1.0. In this way, the use of the figure will reduce the amount of text necessary to describe the preliminary findings as discussed in Tip #2: When Describing Results in a Table or Figure, Point Out the Highlights for the Reviewer.

9.13 TIP #2: WHEN DESCRIBING RESULTS IN A TABLE OR FIGURE, POINT OUT THE HIGHLIGHTS FOR THE REVIEWER

While pictures say a thousand words, it is not sufficient to include preliminary study tables and figures in the proposal without accompanying text. Include text that walks the reader through the tables/figures and points out the important points. In this way, you are guiding the reviewer to what you feel is the **take-home message**.

This can be challenging. One approach is to first look through the tables and circle what you believe are the most important findings in each table. These would be findings that directly show support for your primary hypotheses or some aspect of your hypotheses.

In the text, avoid repeating each value that appears in the tables/figures. Remember that the reader can see all of these data. Instead, limit yourself to **highlighting two to three data points per table**. This is a critical exercise and much more challenging than it originally appears. However, it is an integral exercise not only for describing preliminary studies in a proposal but also subsequently when you are writing up a journal article submission of your findings.

In your text description, be sure to point out the **magnitude of your findings** (e.g., mean differences or relative risks) with their accompanying measures of variation (e.g., standard deviations or confidence intervals) and not just their statistical significance (e.g., p-values). Presenting p-values alone is not informative in the Preliminary Studies section because preliminary data are usually, by definition, underpowered to detect a statistically significant effect.

Example of Pointing Out the Highlights of Preliminary Data
Original Version Needs Improvement
We did not observe a statistically significant association between coffee drinking and risk of melanoma in our pilot study.
Improved Version
As compared to those with no coffee consumption, the RR was 1.30 (95% CI = 0.54–1.35) for those who with the highest level of coffee consumption (>4 cups/day). Lack of a statistically significant trend of increasing risk with increasing coffee consumption (p_{trend} = 0.20) may have been due, in part, to the small sample size, particularly among those with the highest levels of coffee consumption (n = 2 cases).

Note that this example above also follows the principles of presenting the magnitude of study findings (i.e., selected RRs and 95% CIs) and highlights two to three main points for the reviewers to have as a take-home message.

Finally, the text can also contain one-liners of data that do not justify presentation in a table or figure.

Example: Preliminary Studies Not Meriting a Table or Figure
Although we controlled for diabetes in the prior analysis, we repeated the analysis excluding those with diabetes. Results were virtually unchanged.

9.14 TIP #3: HOW TO CREATE DESCRIPTIVE TABLES OF THE STUDY POPULATION

As noted earlier, when proposing to use an existing dataset, it is common practice to show a table of descriptive characteristics of the study population. In this way, you help the reviewer to *see* or envision your study population. Inclusion of this table also supports that you have access to the data and know how to quantify it.

If space permits, you may also want to include additional columns stratifying the study population by categories of your exposure. For example, if you are proposing to conduct a study of alcohol consumption and risk of bladder cancer, your study population table would not only show characteristics of the total population but also stratify participants according to categories of alcohol consumption (e.g., nondrinker, drinker) (Table 9.2).

Example Summary of Preliminary Data
Original Version Needs Improvement
Drinkers and nondrinkers were similar.
Improved Version
Among the participants, 200 (44.4%) reported that they almost never consumed alcoholic beverages, while 250 (55.6%) drank 5 g or more per day. History of hypertension appeared to be similar among drinkers and nondrinkers. Obesity and a history of high cholesterol and diabetes were less common among drinkers, while smoking and regular physical activity were more common.

Note that the improved example strikes a nice balance between being too general vs. repeating every single value in the table. The improved example is also kind to the reviewer by noting patterns: listing those characteristics that were (1) similar among both exposure groups, (2) less common among the exposed than the unexposed, and (3) more common among the exposed than the unexposed. The reviewer's eye would naturally be trying to do this as they look at your table, so instead you have saved them precious time in their review.

TABLE 9.2 Characteristics of the Study Sample According to Alcohol Consumption

CHARACTERISTICS	TOTAL SAMPLE	DRINKER	NONDRINKER
Total in 2019 (n)	450	250	200
Obesity (%)	25.2	24.3	26.5
History of hypertension (%)	10	11	9
History of high cholesterol (%)	20	15	25
History of diabetes (%)	5	3	7
Cigarette smoking (%)	10	12	8
Regular physical activity (%)	30	40	20

9.15 TIP #4: DESCRIBE PRELIMINARY FINDINGS IN LAYPERSON'S TERMS

As with all grant proposal writing, the key principle in describing your preliminary findings is to avoid professional or epidemiologic jargon. Describing results concisely and in layperson's terms is important as not all your reviewers will be experts in your field. When your study is complete, this skill will also serve you well when you translate your important findings into public health messages.

For example, let's say you conducted an analysis of history of severe sunburns (exposure variable) and melanoma (outcome variable). Melanoma is a dichotomous outcome variable (yes, no), so you chose multivariable logistic regression. Your model yielded an odds ratio (OR) of 1.9.

Example Description of Preliminary Data Avoiding Jargon
Original Version Needs Improvement
The multivariate RR of melanoma was 1.9 (95% CI 1.1–2.5) (Table 1).
Improved Version
After controlling for age, race, and BMI, men who had ever had a severe sunburn had almost two times the risk of melanoma compared to men who had never had a severe sunburn (95% CI 1.1–2.5) (Table 1).

The original version did not articulate who was in the comparison group—that is, who were the exposed (those who had ever had a severe sunburn) and who were the unexposed (those with no history of severe sunburn). A similar example is below.

Example Description of Preliminary Data Avoiding Jargon
Original Version Needs Improvement
The RR of liver cancer was 1.2 (Table 2).
Improved Version
Men who had consumed five or more grams of alcohol per day had a 20% increased risk of liver cancer as compared to never drinkers (95% CI 1.12–1.36) (Table 2).

9.15.1 How to Describe a Beta Coefficient in Layperson's Terms

Students often struggle with how to interpret a beta coefficient in layperson's terms. A beta represents the mean change in the outcome variable for a unit change in the exposure of interest. For example, let's say you conducted an analysis of television watching (exposure variable) and weight (outcome variable). Weight is a continuous outcome variable (pounds [lb]), so you chose multivariable linear regression. Your model yielded a beta coefficient of 0.2.

Example Description of Preliminary Data Avoiding Jargon
Original Version Needs Improvement
The beta coefficient was 0.2 (SE = 0.45) (Table 3).
Improved Version
Every one hour increase in television watching was associated with, on average, a 0.2 lb increase in weight (SE = 0.45) (Table 3).

9.15.2 How to Describe Effect Modification in Layperson's Terms

Effect modification can be challenging to write up in layperson's terms. Let's say that your preliminary data evaluated the possibility of effect modification by gender. Your exposure of interest was hemorrhage size and your outcome of interest was three-month mortality. You have preliminary data that support the presence of effect modification by gender.

Example Description of Preliminary Data Avoiding Jargon
Original Version Needs Improvement
We found that gender modified the association between hemorrhage size and mortality (Table 4).
Improved Version
The association between hemorrhage size and risk of mortality was stronger in women (RR = 2.0) than in men (RR = 1.5) (Table 4).

9.16 TIP #5: DESCRIBE TABLES IN NUMERIC ORDER

The text should describe the tables in numeric order. Avoid going back and forth between consecutive tables. In other words, after you describe Table 2, do not return again to Table 1. If you are having trouble doing this, this may mean that you have to restructure your tables so that the narrative can flow in sequence. At all costs, try to avoid having your reviewer bounce forward and then backward between study tables.

9.17 TIP #6: TRY TO DESCRIBE TABLES FROM TOP TO BOTTOM

Within a table, try to -describe it from top to bottom. However, keep in mind that this may not always be possible, and it is often better to break this rule than to have to reorder the table. As mentioned above, your top priority when describing a table is to identify patterns for the reviewer. For example, in the alcohol table (Table 9.2), it would not be appropriate to reorder the table rows according to the post hoc observance of study findings, because tables are meant to be structured *a priori* (e.g., before findings are known). However, all other things being equal, try to describe the key results in order from top to bottom as they appear in the table.

9.18 TIP #7: SPELL OUT NUMBERS THAT START SENTENCES

Sentences should never start with a number in digit form. Instead, numbers should be spelled out if they start a sentence.

Example Description of Preliminary Data Using Numbers
Original Version Needs Improvement
25 adolescents agreed to participate in our pilot study.
Improved Version
Twenty-five adolescents agreed to participate in our pilot study.

In the case of large numbers, it is best to restructure the sentence so that you avoid spelling out the number (which is cumbersome to the reader and takes up valuable space). Instead, write the sentence so that the number is not the first word.

Example Description of Preliminary Data Using Numbers
Original Version Needs Improvement
Seven thousand six hundred thirty-four women are included in the National Health Survey dataset.
Improved Version
A total of 7634 women are included in the National Health Survey dataset.

9.19 TIP #8: AVOID PRESENTING CONFIDENCE INTERVALS *AND P*-VALUES

Like a *p*-value, a CI provides information about the statistical significance of a finding. However, the 95% CI has the additional advantage of providing the range that will include with a 95% probability the true measure of association. Therefore, presenting CIs as well as *p*-values is repetitive.

How can we tell if a finding is statistically significant by looking at the CI? If the CI includes the null value for the association being calculated, then the observed association is not statistically significant.

- If the CI spans the null value of 1.0, then the RR is not statistically significant. The *p*-value is >0.05.
- If the CI does not span 1.0, the RR is statistically significant. The *p*-value is <0.05.

Example Determination of Statistical Significance from Confidence Intervals
RR = 1.75, 95% CI = (1.12–2.75): statistically significant
RR = 1.43, 95% CI = (0.92–2.25): *not* statistically significant
RR = 0.35, 95% CI = (0.14–0.89): statistically significant

9.20 TIP #9: AVOID REFERRING TO YOUR TABLES AS ACTIVE BEINGS

Tables should not be the subject of sentences and instead should simply be referred to in parentheses within sentences describing the table contents. This approach is also more space efficient.

Example Description of Preliminary Data Tables
Original Version Needs Improvement
Table 1 shows that cases were older than controls.
Improved Version
Cases were older than controls (Table 1).

Another space-saving technique is to avoid including sentences that say what tables *will* present. Instead, jump straight to describing the table contents.

Example Reference to Tables in Preliminary Data
Original Version Needs Improvement
Table 1 shows characteristics of cases and controls in our dataset. Cases were on average older than controls (mean 35 years vs. 30 years, respectively).
Improved Version
Cases were on average older than controls (mean 35 years vs. 30 years, respectively) (Table 1).

9.21 TIP #10: TIPS FOR TABLE TITLES

Table titles should be concise yet be **freestanding** such that the title and table could stand alone from the remainder of the proposal and still be understandable.

Specifically, a well-written table title should include the following information:

- The study name and dates of conduct
- The statistics presented in the tables (e.g., means and SDs or RRs and 95% CIs)
- The variables that were measured

If there are too many variables to fit concisely in the title, then the corresponding umbrella terms should be used. For example, if your preliminary data present information on markers of cardiovascular disease such as HDL, LDL, and triglycerides, it would be more efficient to simply use the umbrella term *cardiovascular disease risk factors*. Similarly, if your preliminary data involves lifestyle behaviors such as diet, exercise, and weight management, instead using the term *lifestyle behaviors* would be preferable.

Example Description of Preliminary Data Tables
- Table 1. Number of Participants by Gender and Grade Level; the Idaho Women's Health Study, 2015–2020.
- Table 2. Means and Standard Deviations of Reading and Mathematics; the Idaho Women's Health Study, 2015–2020.
- Table 3. Analysis of Variance for Reading Scores; the Idaho Women's Health Study, 2015–2020.

Note that all three examples follow the titling guidelines by naming the variables, statistics, and study name and dates.

9.22 PRELIMINARY STUDY EXAMPLES

Below are two preliminary studies to support *A Proposal to Conduct a Lifestyle Intervention in Hispanic Women*. Note that the first preliminary study focuses more on supporting the feasibility and acceptability of the intervention, while the second preliminary study focuses more on supporting the proposed hypotheses that the intervention will be efficacious.

9.22.1 Preliminary Study #1

Estudio Salud *(Pilot Grant # xxxx*, PI: Smith). We conducted a series of focus groups to evaluate the acceptability of the proposed intervention materials among our target population (overweight/obese Hispanic women). Participants (n = 25) reported that having materials that addressed culture-specific barriers was helpful in terms of setting realistic goals (87%), reported reading most/all of the physical activity information (85%), gaining knowledge about exercise via reading the materials (97%), finding it enjoyable (95%), and wearing the pedometers (90%). **These data support the** *feasibility and acceptability* **of the study protocol for a high-reach, low-cost, individually tailored mailed intervention among at-risk Hispanic women and therefore directly support the proposed intervention outlined in Specific Aim #1.**

9.22.2 Preliminary Study #2

Estudio Salud *(Small foundation grant # xxxx*, PI: Smith). We conducted a pilot study to test the proposed intervention among overweight/obese Hispanics (n = 50). Moderate-intensity (or greater) activity increased from an average of 16.6 min/week (SD = 25.8) at baseline to 147.3 (SD = 241.6) at 6 months in the intervention arm and from 11.9 min/week (SD = 22.0) to 96.8 (SD = 118.5) in the wellness contact control arm. Retention rates were high (87%) for this hard-to-reach Hispanic group, and there were no differences in the follow-up according to participant characteristics or study arm. Recruitment and retention rates were used to inform the proposed power calculations (see c3. Power). **These data support the** *efficacy* **of a high-reach, low-cost, individually tailored mailed intervention among at-risk Hispanic women and therefore directly support the proposed intervention outlined in Specific Aim #1.**

Pilot Grants
Reproducibility and Validity Studies

10

A reproducibility and validity study of your proposed methods is an excellent topic for an early grant in your grantsmanship trajectory. Due to their fairly small size and delineated methods, reproducibility and validity studies are quite feasible for early-stage investigators. Validation studies can provide assurance that a larger study based upon these methods will work; thus, such studies are the first step toward answering a larger etiologic question. The fact that reproducibility and validity studies play a critical role in the development of a larger project makes them particularly appealing for reviewers.

Demonstrating the reproducibility and validity of your measures is one way of assuring your reviewers that a larger proposal based upon these measures will work. Remember that showing that you can *pull it off* is one of the "Ten Top Tips for Successful Proposal Writing," as presented in Chapter 1. This approach is critical as grant review panels often see a large grant as the culmination of a growing body of work progressing from small seed grants to larger and larger awards in a cumulative fashion.

As noted in Chapter 1, applying for a seed grant or foundation grant to support such validation work is often a key first step toward applying for a larger grant designed to use these measurement tools to evaluate etiologic associations between exposures and diseases. Indeed, a proposal to conduct a reproducibility and validity study is typically the first proposal written by a graduate student or early-career faculty.

As discussed below, the need for reproducibility and validity studies remains even if the tools that you are proposing to use have been validated previously, but you are proposing to use them in a **new study population** or **modify** them in any way.

Therefore, this chapter will describe methods for designing and conducting reproducibility and validity studies, issues to consider in the analysis and interpretation of findings from these studies, as well as strategies for writing their corresponding limitations sections.

10.1 WHY CONDUCT A REPRODUCIBILITY OR VALIDITY STUDY?

The majority of proposals in epidemiology propose to measure the association between some type of exposure and risk of some outcome. These studies are termed *etiologic studies*, and they rely upon tools to measure exposure and disease.

It is critical that these tools be *reliable and valid*. When tools have low reproducibility and validity, their use may lead to failure to observe an association when one indeed exists. At worse, their use may lead to the finding of a biased association between exposure and disease.

For these reasons, grant reviewers and committee members may consider a proposal to be **fatally flawed** if it does not provide evidence on the reproducibility and validity of the proposed measurement tools.

An important caveat
Earlier, in more economically advantaged times, it was considered acceptable for a large NIH R01 grant to include pilot studies within its aims. However, in the current climate, reviewers do not look favorably upon this approach. They naturally ask, "What if the pilot study finds that the methods are not successful?" and "How would the investigator accomplish the subsequent aims of the project?" For example, suppose Specific Aim #1 proposes to conduct a validation study of the questionnaire to be used in Specific Aims #2 and #3. If Specific Aim #1 subsequently fails to find that the questionnaire is valid, then how can the remainder of the project proceed? As noted in Chapter 6, "Specific Aims," these are termed interdependent aims and reviewers often consider such aims to be a fatal flaw of a proposal.

10.2 WHAT IS REPRODUCIBILITY?

Reproducibility is defined as the ability of the measurement tool to produce the same results over repeated administrations. Reproducibility answers the question, "Does the questionnaire consistently provide the same results under the same circumstances?" Therefore, a *reproducibility study* is typically designed to compare data from repeated administrations of a measurement tool.

Reproducibility is the consistency of measurements:

- On more than one administration
- To the same people
- At different times

A perfectly reproducible method will yield the same results on repeated administrations. However, in reality, a measurement method will always be subject to error.

10.3 WHAT IS VALIDITY?

In contrast, validity answers the question, "How well does the tool measure what it is designed to measure?" Therefore, validation studies are designed to compare data collected by some type of proxy measure (e.g., your proposed measurement tool) against a *gold standard*. In practice, *gold standards* often do not exist, and in their place, a superior, although typically imperfect, comparison measure is utilized.

Validity is the degree to which the tool actually measures what it was designed to measure.

10.4 RELATIONSHIP BETWEEN REPRODUCIBILITY AND VALIDITY

In Figures 10.1 and 10.2, the *bull's-eye* center of the dartboard reflects the truth, that is, the true value that you are trying to measure. The dots represent the values observed by your measurement tool over repeated administrations of the tool.

The degree of **validity** is indicated by the proximity of these dots to the bull's eye.

The degree of **reproducibility** is indicated by the proximity of these dots to each other.

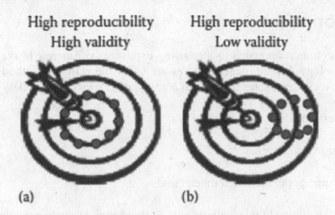

FIGURE 10.1 The relationship between reproducibility and validity: high reproducibility and high (a) and low (b) validity.

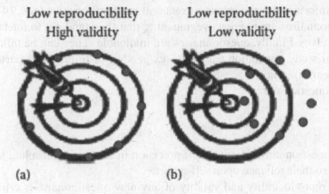

FIGURE 10.2 The relationship between reproducibility and validity: low reproducibility and high (a) and low (b) validity.

Figure 10.1 demonstrates high reproducibility because the dots are in a tight circle—showing that repeated measurements are consistent with each other over time. Figure 10.1a demonstrates high validity because the dots encircle the center of the circle (the truth), while Figure 10.1b demonstrates low validity because the circles do not encircle the truth.

The take-home message here is that *high reproducibility does not ensure high validity.*

Figure 10.2 demonstrates low reproducibility because the dots are in a wide circle—showing that repeated measurements are not consistent with each other over time. However, Figure 10.2a demonstrates high validity because the dots still encircle the center of the circle (the truth). Figure 10.2b demonstrates low validity because the circles do not encircle the truth.

In summary, because reproducibility studies are usually quick and inexpensive to conduct, they are an appropriate part of the measurement tool evaluation but cannot substitute for validity studies. Ideally, studies should propose to assess both reproducibility **and** validity.

10.5 BOTH SUBJECTIVE AND OBJECTIVE MEASUREMENT TOOLS REQUIRE EVIDENCE OF REPRODUCIBILITY AND VALIDITY

Because there are typically no true *gold standard* measurement methods, the need for reproducibility and validity studies is critical whether you are using subjective measures (e.g., questionnaire-based) or using more *objective* measures (e.g., laboratory assays, medical records).

10.5.1 Questionnaires

Questionnaires are a common approach to measuring exposures of interest in the fields of preventive medicine and epidemiology. Indeed, questionnaires are often the primary method for measuring such behavioral and psychosocial exposures as physical activity, diet, stress, and anxiety in large population-based studies.

Advantages of questionnaires

- Practical for large sample sizes
- Nonreactive
- Tailored to specific populations and time periods

As epidemiologic studies typically involve hundreds to thousands of study participants, questionnaires are extremely practical and cost-efficient. They are easy for study participants to complete and can be self-administered or interviewer-administered, both in person and over the telephone. They can ask participants to recall past information or to report current real-time information (e.g., 24-hour logs or diaries).

In addition, questionnaires are nonreactive, meaning that they tend not to interfere with the conduct of the behaviors themselves. Finally, questionnaires are malleable. They can be tailored to the characteristics of your particular study population (e.g., age, sex/gender) or limited to a particular period of time (e.g., past week, past year, lifetime).

Disadvantages of questionnaires

- Precision

The disadvantages of questionnaires involve their precision in measuring absolute levels of the exposure of interest, due in part to their reliance upon self-report.

Documenting the reproducibility and validity of any new questionnaire is critical (Table 10.1). For existing questionnaires, even small changes in the design of instruments may affect their performance. Therefore, the validity and reproducibility of any modified instrument should be evaluated independently. In addition, when a questionnaire will be administered to a study population that differs from the one in which it was developed, its reproducibility and validity should again be evaluated. Questionnaire performance will differ according to the age, sex/gender, race/ethnicity, and culture of the study population.

Example Need for a Validity Study

Consider a proposal to use a questionnaire to evaluate diet in Asian youth. Ideally, you would want to cite studies showing that the questionnaire was valid not only among children but also among Asian children. If such studies are not available, you may want to consider conducting such a validation study yourself.

TABLE 10.1 When to Perform Reproducibility/Validity Studies

- For new questionnaires
- When a questionnaire is modified
- When questionnaires will be used in a different population according to:
  - Age
  - Sex/gender
  - Race/ethnicity
  - Culture
  - Other socioeconomic, medical, or behavioral factors

10.5.2 Particular Challenge of Behavioral Questionnaires

Questionnaires have become the primary method for measuring behaviors (e.g., physical activity, diet, substance use) in epidemiologic studies. Such human behaviors are complex and difficult to measure accurately. In addition, because epidemiologic questionnaires are based upon self-reported data, documenting the reproducibility and validity of any new behavioral questionnaire is critical.

The particular challenges of behavioral questionnaires include:

- Behaviors have multiple components
- Reliance on self-report
- Unstructured nature of many behaviors
- Rare nature of many behaviors

Many behaviors have **multiple components** that make up the total *dose* of behavior (i.e., type, frequency, and intensity/content). Each of these individual components may vary from person to person. Furthermore, individuals rarely make clear changes in their behaviors at identifiable points in time. Instead, behavioral patterns typically evolve over periods of years.

Questionnaires designed to assess such behaviors are based upon **self-report** and therefore face the additional challenges of relying upon a participant's memory and accuracy in reporting.

Because many human behaviors are **unstructured**, they are even more difficult for study participants to report accurately. In addition, unstructured activities are less memorable than behaviors that require planning or effort.

Behaviors that are **rare** may be more or less difficult to report accurately. On the one hand, the planned nature of rare activities may make them easier to accurately report. In addition, salient events (e.g., key life events) may be easier to recall and lead to higher estimates of validity and reproducibility as compared to routine day-to-day events. On the other hand, activities that are rarely engaged in may be more difficult to reliably recall.

Example Challenges to Validity

Physical activity is a complex behavior made up of type, frequency, duration, and intensity of activity. "Types" of physical activity can include sports/ exercise, occupational activity, and household activity. Physical activity also spans different intensities including light intensity, moderate intensity, and vigorous intensity. Perceived intensity may also vary from person to person.

Studies have found that vigorous physical activity is more accurately reported from memory than moderate and nonvigorous activity since it may require planning or an effort that moderate activities do not require. In addition, vigorous activities like skiing or running may be reported more accurately if they are part of a participant's exercise schedule. In contrast, moderate activities such as walking and playing with children tend to be much more difficult to accurately report from memory yet may still constitute an important component of one's total physical activity.

Example Challenges to Validity

Dietary consumption is also a complex behavior made up of type, portion size, number of servings, and the nutrient content of the food consumed. The same food may have a different nutrient content depending upon the preparation technique and other factors. In addition, mixed foods such as casseroles and stews may contain many individual food components that are often difficult to tease apart. Unstructured behaviors such as snacking may be difficult for study participants to report accurately.

10.5.3 Objective Measures Also Require Reproducibility and Validity Studies

Objective measures are also subject to error. Examples of objective outcome measures can include biomarkers, medical records, and monitors. Each of these measures, although termed *objective,* faces potential errors as described below.

Biomarkers are measurable chemical, physical, or biological characteristics that aim to represent the severity or presence of some disease state. They are often obtained via blood or urine samples or biopsy. However, biomarkers face several limitations. First, biomarkers may not reflect the etiologically relevant time period for the impact of your exposure on your outcome of interest. For example, a cholesterol measure obtained after diagnosis of heart disease may not be representative of the cholesterol levels that preceded the heart disease. Second, degradation over time in frozen samples could reduce their validity. In addition, the biomarker may be influenced by other factors. For example, blood levels of vitamin D are influenced not only by diet but also by sunlight exposure.

Medical records or **ICD codes** are often considered the gold standard. However, medical records may be completed by a variety of personnel including residents, attending physicians, and nurses. Any of these personnel can make an error in recording key information in the medical record or in selecting the appropriate code. There may also be error on the part of the medical record abstractors in terms of their ability to abstract data.

Monitors can include physical activity monitoring systems such as actigraphs. Monitors face several sources of error. Participants may not be compliant in consistently wearing the monitors or may wear them incorrectly. Such devices can be reactive such that participants change their activity when they are wearing them. Lastly, the monitors themselves may have difficulty measuring particular types of activity. For example, waist-worn physical activity monitors have difficulty measuring upper body movements and may have to be removed during swimming.

Therefore, providing evidence for the reproducibility and validity of objective measures is just as important as doing so for subjective measures.

10.6 STUDY DESIGN OF REPRODUCIBILITY STUDIES

The goal of a reproducibility study is to assess variation in questionnaire performance from one administration to the next.

The first step in designing a reproducibility study is to consider the **time interval** between administrations of the measurement tool (Figure 10.3).

Both short and long time intervals have advantages and disadvantages:

Short intervals (i.e., days or weeks) between questionnaire administrations may result in participants recalling their previous responses as opposed to truly considering the questions. This will lead to artificially increased reproducibility.

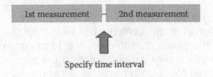

FIGURE 10.3 Reproducibility studies: consider the time interval between administrations of the measurement tool.

Long intervals of time between questionnaire administrations (i.e., one year) may encompass true changes in behaviors and lead to reduced reproducibility.

One approach to address these problems is to administer the questionnaire over both short and long intervals of time to provide an estimate of both the lower and the upper level of reproducibility.

10.7 STUDY DESIGN OF VALIDITY STUDIES

The goal of a validity study is to compare your measurement tool with the *gold standard*—a perfect measure of your variable of interest. In the absence of a true gold standard, you will want to select a superior method that has few, if any, shared sources of error with your measurement tool. Therefore, the first step in conducting a validity study is to choose your comparison measure.

All measures have errors; however they differ in magnitude and type. Given that neither your measure nor the comparison measure will be perfect, the error of both should be as uncorrelated as possible to avoid falsely high estimates of validity.

10.7.1 Subjective Comparison Measures

Among subjective comparison measures, logs or diaries are likely to have the least correlated errors with questionnaires. Unlike a self-administered questionnaire, a 24-hour log or diary is filled out in real time over the course of the day (Table 10.2). For example, participants could record their actual behavior (e.g., diet, physical activity), or a code corresponding to the type of behavior, every day at prespecified time intervals.

Major sources of errors associated with questionnaires are due to the restricted list of activities, memory, and misinterpretation of questions. These sources of error are not typically shared by logs or diaries that are open-ended and not reliant upon memory (i.e., activities are recorded as they occur) (Figure 10.4). Disadvantages of logs or diaries involve the fact that they rely heavily on subject motivation—they are time-consuming to complete. Completing them may also lead to heightened awareness that may alter normal behaviors (i.e., reactivity). Logs or diaries also share error due to self-report with questionnaires. For example, study participants are often prone to overestimating their physical activity on both questionnaires and diaries.

Table 10.2 provides examples of subjective comparison measures.

10.7.2 Objective Comparison Measures

Objective measures are often the comparison measure of choice for questionnaires as they are not subject to errors associated with self-report. On the other hand, objective measures are typically more expensive to administer and can cause reactivity (i.e., changes in behavior due to the device) (Table 10.3). Lastly, objective comparison measures are not all able to assess typical or long-term exposures, often the more

---

TABLE 10.2   Examples of Subjective Comparison Measures

- Logs or diaries
- 24-h recall
- 7-day recall
- Previous month recall
- Previous year recall

My Physical Activity Diary   Date _____

Day of week	Time of Day	Description of Activity (Type and Intensity Level)	Duration

FIGURE 10.4   Example excerpt from a seven-day activity diary.

TABLE 10.3   Examples of Objective Comparison Measures for Physical Activity

- Monitors (e.g., actigraph, heart rate monitors)
- Biomarkers
- Doubly labeled water
- Direct observation

important predictor of disease outcomes. In other words, while a questionnaire could query typical exposure over the past year, certain biomarkers may only be able to assess recent exposures.

Example Choice of an Objective Comparison Measure
Consider that you are proposing to validate a physical activity questionnaire. Examples of comparison measures include subjective measures (based on self-report) and objective measures (based on direct measurement). Subjective comparison measures can ask participants to report current physical activity (24-hour logs or diaries). Objective comparison measures include markers of movement (accelerometers), physiological responses that are affected by physical activity (heart rate), direct measures of energy expenditure (doubly labeled water), and observed or videotaped activity (direct observation).

10.7.3 Number of Administrations of the Comparison Measure

The next step in designing a validity study is to consider the **number of administrations** of the comparison measure. This decision should be based upon:

- Intraindividual variation in the behavior
- The accuracy of the comparison measure
- Participant burden
- Questionnaire time frame

The greater the variation in the behavior being measured, and the lower the accuracy of the comparison measure, the more administrations of the comparison measure needed. On the other hand, the number of administrations of the comparison measure should be tempered by the burden on the participant.

Example Study Design

Consider a proposal to conduct a validation study of a physical activity questionnaire whose goal is to assess usual activity over the past year. To assess reproducibility, you propose to administer the questionnaire at the beginning of the year and then repeat it at the end of the year. As a validation tool, you propose to administer four comparison measures (i.e., seven-day activity diaries) during each season throughout that year to capture day-to-day and seasonal variation in activity levels. In this way, the comparison measure covers the interval of time corresponding to the questionnaire—one year. Each seasonal administration will include a sufficient number of days to represent average energy expenditure (i.e., seven days) (Figure 10.5).

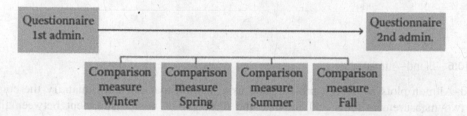

FIGURE 10.5 Study design for a reproducibility and validity study of a physical activity questionnaire.

10.8 WRITING DATA ANALYSIS SECTIONS FOR REPRODUCIBILITY/VALIDITY STUDIES

There are many statistical techniques available that can be used to assess reproducibility and validity. These include:

- Kappa coefficients
- Percent agreement
- Correlation coefficients (e.g., Pearson or Spearman)
- Sensitivity
- Specificity
- Paired comparisons (e.g., paired t-test, Wilcoxon signed rank test)
- Bland–Altman plots

Ideally, these agreement statistics should be accompanied by **confidence intervals (CIs)**, which allow for the interpretation of the precision of the reported estimates.

These measures all have strengths and limitations and the choice of which method to use will depend upon your specific measurement tools and other characteristics of your study design and setting. Consultation with a statistician on which technique to choose is highly recommended.

For example, because kappa is prevalence dependent, it is often viewed in combination with percent agreement and sensitivity to obtain a more accurate overall interpretation of agreement. Sensitivity calculations are especially instructive when a condition is rare. In contrast, specificity may be inflated in the context of rare events as they are less likely to have false-negative findings. Correlation coefficients are largely influenced by the range of the observed values and can be high even when the measurements do not agree (e.g., when there is a systematic difference between measures).

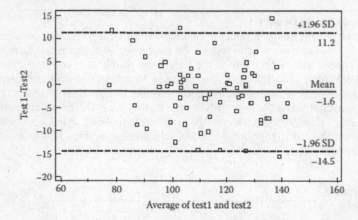

FIGURE 10.6   Bland–Altman plot.

Bland–Altman plots have been promulgated as a method that can both quantify the comparison between two measurement tools and indicate the direction of mismeasurement between the tools. Specifically, for every subject, the **difference** between the two measures (y-axis) is plotted against the **average** of the two measures (x-axis) (Figure 10.6).

Example Data Analysis Section for a Validity Study
Recall the previous example of a proposal to validate a physical activity questionnaire.
Intraclass correlation coefficients will be used to describe the reproducibility of the questionnaire. To evaluate the questionnaire's validity, Spearman correlation coefficients will be calculated between each of the questionnaires and the comparison measure (i.e., the average of the four weekly diaries). Correlations will be calculated for overall activity, as well as activity according to intensity and type.

10.9 WRITING LIMITATIONS SECTIONS FOR REPRODUCIBILITY/VALIDITY STUDIES

Limitations sections for reproducibility/validity studies differ from limitations sections for etiologic studies described in Chapter 14, "Study Limitations to Consider." Specifically, the limitations section for a reproducibility/validity study focuses on factors that may bias the observed measure of agreement—either between repeated administrations of your measurement tool (i.e., reproducibility) or between your measurement tool and a comparison measure (i.e., validity) (Table 10.4).

TABLE 10.4   Study Limitations for a Reproducibility/Validity Study

Threats to observed reproducibility scores
- Correlated error between administrations
- True changes in behavior between administrations
- A heightened awareness of behavior after the first administration

Threats to observed validity scores
- Correlated error between the measurement tool and the comparison

Threats to generalizability

TABLE 10.5 A Four-Part Approach for Presenting
Study Limitations in a Proposal

Step 1: Identify the limitation
Step 2: Describe the impact on your findings
Step 3: Discuss alternatives
Step 4: Describe methods to minimize the limitation

Just as described in detail in Chapter 15, "How to Present Limitations and Alternatives," when presenting limitations in your reproducibility/validity proposal, use the following four-part approach: (1) describe the potential limitation, (2) describe the potential impact of the limitation on your study findings, (3) discuss alternatives and why they were not selected, and (4) describe the methods that you propose to minimize the impact of this limitation (Table 10.5).

10.9.1 Threats to Observed Reproducibility Scores

There are several common threats to observed reproducibility scores as described below:

1. *Correlated error*

Observations of high reproducibility scores for a questionnaire may be caused by consistent errors in the completion of both administrations of the measurement tool. For example, if the participants consistently **misinterpret questions** on each administration of the questionnaire, their scores would be highly (but incorrectly) correlated.

Similarly, if the questionnaire consistently **omitted an important question**, this would also lead to incorrectly high reproducibility scores.

Example Limitations Section for a Reproducibility/Validity Study
Recall our proposal above to conduct a reproducibility and validity study of a physical activity questionnaire. The questionnaire was administered at the beginning of the year. To assess reproducibility, the questionnaire was administered for a second time at the end of the year.
Identify the limitation
It is possible that findings from the first and second questionnaires may be highly correlated but not represent the actual ability of women to recall physical activity. In other words, a high correlation could be due to consistent errors of self-report on both questionnaires or to consistent errors in the questionnaire itself such as omission of a common activity. It is also possible that participants may systematically exaggerate their level of physical activity.
Describe the methods to minimize the limitation
The questionnaire was developed based on a series of focus groups that used open-ended techniques to assemble a comprehensive list of activities engaged in by the study population. Therefore, we feel it is unlikely that the questionnaire will omit any important activities. In addition, the questionnaires will be interviewer-administered and interviewers will be highly trained to provide guidance on interpretation of questionnaire items and to reality check responses with participants. Therefore, we feel that the concerns of misinterpretation and exaggeration will be minimized.

---

2. *True changes in behavior*

Observations of low reproducibility scores may reflect **too long a time period** between administration of the measurement tools such that there are true changes in behavior between the intervals. This would lead to an underestimate of reproducibility between the measures.

On the other hand, **too short a time interval** between administrations of the questionnaire may lead to respondents recalling their previous responses as opposed to truly considering the questions. This would lead to an overestimate of reproducibility between the measures.

Low reproducibility scores may also reflect *differences in the reference time period* of recall. For example, consider a questionnaire that asks respondents to recall their behavior over the past three months and then is repeated three months later. By definition, the participants are being asked to recall behaviors over a different time period on the first questionnaire than on the second questionnaire. If the participants truly changed their behavior over this time period, this would lead to an underestimate of reproducibility between the measures due to this true variation in behavior.

This concern can be minimized in several ways:

If the measurement tool is querying **usual behavior**, this concern is reduced. For example, if the questionnaire is asking about *usual* dietary consumption and is repeated one week apart, then differences between the recalled time periods are no longer relevant. In addition, true changes in diet over that past week should not substantively influence the responses regarding *usual* diet on the second administration of the questionnaire.

This is also less of a concern if the behavior tends to be **stable over time**. For example, if the respondent tends to eat the same foods from week to week, then any true changes in diet over the week are likely to be minimal.

Finally, this concern is also minimized if participant responses are categorized in fairly **broad categories**. In this situation, for bias to occur, it would have to be substantial enough to move participants from one category of, for example, dietary consumption (e.g., the lowest quartile) to a higher category (e.g., the second or higher quartile).

Example Limitations Section for a Reproducibility Study

Consider a proposal to conduct a reproducibility study of a dietary questionnaire among middle-aged men. The dietary questionnaire asks about usual diet and is repeated three months apart.
Identify the limitation
Random within-person error may lead to underestimates of the true reproducibility of the questionnaire.
Describe the methods to minimize the limitation
Because the questionnaire asks men to integrate diet over the course of an entire year, we expect that random within-person error will be minimal. In addition, actual dietary patterns are unlikely to change substantially for men of that age range between questionnaire administrations. It is also unlikely that participants will have changed their dietary consumption levels so dramatically as to move from quartile 1 (lowest) to quartile 4 (highest) of total energy intake.

---

3. *A heightened awareness of behavior*

Low reproducibility scores may also reflect heightened awareness of behavior due to the first administration of the questionnaire. That is, the completion of the first questionnaire may lead respondents to be more aware of their behaviors during the following time interval such that on the administration of the second questionnaire, they will report their behavior differently even if it has not changed.

Example Limitations Section for a Reproducibility/Validity Study

Consider again a proposal to assess the reproducibility and validity of a physical activity questionnaire.
Identify the limitation
The experience of completing the first questionnaire may influence participants in completing the second questionnaire. It is possible that participants will be more likely to accurately report their physical activity on the second questionnaire due to an increased knowledge and understanding of the questions gained from completing the first questionnaire. In addition, the questions asked on the first questionnaire may lead participants to be more aware of their physical activity over the intervening time period.
Describe the impact on your findings
This would result in lower agreement between the first and the second questionnaires and produce an underestimation of the intraclass correlation coefficient.
Describe the methods to minimize the limitation
Therefore, in interpreting our findings, we will consider the observed reproducibility as a lower bound of the questionnaire's true reproducibility.

10.9.2 Threats to Observed Validity Scores

A common threat to observed validity scores is correlated error between the measurement tool and the comparison measure.

   1. *Correlated error*

Observations of high validity between your measurement tool and comparison measure may reflect correlated error. For example, if both your measurement tool and the comparison measure omit an item, they will be highly correlated, but they will both be similarly incorrect (invalid). Similarly, if both your measurement tool and the comparison measure include questions that are misinterpreted, they will also be likely highly correlated but again less than valid. Third, if both your measurement tool and the gold standard rely upon self-report, then both will be similarly influenced by limitations of memory and social desirability bias (e.g., the tendency of respondents to report what they think they should be doing or what they feel would be the correct behavior but not what they are truly doing).

   In other words, high validity scores may simply indicate that error in the questionnaire and the comparison measures are correlated. As noted above, given that neither method will be perfect, it is critical that the errors of both methods be as independent (uncorrelated) as possible. To the extent that errors in a comparison measure are uncorrelated with error in the questionnaire, the correlation between the two tends to be underestimated. Alternatively, correlated errors will result in spuriously high estimates of validity.

Example Limitations Section of a Reproducibility/Validity Study
Recall the proposal above to conduct a reproducibility and validity study of a physical activity questionnaire. The questionnaire was administered at the beginning of the year. As a validation tool, four comparison measures (e.g., 7-day activity diaries) were then administered during each season to capture day-to-day and seasonal variation in activity levels. At the end of the year, the questionnaire was administered for a second time.
Identify the limitation
Diaries are not a gold standard because they share several sources of errors with the questionnaires. While diaries, unlike questionnaires, are not subject to errors due to restrictions imposed by a fixed list of activities, memory, and interpretation of questions, both diaries and questionnaires likely elicit socially desirable responses. Also, if the diaries are not filled out properly (e.g., in real time), they may rely upon memory in the same way that questionnaires do.
Describe the methods to minimize the limitation
In spite of these concerns, diaries are judged to be superior to questionnaires and are considered an acceptable method to validate questionnaires.[1] Because errors associated with the questionnaires and diaries will be largely independent, our validity scores will likely be underestimated.

10.9.3 Threats to Generalizability

As with any research study, participants in reproducibility/validity studies tend to be convenience samples, that is, people who are available and volunteer to be in the study as opposed to a random sample of the study population. These volunteers may differ in important ways from those who do not volunteer. In turn, these differences may be responsible for your observed reproducibility and validity scores. For example, volunteers may be healthier or more likely to have higher levels of education than those who do not volunteer. As such, they may be more likely to accurately report their behavior or be more aware of their behaviors than the general population.

However, this *concern is minimized* if the measurement tool is actually intended for use in the same population that healthy volunteers are likely to arise from. In this situation, your findings for reproducibility and validity would be relevant for epidemiologic studies among this population.

In addition, the fact that people who participate in this study may be different from those who could not or would not participate does not necessarily mean that findings cannot be generalized. Generalizing depends on whether you think the *ability to self-report such information would be different* among participants as compared to those who did not participate.

If you have any concerns about generalizing, you can consider repeating your reproducibility/validity study among participants who share the characteristics of the population for whom the measurement tool is intended.

10.10 HOW TO INTERPRET FINDINGS FROM REPRODUCIBILITY/VALIDITY STUDIES

It is important to note that the range of acceptable reproducibility and validity measures for a questionnaire will tend to be lower than the acceptable range for a laboratory measure. For example, measures of agreement ranging from 0.5 to 0.7 are not unusual for behavioral questionnaires. Indeed, dietary and physical activity questionnaires with these ranges of reproducibility and validity have been found to be strong and consistent predictors of disease.

Various recommendations have been published for interpreting measures of reproducibility and validity. These recommendations vary slightly but in general are consistent with the following:

* <0 poor
* 0–0.20 slight
* 0.21–0.40 fair
* 0.41–0.60 moderate
* 0.61–0.80 substantial
* 0.81–1.00 almost perfect

Once you have conducted your reproducibility and validity study, you will need to consider these ranges in deciding whether you want to rely upon these measurement tools in your subsequent proposals.

It is important to note that there are no generally accepted thresholds below which agreement is considered too low. However, if you find that your reproducibility and validity are poor to slight, you may want to consider modifying your assessment tool for future use. In the case of a questionnaire, focus groups on the acceptability and interpretability of the questionnaire could be considered. On the other hand, as described above, there may be other explanations for low reproducibility and validity (e.g., true changes in behavior, error in the reference method). All these factors need to be considered in deciding whether or not to accept your measurement tools. Therefore, interpret your findings with caution!

10.11 ISSUES OF SAMPLE SIZE AND POWER FOR A REPRODUCIBILITY AND VALIDITY STUDY

The number of study participants to be included in a reproducibility and validity study varies and depends upon the following:

- The expected correlation between the measurement tool and the comparison measure
- The degree of desired precision

For example, if the goal is to observe a correlation between a dietary or physical activity questionnaire and a comparison measure of 0.5–0.7, it is generally recommended that the study population include 100–200 study participants. Often, power calculations are not included in proposals for reproducibility and validity studies as the goal of these studies is to generate findings that will be used for power and sample size calculations for future proposals.

However, if conducted, power calculations should not rely entirely upon significance testing, because whether or not a measure of agreement is statistically significant depends largely on the number of participants, typically a small number in such studies. In addition, power calculations for a correlation coefficient only indicate the ability of the correlation coefficient to differ from 0, which is not particularly informative.

Instead, it is possible to present the reviewer with a range of desired measures of agreement and the corresponding CIs that you will be able to detect at 80% power. That is, power the study to achieve a particular range of CIs for a desired measure of agreement.

Example Sample Size and Power for a Reproducibility/Validity Study
The study was powered to achieve 95% CIs of 0.66–0.90 for a sensitivity of 0.80.

10.12 SUMMARY

Evaluating the reproducibility and validity of your proposed measurement tools is critical and often serves as an excellent topic for an early-career grant. A variety of comparison measures are available and the design of a reproducibility and validity study should be tailored to your specific population. Interpretation of results should be informed by a comprehensive understanding of the possible reasons for over- or underestimates of your observed reproducibility and validity scores. Finally, because there is typically no gold standard comparison measure, interpretation of results of validity/reproducibility studies should be informed by an understanding of the sources of error associated with both the measurement tool and the comparison measure.

10.13 EXAMPLE

A PROPOSAL TO EVALUATE THE REPRODUCIBILITY AND VALIDITY OF AN EXERCISE QUESTIONNAIRE FOR USE IN THE ELDERLY

I. *Study design*

Participants will complete the exercise questionnaire and then wear an actigraph as a validation tool for the following seven days. At the end of the seven-day period, the exercise questionnaire will be repeated.

II. *Methods*

The actigraph detects vertical accelerations ranging in magnitude from 0.05 to 2.00 G with frequency response from 0.25 to 2.50 Hz. The above parameters will detect normal human movement while filtering out high-frequency movements such as vibrations. The filtered acceleration signal is digitized, and the magnitude is summed over a user-specified time interval (epoch). At the end of each epoch, the activity count is stored in memory, and the accumulator is reset to zero. A one-min epoch will be used in this study.

The actigraph will be affixed with an adjustable belt on the right hip under clothing during the waking hours of the following seven days. While wearing the actigraph, participants will be given a form on which to note whether they removed the actigraph during the day for longer than one hour to swim, shower, or nap.

Total energy expenditure will be calculated from both the questionnaire and the actigraph. In addition, data from the questionnaire and the actigraph will be classified by intensity: light, moderate, or vigorous.

III. *Statistical analysis*

The reproducibility between the two administrations of the exercise questionnaire will be described by intraclass correlation coefficients. We will calculate reproducibility for total energy expenditure as well as according to activity intensity (i.e., light, moderate, and vigorous).

To evaluate the validity of the exercise questionnaire, we will calculate Spearman correlation coefficients between the exercise questionnaire and the actigraph values for total energy expenditure as well as according to activity intensity (i.e., light, moderate, and vigorous).

IV. *Study limitations*

This study will be subject to several limitations. Wearing an activity monitor during the one-week interval between the administrations of the questionnaires may lead to a heightened awareness of activity among participants. In addition, although less likely, true changes in activity patterns may have occurred during the one-week interval. However, as the exercise questionnaire assesses usual activity, which is less likely to have changed over a one-week time period, we believe that the correlations will largely reflect the reproducibility characteristics of our questionnaire. Given these changes in awareness or true activity over the week, the correlations we observe will provide a lower limit on the questionnaire's actual reproducibility.

As our comparison measure of usual activity, we will utilize estimates of physical activity from an actigraph worn for a one-week period. A number of studies have been conducted to determine how many measurement days are needed to reliably estimate habitual physical activity from the actigraph. In these studies, the number of days has varied between 4 and 12 depending on the precision that is required, the accuracy of the reference method, and the intraindividual variation in activity. In light of these factors, we feel that seven days of actigraph use will be appropriately conservative.

The validity results will be impacted by errors in the actigraph data as well as in the exercise questionnaire measures. For example, when the actigraph is worn on the hip, error results from the inability of the actigraph to accurately measure activities involving upper body movement, pushing or carrying a load, stationary exercise (e.g., cycling), and weight lifting. In contrast, errors in the exercise questionnaire may result from subject inaccuracy in self-reporting physical activity. Given that neither method is perfect, it is critical that the errors inherent in each method be as independent as possible, as correlated errors will result in spuriously high-validity coefficients. Therefore, because errors associated with the actigraph and exercise questionnaire are largely independent, our correlation coefficients will not likely be overstated.

Study Design and Methods

11

The Study Design and Methods section falls within the Approach section of the proposal immediately after the Preliminary Studies (if applicable) and the Significance and Innovation sections. A well-written Significance and Innovation section will "warm the reviewer up" for this section by highlighting the existing research gap, and therefore implicitly justifying the need for the study design and methods you are proposing.

National Institutes of Health (NIH) has called for grant applications to "Enhance Reproducibility through Rigor and Transparency," and the Study Design and Methods section (along with the Data Analysis Plan described in Chapter 11) is where you can show that you are meeting this call. Therefore, this chapter will walk you through addressing rigor and reproducibility in your grant application such that you can address what reviewers will be looking for as they evaluate the application for scientific merit.

11.1 OUTLINE FOR THE STUDY DESIGN AND METHODS SECTION

The following outline displayed in Table 11.1 is particularly well suited to a grant proposal whose overall goal is to conduct an etiological study of an exposure–outcome relationship, as this is most typical of

TABLE 11.1 Outline for the Study Design and Methods

II. Approach
  A. Preliminary Studies (Chapter 9)
  B. Study Design and Methods
    i. Study Design
    ii. Study Population Characteristics
      a. Setting
      b. Eligibility criteria
      c. Recruitment and retention plan
    iii. Exposure Assessment
      a. How exposure data will be collected
      b. Exposure parameterization
      c. Validity of exposure assessment
    iv. Outcome Assessment
      a. How outcome data will be collected
      b. Outcome parameterization
      c. Validity of outcome assessment
    v. Covariate Assessment
      a. How covariate data will be collected
      b. Covariate parameterization
      c. Validity of covariate assessment
    vi. Variable Table

DOI: 10.1201/9781003155140-13

grants in epidemiology and preventive medicine. However, the outline can be modified for other study aims as well.

Below, I provide strategic tips for the Study Design and Methods section.

11.2 OVERALL STRATEGY

In Chapter 6, "Specific Aims," I emphasized that one way of being kind to your reviewer is to insert a brief summary paragraph at the very beginning of this section of the proposal that encapsulates all the key features of the study design. Such a synopsis will serve as "speaker notes" for the reviewer when they are presenting your study to the review panel. By writing this section for your reviewers, you are increasing the probability that they will share what you consider to be the key and novel aspects of your study design and methods with the rest of the panel, and not overlooking anything that you feel is important.

A well-written paragraph on "overall strategy" should ideally state the sample size, study population, study design (e.g., prospective cohort case-control study, cross-sectional study), assessment tools (e.g., self-reported questionnaire, biomarker assays, medical record data), and any other key features.

The following example corresponds to a proposal to evaluate the association between physical activity, psychosocial stress, and risk of gestational diabetes mellitus (GDM). (Underlining is for emphasis here but is not typically included.)

Example Overall Strategy

Using a prospective cohort design, 2300 Latina prenatal care patients will be recruited from Valley Medical Center at their first prenatal care visit. At this time, bilingual interviewers will use the validated Pregnancy Physical Activity Questionnaire to obtain detailed information on physical activity patterns (household/childcare, occupational, and sports/exercise) as well as Cohen's Perceived Stress Scale to obtain information on psychosocial stress. Information on covariates including pregravid body mass index (BMI), medical and obstetric history, acculturation, and sociodemographic factors will also be queried. Two subsequent interviews, conducted in the second and third trimesters of pregnancy, will update information on these variables. Laboratory reports will be abstracted for gestational diabetes. Multivariable logistic regression will be used to assess the relationship between physical activity, psychosocial stress, and gestational diabetes risk while adjusting for important risk factors.

11.2.1 Note for Applications Which Use Substantively Different Methods for Each Specific Aim

Note that if your methodology differs *substantively* for each specific aim (e.g., in terms of the dataset used, sample size, and methodology), then NIH notes that you may "address the Significance, Innovation, and Approach either for each Specific Aim individually or for all of the Specific Aims collectively." Therefore, an alternative approach is to intersperse your methods below each specific aim.

11.3 IDENTIFY BENCHMARKS FOR SUCCESS

An important goal of the Study Design and Methods section is to identify benchmarks for success anticipated to achieve the specific aims. This will help your reviewer to clearly envision the potential products of your grant and its impact on the field.

The following example shows the benchmark for success from a proposal to evaluate the efficacy/impact of a pregnancy physical activity intervention on risk of gestational diabetes. In this example, the benchmark for success is whether the intervention can increase physical activity levels to a sufficient threshold to impact risk of gestational diabetes.

Example Benchmark for Success

Consider a proposal to evaluate the efficacy/impact of a pregnancy physical activity intervention on risk of gestational diabetes.

Based on prior literature[23, 24] and our preliminary studies,[20,21] women participating in 10 MET-hours/week of physical activity experience a clinically significant 30% reduction in risk of gestational diabetes. To achieve a goal of 10 MET-hours/week requires that the intervention leads to an increase in physical activity of 3.8 MET-hours/week over and above their baseline levels. This increase represents 0.19 of a standard deviation or a "small effect" according to Cohen's effect size.[25] In practical terms, this translates to an additional hour per week or 10 min per day of brisk walking. The following sections of the proposal demonstrate that the exercise intervention will be well capable of achieving this increase (Figure 11.1).

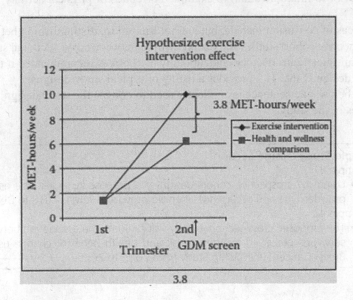

FIGURE 11.1   Benchmarks for success.

11.4 SECTION i: STUDY DESIGN

Before writing this section of the proposal, it is critical to consider what study design you are planning to utilize. This often seems like an easy question, but there are opportunities for confusion.

For example, let's say that you are proposing to use data from an existing study. While this existing study (also known as the *parent study*) may have one study design, this does not necessarily mean that your project shares the same design. For example, the parent study may be a prospective cohort study, but you may be proposing to conduct a nested case-control study, case-cohort, or cross-sectional design within that cohort. One typical study design seen in many early-career proposals is to propose to conduct

TABLE 11.2   Typical Epidemiologic and
Preventive Medicine Study Designs

- Cohort study
  - Prospective
  - Retrospective
- Case-control study
- Cross-sectional study
- Ecologic or correlational study
- Other types
  - Case-cohort
  - Case-crossover

a cross-sectional study using baseline data from a prospective study. For example, within a prospective randomized trial with follow-up over pregnancy and postpartum, an investigator could propose to use their baseline data (prior to randomization) to examine correlates of physical activity at baseline (cross-sectional design)

Other typical areas of confusion include, but are not limited to, distinguishing between case-control studies versus retrospective cohort studies and distinguishing between cross-sectional studies versus case-control studies. Consulting an introductory epidemiology textbook is recommended if there is any confusion with your study design. Table 11.2 provides a listing of typical study designs.

In the examples below, one sentence is efficiently used to convey the study design, the association of interest, and the dates of the study:

Example Study Design Section
Example #1
- Using a retrospective cohort design, we propose to assess the association between provider type and occurrence of episiotomy from July 1, 2018 to December 31, 2019.
Example #2
- The proposed cross-sectional study will evaluate the association between breast cancer survivors' perceived recurrence risk and health behavior change using data from the Breast Cancer Survivorship Study from 2015 to 2020.

11.4.1 Consider a Study Design Figure

As noted in Chapter 1, "Ten Top Tips for Successful Proposal Writing," I have never met a proposal with too many tables and figures. I would strongly suggest including a study design figure to complement the text in this section of the proposal. The old adage that "a picture can tell a thousand words" is particularly relevant here.

Example Study Design Figures Corresponding to Specific Aims
Consider a study whose overall goal is to evaluate the association between physical activity and GDM.
Specific Aims
Specific Aim 1. To determine whether physical activity is prospectively associated with risk of GDM using a prospective cohort study design.
Specific Aim 2. To determine whether psychosocial stress measured via cortisol is prospectively associated with risk of GDM using a nested case-control study design (Figure 11.2).

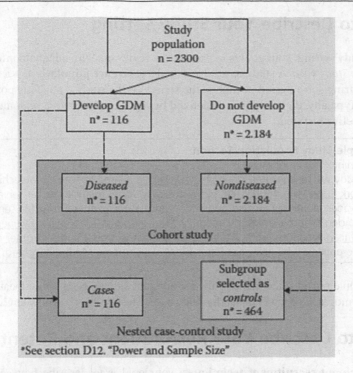

FIGURE 11.2   Study design for Aims #1 and #2.

Figure 11.3 encircles the baseline data that will be evaluated in a proposed study to evaluate the correlates of physical activity at baseline using data from a prospective randomized trial with follow-up over pregnancy and postpartum.

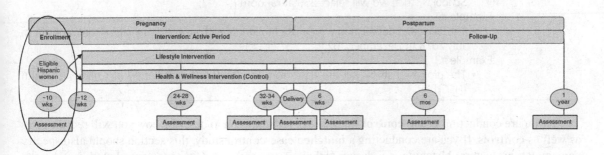

FIGURE 11.3   Study design for a proposal to use baseline data only.

11.5 SECTION ii: STUDY POPULATION CHARACTERISTICS

After describing the study design, the proposal should next describe your study population, specifically: (1) the setting for the proposed study, (2) your recruitment and retention plan (if relevant), and (3) your eligibility criteria.

11.5.1 How to Describe Your Study Setting

In describing the **study setting**, your goal is to provide the reviewers with adequate information such that they can picture your *study base*. A study base, also called a **reference population**, is a defined population whose experience during some period of time is the source of the study data. This population gives rise to study outcomes. Typically, the study base is defined by a geographical area or some other identifiable entity like a health delivery system.

Example Study Population Section
(Underlining for emphasis)
The study will be based at <u>Jones Medical Center</u>, a large tertiary care teaching hospital in <u>New York State</u>, with <u>4500–5000</u> births annually. Jones Medical Center serves an ethnically and socioeconomically diverse population and is the perinatal transfer center for the region. Among the pregnant population, <u>22% are Hispanic (predominantly Puerto Rican), 11% are African American, 65% are non-Hispanic white, and 2% are of other ethnicity</u>. A third of the patients who deliver at Jones Medical Center are <u>Medicaid insured</u>.

The above example provides the name of the recruitment site, its geographic location, a sense of the size, and key sociodemographic factors about the study base. The reviewer can now *envision* the study base.

11.5.2 How to Describe Your Recruitment and Retention Plan

In describing **participant recruitment techniques**, your goal is to describe how you will locate and enroll the participants in your study. For example, will you post fliers or advertise in some other manner? Will you enroll patients in a hospital? Will you be selecting participants from an existing database? Will you use random sampling? Below are several examples:

Example Participant Recruitment Techniques
Example #1
- From the population of all seniors enrolled in high schools in the Los Angeles Unified School District, we will select 250 at random.

Example #2
- The labor and delivery log will be used to identify all patients with vaginal deliveries from July 2018 to December 2021.

Example #3
- The proposed study will use data from the 2020 National Survey of Children's Health (NSCH).

If you are conducting a **case-control** study, it will be important to describe how you will recruit cases as well as **controls**. If you are conducting a **matched** case-control study, this section should also specify your matching factors. Matching is a design technique typically used in case-control studies, whereby cases are matched to controls on several key confounding factors (e.g., age, sex/gender, study site). In this way, the cases and controls will not differ on these factors, and in turn these factors cannot be responsible for the observed association between exposure and disease (see Chapter 12, "Data Analysis Plan," for more details on the use of matching).

Example Participant Recruitment Technique for a Case-Control Study
The cancer registry will be used to identify all bladder cancer *cases* from 2010 to 2020. *Control group participants* will be identified from lists of licensed drivers in the state during the same time period and matched to cases on age, race, and family history of breast cancer.

11.5.3 How to Describe Eligibility Criteria

In describing **eligibility criteria**, your goal is to describe who will be eligible to participate in your study. This involves describing both inclusion and exclusion criteria. Typically, inclusion criteria are listed first.
   Examples of inclusion criteria required by NIH include specifying

- Age range
- Sex/gender
- Race/ethnicity
- Dates

Other inclusion criteria may include:

- Geographic area

Examples of exclusion criteria include specifying

- Prevalent disease (for a prospective cohort study)
- Comorbidities

The example below is excerpted from a proposal designed to evaluate the association between provider type (i.e., certified nurse midwife vs. obstetrician) and episiotomy use.

Example Eligibility Criteria Section
(Underlining only for emphasis)
The study population will consist of 1200 <u>women aged 18–40 years</u> having spontaneous vaginal delivery of a living, singleton, vertex-presenting fetus of 35 weeks gestation at the <u>Valley Hospital in Western Massachusetts</u> from <u>July 1, 2018 to December 31, 2020.</u> We will exclude forceps and vacuum extraction deliveries, vaginal breech and multiple gestation deliveries, and preterm fetuses <35 weeks gestation as certified nurse midwives rarely are involved in delivery decisions in these cases, and these delivery situations have historically involved an increased indication for episiotomy.

   A strength of the above example is that the writer provided a brief justification for the exclusion criteria of <35 weeks gestation. This can be helpful for the reviewer, particularly when the reason for the exclusion criteria is not self-evident.
   Also note that, in most proposals, you may not know the exact final sample size of participants who will be eligible after considering all exclusion criteria including those missing data on your key exposure or outcome variables. However, for the purposes of ensuring feasibility, it will be critical to estimate these numbers in the section on power and sample size (see Chapter 13, "Power and Sample Size").

11.6 SECTION iii: EXPOSURE ASSESSMENT

This section focuses on your **exposure of interest** (Table 11.3).

TABLE 11.3   Exposure Assessment Excerpt from Study Design and Methods Outline

iii. Exposure Assessment
a. How exposure data will be collected
b. Exposure parameterization
c. Validity of exposure assessment

11.6.1 How Your Exposure Data Will Be Collected

The first step is to describe how you plan to collect data on your exposure of interest. Remember that "exposure" is broadly defined as the independent variable—the variable whose effect you are interested in. Examples of exposure assessment tools include questionnaires, medical records, biomarkers, or other methods. If you will be using a preexisting dataset, describe how the exposure data were originally collected regardless of the fact that you will not be collecting it yourself.

If your exposure is assessed via questionnaire, describe the following:

- Name of the questionnaire
- Number of questions
- Scale used

In describing the exposure assessment tool, provide some details about the instrument. In other words, if a questionnaire is to be used, it is not sufficient to simply state the name of the questionnaire without giving a sense of the number of questions and the scale used. On the other hand, it is too detailed to restate every single question on the questionnaire. Stating a question verbatim is only warranted if your exposure was assessed via one or two specific questions and these were so complex that it would help the reviewers to see them, in their entirety, in the proposal. According to the most recent NIH guidelines, data collection instruments such as blank surveys and questionnaires may be included in the Appendix of the proposal, so that reviewers can access these if necessary.

Example Exposure Assessment Section for a Questionnaire
(Underlining for emphasis)
Attitude toward school was measured with the <u>Jones Attitude Survey</u> (Appendix A). The survey contains <u>nine questions</u>. The first three questions measure attitudes toward academic subjects; the next three questions measure attitudes toward teachers, counselors, and administrators; the last three questions measure attitudes toward the social environment in the school. Participants will be asked to rate each statement on a <u>five-point scale</u> from one (strongly disagree) to five (strongly agree).

The example above follows the guidelines by providing not only the name of the questionnaire but also a sense of the types of questions and the numerical range of responses.

If your exposure is assessed via **biomarker** (e.g., laboratory tests of blood, urine, and/or tissues), describe the following:

- Collection methods (e.g., phlebotomist)
- Processing methods
- Assay used
- Laboratory name and location

Example Exposure Assessment Section for a Biomarker (Underlining for emphasis)
<u>Fasting blood samples</u> will be collected at home visits by study assessors at six months and one year. Assessors will collect whole blood and centrifuge the samples either immediately (to obtain plasma) or after allowing the blood to clot (to obtain serum). Samples will then be placed on dry ice and brought daily to the <u>Franklin Laboratory in Western Massachusetts</u> and immediately <u>stored at −80°C in a dedicated freezer</u> with a temperature monitor, alarm, and backup power system. Samples will be <u>assayed by Dr. Smith (Department of Laboratory Medicine, Johnson University, Boston, MA)</u> (letter of collaboration attached). Fasting glucose (FG) will be <u>measured enzymatically on the Roche P Modular system</u> using Jones Diagnostics reagents (Boston, MA).[1]

11.6.2 Exposure Parameterization

Next, provide information on how your exposure will be parameterized for analysis.

- *Categorical* = a categorical variable with two or more categories
  - *Dichotomous* = a categorical variable with two categories (e.g., *exposed, unexposed*)
- *Continuous* = a variable that take on any value within a range of plausible values (e.g., total serum cholesterol level, height, weight)

It is also possible to propose that you will use several exposure scales (e.g., both categorical and continuous).

One important factor in deciding how to parameterize your exposure variable is the state of science in the field. For many variables, cut points are already established. For example, the accepted World Health Organization (WHO) cut point for obesity is a BMI ≥ 30 kg/m^2. Look over the prior literature in your proposed area to see how prior studies have parameterized your exposure variable. The advantage of using the same parameterization as prior studies is that it will enable you to directly compare your findings to the prior literature. This does not, however, rule out your option of using additional parameterizations to extend the prior research.

If you are proposing to use an existing dataset, you will likely have little choice in how to parameterize your exposure variable and will be limited to the level of detail that was already used. For example, the existing dataset may use a questionnaire that only asked respondents to check off age categories (e.g., <24, 25 to <35, 35 to <45) instead of asking them to write in their actual age.

In most cases, you will have some flexibility. For example, you could choose to parameterize your exposure variable as **both** a categorial variable **and** a continuous variable. For example, you could categorize BMI (e.g., underweight, normal weight, overweight, obese) **and** also evaluate BMI continuously (kg/m^2). The categorical variable has the advantage of generating findings that are translatable into public health messages (e.g., the impact of being obese on your outcome). The continuous variable, in contrast, allows you to assess if a one-unit increase in BMI has an influence on your outcome in a dose–response manner. However, note that assumptions of linearity should be assessed first (e.g., utilizing a continuous variable assumes a linear dose–response relationship between your exposure and outcome such that each unit change in exposure is associated with the same increment of increased risk; see Chapter 12, "Data Analysis Plan").

Other possibilities, in the absence of established published cut points, are to divide your exposure variable into quartiles, quintiles, or tertiles. Ideally, this division should be based on the exposure distribution among the nondiseased. In other words, exclude cases of your outcome when deriving cut points. This approach has the disadvantage of being data dependent, in that the cut points will be dependent on the distribution of the data in your study population. On the other hand, if you are conducting your study in a new study population, it may actually be preferable to have the cut points be study specific.

Ultimately, the decision for how to parameterize your exposure of interest will depend on your sample size and corresponding power to detect an effect (as described in Chapter 13, "Power and Sample Size"). Each of your parameterization choices will also impact your Data Analysis section later in the proposal (as described in Chapter 12, "Data Analysis Plan").

11.6.3 Validity of Exposure Assessment—Subjective Measures

Your goal in this section is to establish the validity of the technique that you will be using to assess your exposure. This is important whether you are using subjective measures (e.g., questionnaire-based) or objective measures (e.g., blood samples, medical records).

In the case of **subjective measures**, this section should cite prior validation studies of the assessment tool. Ideally, you will want to cite those validation studies conducted in a study population as similar as possible to your own. For example, let's say you are proposing to assess diet in Puerto Rican youth. Ideally, you would want to cite studies showing that the questionnaire was valid among Puerto Rican youth. If these are unavailable, validation studies of this questionnaire among a general population Hispanic youth, or as close a group as possible to your study population, will still serve to reassure the reviewers to some degree.

Questionnaires face the limitation of self-report. Validation studies compare these self-reported findings to those of *gold standards*. When these validation studies are available, provide the reviewer with the specific **magnitude** of findings for validity and reliability as opposed to simply their statistical significance.

Example Section on Validity of a Questionnaire
(Underlining for emphasis)
The Cleveland Sleep Questionnaire also has high validity, with analyses showing a correlation of **r = 0.81** between the Cleveland Sleep Questionnaire and sleep log data and lower correlations with polysomnography data, ranging from **r = −0.32 to r = 0.28**.[20]

This section on validity is relevant even if your exposure assessment is based on what is typically considered a *gold standard*. For example, obtaining exposure information via **medical record abstraction** is often considered a gold standard. However, medical records may be completed by a variety of personnel including residents, attending physicians, and nurse midwives. Any of these personnel can make an error in abstracting key information from the medical record.

Example Section on Validity of Medical Record Abstraction (Underlining for emphasis)
Patients with ICD-9-CM codes for obstetric trauma/laceration, infection, hemorrhage, episiotomy, or obesity discharged between January 2019 and March 2020 were identified in the study hospital's administrative data. One hundred medical records with ICD-9-CM codes of interest were randomly selected for review from each of the five categories. An additional 60 medical records without the ICD-9-CM codes of interest served as controls for each category. Weighted sensitivities ranged from 0.15 [95% CI 0.11, 0.20] for obesity to 1.00 for overall infection while specificities ranged from 0.994 [95% CI 0.987, 0.998] for obesity to 0.999 [95% CI 0.996, 1.000] for episiotomy.[1]

11.6.4 Validity of Exposure Assessment—Objective Measures

In the case of **objective measures** such as biomarker assessments, provide the laboratory coefficient of variation. Additionally specifying how you will assess quality control in the laboratory will also serve to reassure the reviewer of the validity of your biomarker assessment. Example quality control measures involve including blinded quality control samples in assays and blinding the laboratory personnel to participant characteristics (e.g., to case and control status in the context of a case-control study).

Example Section on Validity of a Biomarker
(Underlining for emphasis)
C-reactive protein will be measured using a high-sensitivity assay with latex-enhanced nephelometry on a nephelometer at the University of Washington Medical Center, Seattle, Washington. Day-to-day coefficients of variation range from 4.93 to 7.84. Quality control for specimen handling will be performed monthly by the head lab technician. All lab technicians will be blinded to case/control status.

Even though they are considered objective measures, biomarkers have limitations. First, they may not be truly reflective of your exposure of interest. Second, biomarkers may not reflect the etiologically relevant time period for the impact of your exposure on your outcome of interest. Third, degradation over time in frozen samples could reduce their validity. Fourth, biomarkers may be influenced by other factors. Therefore, the validity section should reassure the reviewer regarding these concerns when relevant, as in the example below.

Example Section on Validity of a Biomarker
(Underlining for emphasis)
Consider a proposal of the impact of dietary vitamin D on a disease outcome:
Plasma vitamin D levels will be determined by laboratory assay of the participants' stored plasma samples for levels of $25\text{-}(OH)D_3$. We chose to analyze $25\text{-}(OH)D_3$ rather than its metabolite, 1,25-dihydroxyvitamin D_3 for several reasons. First, $25\text{-}(OH)D_3$ <u>better reflects combined exposure from sunlight and dietary intake and is more easily influenced by behavioral interventions than its metabolite.</u>[1] Second, $25\text{-}(OH)D_3$ is <u>less closely regulated by other hormones and exists at substantially higher concentrations in the blood than its metabolite.</u>[2] Finally, the $25\text{-}(OH)D_3$ assay requires less plasma than does the assay for its metabolite.[3]

In summary, it is critical to provide as much information to support the validity of your questionnaire-based measure as possible. Later, in Chapter 15, "How to Present Limitations and Alternatives," I provide tips on how to strategically describe the limitations of these measures. In this way, you will indicate to the reviewers that you have carefully weighed both the strengths and limitations of your selected exposure assessment technique.

11.6.5 What to Do if There Are No Prior Validation Studies

There are several strategies for addressing validity in the absence of prior validation studies:

* Conduct your own validation study.
* Search for prior validation studies in similar study populations.
* Search for prior validation studies in any study population.
* Cite prior studies showing significant associations **between** your exposure measured via your proposed assessment tool and your outcome of interest.

If you find that there are no prior validation studies on your measures of interest, you may want to conduct a validation study yourself. Indeed, applying for a seed grant or foundation grant to support validation work is often the topic of the first small grant in an early-career faculty's funding portfolio. Recall in Chapter 10, "Pilot Grants: Reproducibility and Validity Studies," that this type of validity study can provide critical preliminary data toward applying for a larger grant designed to use the proposed tool to evaluate associations with key outcomes of interest.

If time constraints or other limitations prevent you from conducting your own validation study, search the literature for prior published validation studies in a study population as similar as possible to your own. In the absence of such work, try to find prior studies that found significant associations between your exposure, **as measured via your proposed tool**, and your outcome of interest. Such studies can help to reassure reviewers that your tool has sufficient precision to predict disease outcomes. In the example below from a proposal examining the association between food insecurity and risk of diabetes, there were no validation studies of the food security. However, prior studies measuring food insecurity via the same questionnaire found significant associations with diabetes.

Example Section on Validity of a Questionnaire in the Absence of Prior Validity Studies
(Underlining for emphasis)
While there are no published data on the validity of the six-item Smith Food Security Questionnaire, <u>food insecurity measured by this questionnaire was predictive of incident diabetes</u> in previous studies.[3,10]

11.7　SECTION iv: OUTCOME ASSESSMENT

This section focuses on your **outcome of interest**. Note that the structure and content of the Outcome Assessment section mirrors that of the Exposure Assessment section but instead focuses on your outcome of interest. Remember that "outcome" is broadly defined as the dependent variable—the variable that you are proposing may be "dependent" on the independent variable (Table 11.4).

TABLE 11.4　Outcome Assessment Excerpt from Study Design and Methods Outline

iv. Outcome Assessment
    a. How outcome data will be collected
    b. Outcome parameterization
    c. Validity of outcome assessment

First, describe how your outcome data will be collected. Specifically, in this section, describe the tools by which you are assessing your outcome variables and provide relevant citations. Such tools could include medical record abstraction, questionnaires, biomarkers, or other methods.

If you are conducting a **case-control** study, delineate clear diagnostic criteria that you will use to identify disease outcomes (e.g., based on published consensus guidelines). You can strengthen this section by stating that diagnoses will be confirmed by a clinician or medical review panel through the review of medical record and/or pathology reports. Clarify how the controls will be defined as well.

The decision for how to parameterize your outcome variable will affect your choice of regression model (see Chapter 12, "Data Analysis Plan"). For a case-control study, your outcome variable will be dichotomous (case vs. control), while for other study designs, there may be several options for how to parameterize your outcome variable (e.g., continuous). Regardless, the outcome parameterization should be specified in this section of the proposal.

Finally, the **validity** of the Outcome Assessment section should cite relevant studies and their findings as to the validity of the tool used to assess your proposed outcome. The same cautions with both subjective and objective measures apply as described in the Exposure Assessment section.

Example Section on Validity of Case/Control Status
(Underlining for emphasis)
    Breast cancer <u>cases will be confirmed through medical record review</u> by a study physician; invasive versus *in situ* and hormone receptor status will be abstracted from the medical record. Controls will be those with no personal history of breast cancer.

11.8　SECTION v: COVARIATE ASSESSMENT

The Covariate Assessment section mirrors the section on exposure and outcome assessment but is typically briefer (Table 11.5).

TABLE 11.5　Covariate Assessment Excerpt from Study Design and Methods Outline

v. Covariate Assessment
    a. How covariate data will be collected
    b. Covariate parameterization
    c. Validity of covariate assessment

In the Covariate Assessment section, state which variables you will consider as possible confounders of your exposure–outcome relationship, how you will collect information on each of these covariates, how you will parameterize them, and provide information regarding their validity.

Chapter 14, "Study Limitations to Consider," provides a detailed overview of confounding and Chapter 12, "Data Analysis Plan," will assist you in determining which possible confounding factors to consider.

Briefly, a typical first step is to consider **prior established risk factors** for your outcome of interest as potential confounding factors. Provide a citation supporting that these variables are indeed established risk factors for your outcome—a review article can be a useful reference.

Secondly, look back at your **summary table** of the literature which you created as part of Chapter 3, "Identifying a Topic and Conducting the Literature Search," and consider covariates that were included in these prior studies. This will improve your ability to compare your findings to those of the prior studies.

Further techniques for covariate selection, such as creating directed acyclic graphs are described in Chapter 12, "Data Analysis Plan." These diagrams are a quick, visual way to assess confounding that can aid in covariate selection

Example Section on Covariate Assessment
Consider a proposal designed to evaluate the association between provider type (certified nurse midwife vs. obstetrician) and episiotomy use:
Data for covariates will be collected via self-report as well as through postdelivery medical record abstraction (Variable Table 1). Specifically, education, income, smoking and drug use, and acculturation will all be obtained via interview. Physical activity data were assessed via the Frances Physical Activity Survey.[8] Acculturation was measured both via language preference (English or Spanish) and through birthplace (United States or elsewhere). Data on physical characteristics, such as prepregnancy weight and height, and obstetric and medical history, such as parity, will be abstracted from the medical record.

If you plan to consider any of your covariates as possible effect modifiers of the relationship between your exposure and disease, specify those variables in this section, as well as how they will be parameterized.

Example Section on Effect Modifier Assessment
We will investigate established risk factors for type 2 diabetes as potential effect modifiers.[1] These include study site, BMI (i.e., normal weight vs. overweight/obese), and age (i.e., <40, ≥40 years of age).

11.9 SECTION vi: VARIABLE TABLE

As mentioned in Chapter 1, "Ten Top Tips for Successful Proposal Writing," I've never met a grant with too many tables and figures. One of the most important tables is a variable table. This table lists the key study variables (exposure, outcome, and covariates) corresponding to each specific aim. The table can also include additional details as relevant (e.g., assessment tool, timing of variable collection). Including such a table in a grant proposal is an example of being kind to your reviewer. It demonstrates to the reviewer that you have *a priori* thought through your variables of interest and have an organized plan. It removes

TABLE 11.6   Variable Table for a Proposal to Evaluate the Association between Mental Health in Pregnancy and Risk of Adverse Birth Outcome Complications (Specific Aim #1) and Postpartum Sleep (Specific Aim #2)

VARIABLE NAMES	PREGNANCY			DELIVERY	POSTPARTUM
	EARLY	MID	LATE		
Key Variables					
Exposures: Mental Health					
Chronic physiologic stress (hair cortisol concentrations)				×	
Depression	×	×	×		
Psychosocial stress	×	×	×		
Anxiety	×	×	×		
Outcomes (Specific Aim #1: Pregnancy Complications)					
Preeclampsia				×	
Small for gestational age				×	
Preterm birth				×	
Outcomes (Specific Aim #2: Sleep)					
Sleep	×	×	×		×
Physical activity	×	×	×		×
Potential covariates, effect modifiers					
Sociodemographic status	×				
Medical and obstetrical history	×				
Gestational weight gain	×	×	×		
Cigarette smoking, alcohol consumption, and substance use	×	×	×		

any concerns that you will be conducting a *fishing expedition*. After the proposal is approved, the variable table continues to be useful by serving as a *cookbook* for your data analysis.

Regardless whether you include such a table in your proposal, you will find that the act of creating such a table helps avoid certain pitfalls. First, it ensures that you don't include extraneous variables that are not directly relevant to your analysis and, vice versa, that your proposal does not omit any variables integral to your analysis. In the same spirit, be sure to cross-check that your text description of your methods does not contradict the information included in your variable table. For example, I have seen proposals that list key variables in tables that are not mentioned in the text or, vice versa, that mention key variables in the text that cannot be found in the tables.

Table 11.6 is an example variable table for a proposal designed to evaluate the association between mental health in pregnancy and risk of (1) adverse birth outcomes (Specific Aim #1) and (2) postpartum sleep (Specific Aim #2). Note that the variable names are listed underneath the corresponding specific aims according to assessment time period.

11.10 NIH GUIDANCE ON RIGOR AND REPRODUCIBILITY

NIH has called for grant applications to "Enhance Reproducibility through Rigor and Transparency," https://grants.nih.gov/grants/Rigor-and-Reproducibility-Chart-508.pdf. Throughout the Study Design and Methods section, be mindful of the following NIH guidelines:

1. **Rigor of the Prior Research**: Describe plans to address weaknesses in the rigor of the prior research that serves as the key support for the proposed project.

   In other words, articulate through your study design, how you are filling the research gap that you identified in your section on Significance and Innovation (Chapter 8).

2. **Scientific Rigor (Design)**: Emphasize how the experimental design and methods proposed will achieve robust and unbiased results.

   Note that resources and tools for rigorous experimental design can be found at the Enhancing Reproducibility through Rigor and Transparency website: https://grants.nih.gov/policy/reproducibility/guidance.htm.

3. **Biological Variables**: Explain how relevant biological variables, such as sex, age, weight, and underlying health conditions, are factored into research designs, analyses, and reporting. Strong justification from the scientific literature, preliminary data, or other relevant considerations must be provided for applications proposing to study only one sex.

   Refer to the NIH Guide Notice on Sex as a Biological Variable in NIH-funded Research for additional information: https://orwh.od.nih.gov/sex-gender/nih-policy-sex-biological-variable.

11.11 PITFALL TO AVOID

As mentioned in Chapter 1, "Ten Top Tips for Successful Proposal Writing," one of the classic pitfalls to avoid is to be overly ambitious in study aims. This leads to a proposal with a large number of exposure and outcome variables and covariates. As this chapter demonstrates, the level of detail required for the Study Design and Methods section (e.g., assessment tool, parameterization, validation) underscores the importance of being focused in your specific aims.

11.12 EXAMPLE STUDY DESIGN AND METHODS SECTIONS

11.12.1 Example #1

A PROPOSAL TO PROSPECTIVELY EXAMINE THE ASSOCIATION BETWEEN PSYCHOSOCIAL STRESS AND HYPERTENSIVE DISORDERS OF PREGNANCY: STUDY DESIGN AND METHODSOVERALL STRATEGY

Using a *prospective cohort design*, 2300 Latina prenatal care patients will be recruited from Valley Medical Center at their first prenatal care visit. At this time, bilingual interviewers will use the validated *Pregnancy Physical Activity Questionnaire* to obtain detailed information on physical activity patterns (household/childcare, occupational, and sports/exercise) as well as *Cohen's Perceived Stress Scale* to obtain information on psychosocial stress. Information on *covariates* including pregravid BMI, medical and obstetric history, acculturation, and sociodemographic factors will also be queried. Two subsequent interviews, conducted in the second and third trimesters of pregnancy, will update information on these variables. *Laboratory reports* will be abstracted for hypertensive disorders of pregnancy. *Multivariable logistic regression* will be used to assess the relationship between physical activity, psychosocial stress, and hypertensive disorders of pregnancy while adjusting for important risk factors.

Study Population

Women who self-identify as Latina and are less than 24 weeks gestation will be recruited by trained, bilingual (English/Spanish) interviewers from the prenatal health clinic at Valley Medical Center from January to December 2020. Study exclusions will include: age<16 or >42, multiple gestation, chronic hypertension, preexisting diabetes, heart disease, and chronic renal disease.

Exposure Assessment

Psychosocial stress will be measured using the 14-item Perceived Stress Scale, a validated and widely used measure of perceived stress (Variable Table 1).[1] The scale includes questions such as the following: "How often have you felt you were unable to control the important things in your life?" and "How often have you felt difficulties were piling up so high that you could not overcome them?" The scale was interviewer-administered so literacy and/or language barriers were minimized. This measure will be dichotomized at the median for this analysis, as has been done by others (Variable Table 1).[2] Perceived stress scores will also be analyzed continuously to evaluate a potential dose–response effect.

Validity of Exposure Assessment

The Perceived Stress Scale has been shown to have adequate reliability (r=0.78) and to be correlated with physical symptoms (r=0.52–0.70) and depressive symptoms (r=0.65–0.76).[3] Additionally, in a random sample of adults residing in the United States, there was little variance between responses when questions were analyzed by sex/gender, race, and/or education suggesting that the test provides a meaningful measure regardless of these factors.[4] The Spanish version of the Perceived Stress Scale (10-item version of the questionnaire) has been shown to have adequate reliability (a=0.82, test–retest, r=0.77, $p < 0.001$) and validity (r=0.71 for distress score and r=0.66 for anxiety score).[5]

Outcome Assessment

Hypertensive disorders of pregnancy will be diagnosed using American College of Obstetricians and Gynecologists (ACOG) criteria (Variable Table 1).[6] Cases will be identified through postdelivery review of medical records, as well as through International Classification of Disease (ICD) codes. Further, all cases identified through these mechanisms will then be confirmed and classified into a subgroup (gestational hypertension or preeclampsia) by the study obstetrician.

Gestational hypertension is defined as two blood pressure measurements greater than 140/90 after 20 weeks gestation in previously normotensive women, with no lab evidence or symptoms of preeclampsia. Preeclampsia is defined as blood pressure greater than 140/90 on two occasions, with proteinuria, also after 20 weeks gestation and in women who were previously normotensive.[7]

Validity of Outcome Assessment

A trained medical record abstractor will abstract diagnoses of hypertensive disorders from medical records which will then be confirmed by the study obstetrician. A reliability study of medical record abstractors at Valley Medical Center conducted in 2017 using a random sample of 100 medical records found coefficients of 0.77 across abstractors for hypertensive disorders of pregnancy.

Covariate Assessment

Data for covariates will be collected via self-report as well as through postdelivery medical record abstraction (Variable Table 1). Specifically, education, income, smoking and drug use, and acculturation will all be obtained via interview. Physical activity data will be assessed via the Frances Physical Activity Survey.[8] Acculturation was measured both via language preference (English or

Spanish) and through birthplace (United States or elsewhere). Data on physical characteristics, such as prepregnancy weight and height, and obstetric and medical history, such as parity, will be abstracted from the medical record.

11.12.2 Example #2

A PROPOSAL TO EXAMINE THE ASSOCIATION BETWEEN COFFEE CONSUMPTION AND RISK OF CUTANEOUS MELANOMA *USING AN EXISTING DATASET*: STUDY DESIGN AND METHODS

STUDY DESIGN AND METHODS

Study Design and Population

To examine the association between coffee intake and risk of cutaneous melanoma, we propose to use data from the Mediterranean Observational Study (MOS). MOS recruited women at five centers in the Mediterranean between 2015 and 2016.[1] Postmenopausal women aged 50–79 who had expected survival time greater than three years were eligible to participate in MOS.

A total of 1425 participants were enrolled in the study. Participants were screened at baseline for physical measurements (height, weight, blood pressure, heart rate, waist and hip circumferences), collection of blood specimens, and medication/supplement inventory and completed a questionnaire detailing medical history, lifestyle/behavioral factors, and quality of life. In addition, participants completed a questionnaire regarding other exposures such as residency, smoking status, early life exposures, physical activity, weight, and occupational history. Food frequency questionnaires (FFQs) were administered at baseline screening. All questionnaires were mailed annually to update selected exposures and ascertain medical outcomes. Participants were followed for an average of four years until 2020. For the purposes of our proposed study, women will be excluded if they had history of prior cancers, including nonmelanoma skin cancer, or if they had dropped out prior to first follow-up. Follow-up time was accrued from enrollment to date of diagnosis, death, or date of last follow-up.

Exposure Assessment

Data on coffee consumption were collected at baseline and updated annually on the FFQs. Participants were asked "Do you usually drink coffee each day?" Those who answered "yes" further indicated separately the number of cups of coffee per day. We will create a categorical coffee consumption variable: none, 1 cup/day, 2 cups/day, 3 cups/day, or 4+ cups/day (Variable Table 1).

Validation of Exposure Assessment

Smith et al. assessed the validity of the FFQ used to collect coffee and tea intake using four 24-h diet recalls and one four-day food record.[2] The authors compared 30 nutrients estimated from the FFQ with means from 24-h recalls and the four-day food records. The authors found that most nutrients estimated by the FFQ were within 10% of the records or recalls. The precision of FFQ used for MOS was similar to that of other FFQs.[3]

No study has assessed the validity of the self-report of coffee intake in the MOS. However, a validation study by Taylor et al. found a high correlation coefficient between self-reported FFQ and two 7-day diet records for coffee in the Women's Health Study, a cohort similar to MOS in terms of dietary consumption (4). Correlation coefficients of 0.78 and 0.93 were reported for coffee and tea, respectively.

Outcome Assessment

Melanoma cases were defined as women who had an adjudicated diagnosis of melanoma (over the duration of follow-up). Potential cases were self-reported on the annual questionnaires on various medical outcomes including melanoma. The outcome will be categorized as melanoma (yes, no) (Variable Table 1).

Validity of Outcome Assessment

All diagnoses were centrally adjudicated at the Clinical Coordinating Center. Specifically, cancer epidemiologists and physicians reviewed hospital records, operative reports, history and physical examination, radiology, and oncology consultation reports. If a case was adjudicated, the physician recorded ICD codes, date of the diagnosis, and tumor behavior (invasive, *in situ*, or borderline).

Covariate Assessment

Physical measurements and medical history data on all participants were collected at baseline. Lifestyle factors were collected at baseline as well as during follow-up. Dietary data were collected by the FFQ at baseline and updated during annual follow-up. We will consider the following categorical variables as potential covariates: age (50–54, 55–59, 60–69, 70–79), alcohol intake (no/yes), smoking status (no/yes), race (white, black, Hispanic, etc.), skin reaction to sun, and past sun exposure (Variable Table 1). Continuous variable covariates include BMI and total minutes of physical activity per week (Variable Table 1).

Data Analysis Plan

12

The goal of this chapter is to provide you with **strategies and tips** for writing the data analysis plan of your proposal. This chapter will outline (1) a **framework** for writing a typical data analysis plan for a grant proposal in the field of epidemiology and preventive medicine, (2) a sense of the **scope and depth** required for such a data analysis plan, and (3) *best practices* that should be addressed in a robust data analysis plan within a grant proposal.

This chapter also includes an **example data analysis plan** accompanied by mock tables (also known as *dummy tables*) for illustrative purposes. However, note that while mock tables are highly recommended for conceptualizing your plan, a grant proposal will rarely have space to include them. These tables have the additional benefit of giving you a head start on presenting your grant findings for future publications.

This chapter is not meant to take the place of a statistics textbook that would provide detailed information on statistical techniques for hypothesis testing. Ultimately, this chapter will position you well to know the right questions to ask when meeting with your collaborating statistician, a statistical consulting center, or data analysis core.

12.1 PART I: FRAMEWORK FOR THE PROPOSED DATA ANALYSIS PLAN

12.1.1 Start the Data Analysis Plan by Repeating Your Specific Aims Verbatim

The overall goal of the data analysis plan in a grant proposal is to demonstrate how you plan to directly answer the research questions (i.e., the hypotheses) that you outlined on your Specific Aims page. By tightly tying your data analysis plan to your specific aims, you can avoid the common pitfalls that often occur in the data analysis plan of a proposal.

With this goal in mind, a well-written data analysis plan starts by repeating the specific aims verbatim from the Specific Aims page. Immediately below each aim, insert the relevant data analysis plan that you will use to meet these aims (see Table 12.1). Repeating the specific aims in the data analysis plan has several advantages. Firstly, it makes the proposal more organized and falls under the rubric of being *kind* to your reviewers by reminding them of your specific aims; at this point in your proposal, their memory of your exact specific aims may have faded. Secondly, and most importantly, it ensures that you do not accidentally omit the data analysis plan for any of your aims. Lastly, it ensures that you do not include extraneous analysis plans that do not address one of your aims.

An editorial note   One important caution is to carefully check that the wording of the specific aims in the data analysis plan exactly matches the wording of the aims on your Specific Aims page. Sometimes, in revising the proposal, you may change the wording or even the scope of your specific aims. Be sure to make those changes in the data analysis plan too! Nothing can be more disconcerting to a reviewer than seeing new aims in this plan or aims that contradict those on the Specific Aims page.

DOI: 10.1201/9781003155140-14

TABLE 12.1 Template for the Data Analysis Plan of a Proposal

DATA ANALYSIS PLAN

- Specific Aim #1
  - Data analysis plan
- Specific Aim #2
  - Data analysis plan
- Specific Aim #3
  - Data analysis plan

12.1.2 What If All Your Aims Require the Identical Data Analysis Plan?

Often, the data analysis plan is similar for each specific aim. Consider a proposal evaluating the independent association between three exposure variables on one common outcome, for example, *to evaluate the association between age, education, and marital status on risk of knee injury.* In this situation, it may be repetitive and therefore not an efficient use of space to repeat the same data analysis plan under each aim. In this case, it is fine to list all your aims together and then insert the relevant data analysis plan as in Table 12.2.

Or, as an alternative, the data analysis plan for Aims #2 and #3 can refer back to the plan for Aim #1 and simply state if there are any modifications or additions (Table 12.3).

In this alternative data analysis plan, specify, when relevant, any minor differences in data analysis techniques that are unique to each aim.

Example Data Analysis Plan with Similar Analyses for Each Aim
For Aim #2, we will use the same data analysis methods described for Aim #1. However, for Aim #2, we will also exclude participants with preexisting disease.

TABLE 12.2 Template for the Data Analysis Plan of a Proposal with Similar Analyses for Each Specific Aim

---

DATA ANALYSIS PLAN

- Specific Aims #1, #2, #3
  - Data analysis plan

TABLE 12.3 Alternative Template for the Data Analysis Plan of a Proposal with Similar Analyses for Each Specific Aim

---

DATA ANALYSIS PLAN

- Specific Aim #1
  - Data analysis plan
- Specific Aim #2
  - Refer to data analysis plan for Aim #1 with any modifications
- Specific Aim #3
  - Refer to data analysis plan for Aim #1 with any modifications

---

12.2 PART II: SCOPE AND DEPTH OF PROPOSED ANALYSES

12.2.1 Step #1: Are Your Specific Aims Descriptive or Analytic?

As described in Chapter 6, "Specific Aims," the majority of grant proposals in epidemiology and preventive medicine aim to identify an association between an exposure of interest and an outcome of interest. Therefore, addressing these aims typically requires the calculation of a measure of association. These types of specific aims are *analytic*.

Example of an Analytic Aim
Specific Aim #1: To evaluate the **association** between age and incidence of Lyme disease.

This analytic aim evaluates the association between age (an exposure) and Lyme disease incidence (an outcome).

However, some of your aims, particularly in pilot studies, will simply be *descriptive*:

- To measure the frequency of an outcome, regardless of its association with an exposure
- To measure the frequency of an exposure, independent of its association with an outcome
- To calculate recruitment and retention rates

Example of a Descriptive Aim
Specific Aim #1: To estimate seasonal **trends** in the prevalence of tick-borne diseases during 2015–2019 in the northeastern United States.

In the example above, the descriptive aim is to simply describe the prevalence of an outcome (i.e., tick-borne diseases) regardless of its association with an exposure (e.g., age).

Your data analysis plan will differ depending on whether your aim(s) is descriptive or analytic. If you have a mixture of both types of aims, the data analysis plan should have subsections corresponding to each type of aim. Therefore, the first step is to be clear on the types of aims you are proposing.

12.2.2 Step #2: How Will You Parameterize Your Variables?

The second step in developing your data analysis plan is to consider how your variables of interest will be parameterized. You have already considered this in Chapter 11, "Study Design and Methods," when you created your Exposure and Outcome Assessment sections and corresponding variable categorization table. In this table, you specified whether your variables will be categorical or continuous. These decisions will impact the type of statistics that you propose to calculate in your data analysis plan.

A potential pitfall to avoid   The importance of referring back to your variable categorization table and corresponding Exposure and Outcome Assessment sections cannot be understated.

A common pitfall is to not be consistent in your parameterization of key variables throughout the proposal. For example, if you describe your key outcome variable as *dichotomous* in your Outcome Assessment section but then in your data analysis plan state that you will use linear regression—which is only appropriate for *continuous* outcome variables—then your proposal will be viewed as internally inconsistent. It is very important that the proposal be internally consistent.

12.3 OUTLINE FOR A BASIC DATA ANALYSIS PLAN

Table 12.4 provides a simple outline for a basic data analysis plan. Typically, descriptive aims will require only univariate analyses. Analytic aims will require univariate, bivariate, **and** multivariable analyses. The data analysis plan to accomplish each of these analyses is described below.

Throughout the remainder of this chapter, we will apply this basic plan to an example proposal titled "Project Health" designed to evaluate the association between **hemorrhage size (the exposure)** and **mortality (the outcome)**. In this study, the exposure is considered as both categorical (i.e., small vs. large hemorrhage size) and continuous (hemorrhage size in millimeters) variable. The outcome is a categorical variable (mortality—yes or no).

Specific Aim #1. To evaluate the association between hemorrhage size and risk of mortality

TABLE 12.4 Template Data Analysis Plan

DATA ANALYSIS PLAN
• Specific Aim #1
• Data analysis plan
• Univariate analysis plan
• Bivariate analysis plan
• Multivariable analysis plan
• Other statistical issues as relevant
• Specific Aim #2
• Same as above
• Specific Aim #3
• Same as above

12.3.1 Univariate Analysis Plan

A univariate analysis plan is relevant for proposals with either descriptive or analytic aims.

The goal of the univariate analysis plan is to describe:

- Your response rates, retention rates, and any other relevant **feasibility** rates
- The distribution (and frequency) of any **exposure** variables of interest (e.g., hemorrhage size)
- The distribution (and frequency) of any **outcome** variables of interest (e.g., mortality)

The statistics you choose for the univariate plan will depend on the parameterization of your exposure and outcome variables:

- For categorical variables
  - Number (N) and percent (%)
- For continuous variables
  - If normally distributed: mean and standard deviation (SD)
  - If not normally distributed: median and 25th and 75th percentile interquartile range (IQR)

Example Univariate Analysis Plan
We will present the number and percent of subjects who *refused* and were *excluded*. We will calculate the *number and percent* of those with large and small hemorrhage size as well as the *mean and SD* of hemorrhage size as well as the *number and percent* of patients with mortality.

12.3.2 Bivariate Analysis Plan

A bivariate analysis plan is typically relevant for proposals with analytic aims. The goal of the bivariate analysis plan is to cross-classify two variables:

- To assess if your exposure is related to your outcome variable **prior** *to* adjusting for any confounding factors (e.g., unadjusted analysis)
- To assess if covariates are related to your exposure and outcome variables (e.g., to assess for the presence of confounding)

The statistics you choose for the bivariate plan will depend on the parameterization of your exposure and outcome variables:

- To cross-classify categorical variables
    - Chi-square test or Fisher's exact test (if small sample size) and corresponding p-values
- To cross-classify continuous variables
    - If normally distributed: e.g., *t*-tests or ANOVA or Pearson correlations and corresponding *p*-values
    - If not normally distributed: e.g., Wilcoxon rank-sum tests or Spearman correlations and corresponding *p*-values

Example Bivariate Analysis Plan
We will evaluate the unadjusted relationship between our exposure (hemorrhage size) and our outcome (mortality) by cross-tabulating these variables. We will then assess covariates as potential confounders by cross-tabulating them with both the exposure (hemorrhage size) and outcome (mortality). Chi-square tests will be used to calculate *p*-values for categorical variables. For tables with small cell frequencies, Fisher's exact tests will be used. For continuous variables, *p*-values will be derived from two sample *t*-tests.

12.3.3 Multivariable Analysis Plan

A multivariable analysis plan is relevant for proposals with analytic aims and is typically the focal point of the analysis plan. A well-written multivariable analysis plan should:

A. Select an appropriate **model**
B. Specify how the model will adjust for **potential confounding factors** (i.e., covariates)
C. Specify how you will evaluate **potential effect modifiers** (i.e., interaction) if *a priori* included as a specific aim

12.3.3.1 Select an Appropriate Model

The type of multivariable analysis that you propose depends on the parameterization of your outcome variable. In addition, each model requires a set of **assumptions** that you will want to discuss with a statistician. Below is a list of some of the most common multivariable models:

- If your outcome variable is dichotomous:
  - Multiple logistic regression and corresponding odds ratio (OR) and 95% confidence interval (CI)
- If your outcome variable is categorical with more than two categories:
  - Multinomial logistic regression and corresponding OR and 95% CI
- If your outcome variable is continuous:
  - Multiple linear regression and corresponding beta coefficient, standard error (SE), and p-value
- If your outcome variable is time to an event:
  - Cox proportional hazards models and corresponding hazards ratio (HR) and 95% CI
- If your outcome variable is count data:
  - Poisson regression and corresponding rate ratio (RR) and 95% CI

In general, **dichotomous outcome variables** tend to be the most common in epidemiology and preventive medicine as we are often evaluating the incidence of diseases (e.g., diabetes diagnosis: yes or no), and therefore many proposals will propose to use multiple logistic regression. The multiple logistic regression model will generate an OR and corresponding 95% CI. The OR can be used as an approximation of the relative risk in certain contexts.

Continuous outcomes are also evaluated in epidemiology and preventive medicine (e.g., weight, blood pressure, cholesterol levels), and therefore it is also common to see multiple linear regression models. Linear regression requires that the outcome variable be normally distributed or be transformed to be normally distributed. The linear regression model will generate a beta coefficient and a corresponding SE and p-value. The beta coefficient can be interpreted as the expected difference in mean levels of the outcome variable given a unit change in your exposure variable; for example, the difference in mean blood pressure (outcome variable) with each year increase in age (exposure variable).

A potential pitfall to avoid   As noted, the parameterization of your *outcome variable* dictates the type of regression model that you will propose to use. It is common to become confused on this point and believe that the parameterization of the *exposure variable* dictates this choice. However, that is not correct. For example, a logistic regression model for a dichotomous outcome, such as diagnosis of diabetes, can include continuous exposure variables (age in years). Similarly, a linear regression model for a continuous outcome (blood pressure) can include dichotomous exposure variables (e.g., age <24 years, age ≥24 years).

12.3.3.2 Specify How the Model Will Adjust for Potential Confounding Factors (i.e., Covariates)

The goal of the multivariable analysis plan is to evaluate the independent impact of your exposure on your outcome while adjusting for **potential confounding factors** (i.e., covariates). There are many techniques for regression model building and your proposal should delineate a thoughtful plan for how potential confounding variables (which you already listed in the Covariate Assessment section) will be considered.

A statistician will be an excellent resource in this area, as is the state of the science in your proposed area of interest. In general, epidemiologists and those in preventive medicine put a greater emphasis on physiological mechanisms as well as **prior established risk factors** for their outcome of interest. Your summary table of the prior epidemiologic literature (created as part of Chapter 3, "Identifying a Topic and Conducting the Literature Search") will come in handy in identifying covariates that prior studies included in their models.

Many investigators propose to include covariates in their models that they find to be statistically significantly **associated with both their exposure and outcome** variables of interest in their bivariate analysis (as described in Section 12.3.2). Remember that to qualify as a confounder, the variable has to be independently associated with the exposure as well as the outcome and not be on the causal pathway between the exposure and outcome.

An approach commonly used in epidemiology and preventive medicine is the **change-in-estimate** method of covariate selection. In this method, a potential confounder is included in the model if it changes the coefficient, or effect estimate, of the primary exposure variable by 10%. This method has been shown to produce more reliable models than variable selection methods based on statistical significance.

Directed acyclic graphs: Directed acyclic graphs (DAGs) are also widely used in medical research to help understand the role of covariates. Briefly, a DAG is a graphical representation characterizing causal and temporal relationships between variables via a set of arrows drawn along a timeline (Figures 12.1 and 12.2). These relationships may include confounding, effect modification, or mediation of the exposure–outcome relationship. These diagrams are a quick, visual way to aid in variable selection and can complement the above more traditional methods of evaluating confounding. *Causal inference* methods can inform these considerations and should be discussed with your statistician.

In general, epidemiologists and researchers in preventive medicine tend to rely less upon *automated* forward- and backward-selection model building approaches. These techniques rely more heavily on p-values for inclusion of particular covariates in the model as opposed to an understanding of the underlying physiology. Recall that p-values are influenced by many factors including the size of the study and the variability of your exposure of interest.

A potential pitfall to avoid One important point to keep in mind is that the ability to control for covariates will be limited in part by your proposed sample size. A multivariable regression model adjusting for many covariates may not run successfully in the scenario of a small sample size. Therefore, it will be important that your proposal recognize this limitation and outline a clear plan for thoughtful inclusion of covariates. In addition, adjusting for many covariates can reduce your statistical power to detect an association even if it truly exists. Therefore, depending on your calculated statistical power, you may consider only including those covariates that are established risk factors for your outcome according to the prior literature.

Example Directed Acyclic Graph (DAG)
Consider a proposal of the association between exercise and sleep. The investigators began by drawing the following basic DAG. E = Exercise; An = Anxiety; S = Sleep; G = Gender; Ag = Age.

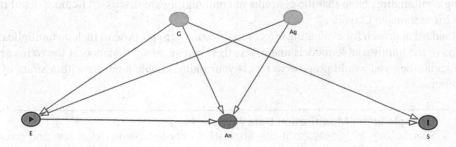

FIGURE 12.1 Example directed acyclic graph (DAG) exploring the relationship between exercise (exposure of interest) and sleep (outcome of interest).

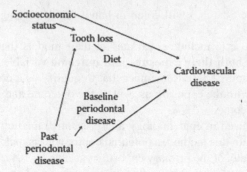

FIGURE 12.2   Example directed acyclic graph (DAG) of the association between periodontal disease (exposure of interest) and cardiovascular disease (outcome of interest).

Example Multivariable Analysis Plan

Multiple logistic regression will be used to model the relation between hemorrhage size and mortality. Those covariates that cause a 10% change in the coefficient for hemorrhage size will be considered confounding factors and included in the model. In addition, because prior studies have shown location of hemorrhage to be strongly associated with mortality, we will also include hemorrhage location in the model. We will calculate unadjusted and multivariable RRs and 95% CIs.

12.3.3.3 Specify How You Will Evaluate Potential Effect Modifiers

If one of your specific aims is designed to determine whether the relationship between your exposure and your outcome differs among different subgroups within your study population—then you are proposing to evaluate effect modification or interaction. Be sure that this corresponds to one of your specific aims (see Chapter 6, "Specific Aims," for best practices for writing effect modification specific aims). This will help to assure your reviewers that you will not be *data dredging* for statistically significant findings if you fail to observe an overall association between your exposure and outcome of interest in your overall analysis.

Often, there is confusion between confounding and effect modification. Confounding variables are considered *nuisance factors* that can be reduced via study design techniques and with careful multivariable modeling. In contrast, **effect modifiers** should be highlighted as they represent groups within which there is a different mechanistic (e.g., physiologic or behavioral) association between your exposure and outcome variables.

Therefore, the data analysis plan to evaluate effect modification differs from data analysis techniques for reducing confounding. Note that the concepts of confounding are discussed in more detail in Chapter 14, "Study Limitations to Consider."

One standard approach for evaluating effect modification is to propose to include multiplicative interaction terms in the multivariable models and assess their statistical significance. If the terms are statistically significant, then you would propose to repeat your multivariable analysis within strata of potential effect modifiers.

Example Effect Modification Data Analysis Plan

Specific Aim #2. To assess if the association between hemorrhage size and three-month mortality differs according to sex.

Multivariable Analysis—Continued

To assess whether sex modifies the relationship between hemorrhage size and three-month mortality, we will include an interaction term (sex X hemorrhage size) in a multivariable logistic model. If this term is statistically significant at $p < 0.05$, we will present results (RR and 95% CIs) for men and women separately (Table 12.5).

TABLE 12.5 Multivariable RR and 95% CI of Three-Month Mortality by Hemorrhage Size According to Sex; Project Health, 2018–2019

	CASES		UNADJUSTED		MULTIVARIABLE[A]	
SEX	N	%	RR	95% CI	RR	95% CI
Females (n=x)						
Small hemorrhage size	N	%	1.0	Referent	1.0	Referent
Large hemorrhage size	N	%	RR	95% CI	RR	95% CI
Males (n=x)						
Small hemorrhage size	N	%	1.0	Referent	1.0	Referent
Large hemorrhage size	N	%	RR	95% CI	RR	95% CI

[a] Multivariable model includes age, ancestry, and location of hemorrhage.

12.3.4 Exploratory Data Analyses

The decision to include exploratory data analyses depends on whether you have decided to include exploratory aims in your Specific Aims. In other words, all exploratory analyses should be *tied to* exploratory aims or hypotheses. As noted in Chapter 6, "Specific Aims," exploratory aims should be limited in number, and while they may require a data analysis plan, they do not typically require power calculations. However, caution should be taken with this approach. Reviewers will carefully examine your application to detect if you are labeling a key aim as *exploratory* as a way to hide poor power.

12.4 PART III: BEST PRACTICES

Throughout the data analysis plan, reviewers will be looking for evidence of *best practices*. Most typically, these include plans to address the following:

1. Model assumptions
2. Model diagnostics
3. Missing data
4. Multiple comparisons
5. Sensitivity analyses to address potential biases

Model Assumptions
All regression models have underlying assumptions. Therefore, your data analysis plan should state: (1) how you will evaluate if these assumptions are met and (2) alternative approaches if any assumptions are not met. For example, linear regression models for the purposes of prediction assume that the relationship between your exposure and your outcome is linear. If model assumptions are violated, then the findings generated by the model may be biased or misleading.

Model Diagnostics
The data analysis plan should also describe how you will assess how well the model fits the data. Techniques to assess model-fit vary according to the type of regression model selected (e.g., linear regression, logistic

regression) and include such techniques as Hosmer–Lemeshow goodness-of-fit tests, R-squared (R^2) statistics, likelihood ratio test statistics, and ROC curves.

Missing Data

Missing data are issues faced by nearly all studies in epidemiology and preventive medicine. Therefore, it is important that your proposal address, even briefly, how you plan to address missing data. Simply stating that you will exclude those with missing data may raise reviewer concerns about biased estimates or reduced power to detect your association of interest. A variety of imputation approaches are available to "fill in" missing data and therefore retain your full sample size. This can be advantageous in terms of reducing potential bias due to loss to follow-up and increased precision. On the other hand, imputation techniques can result in other kinds of bias themselves and also rely upon assumptions including whether you anticipate that data will be missing at random. Alternatively, you may propose to conduct sensitivity analyses which will use weighting to adjust for differences between participants with measured outcomes as compared to those with missing outcomes. In general, stating that you are aware of the limitations of any technique selected is critical in the data analysis plan.

Example Data Analysis Plan for Missing Data

Although every effort will be made to avoid missing data, participants with missing data will be compared to participants with complete data to describe potential bias due to differential loss of data. We will also explore methods for imputing missing data, using propensity score multiple imputation techniques,[1] and apply these in the presence of incomplete and missing data.

Multiple Comparisons

Multiple comparisons arise when a statistical analysis encompasses a large number of formal comparisons, with the presumption that attention will focus on only the strongest differences among all comparisons that are made. For example, if your proposal includes a large number of exposure and outcome variables, you run the risk of raising reviewer concern that some of your findings will be statistically significant due to chance alone. Techniques have been developed to control for the *false positive error rate* associated with multiple statistical tests and should be addressed in a proposal if multiple comparisons are proposed. An alternative technique to minimize this concern is to propose careful consideration of the biologic plausibility of observed findings.

Example Data Analysis Plan for Multiple Comparisons

It is also important to note that we will not be able to rule out chance as an explanation for any observed positive findings given the multiple comparisons we are proposing. However, we will address this issue by carefully considering the biologic rationale of any observed associations.

Sensitivity Analyses to Address Potential Biases

Outlining sensitivity analyses, along with their rationale, in the data analysis plan will help assure the reviewers that you have a plan to address potential biases in your proposal. See Chapter 14, "Study Limitations to Consider," for sources of potential bias.

Examples of sensitivity analyses to address potential bias include:

- Comparing characteristics of participants lost to follow-up to those not lost to follow-up
- Comparing characteristics of cases to controls
- Comparing baseline characteristics of each arm in a randomized trial
- Limiting analyses in a randomized trial to those adherent with the intervention

Comparing the baseline characteristics of those **lost to follow-up versus those not lost to follow-up**, in the context of a cohort study, would help to address the presence and potential magnitude of selection bias (also termed differential loss to follow-up and described in detail in Chapter 14, "Study Limitations to Consider").

Comparing the characteristic of **cases versus controls**, in the context of a case-control study, can help to assess whether the control population adequately represents the source population that led to the cases. Remember not to include your exposure of interest in this table, as you would not want or expect it to be similar between the two groups. Instead, evaluating whether the exposure odds differ between the cases and controls will address the primary specific aim of a case-control study.

Comparing the baseline characteristics of **each study arm** in a randomized trial will help to assess whether the randomization was successful.

Limiting the analysis in a randomized trial to participants who were **adherent** with the intervention defined via their attendance at intervention sessions and/or by other behaviors is another potential sensitivity analyses.

Example Sensitivity Analyses
We will present the characteristics of participants lost to follow-up as compared to those not lost to follow-up according to sociodemographic characteristics to address the possibility of differential loss to follow-up.

12.5 EXAMPLE DATA ANALYSIS PLAN

A Proposal to Examine the Association between Psychosocial Stress and Hypertensive Disorders of Pregnancy: Data Analysis Plan
Data Analysis Plan
Specific Aim #1: We propose to evaluate the association between early pregnancy stress levels and risk of hypertensive disorders of pregnancy in a population of African American women.
Univariate Analysis
The number and percent of subjects excluded according to each exclusion criteria will be calculated. We will calculate the percent distribution of early pregnancy stress and the percent distribution of hypertensive disorders of pregnancy.
Bivariate Analysis
Covariates will be cross-tabulated with hypertensive disorders and early pregnancy stress levels using chi-square tests and corresponding *p*-values to determine whether the observed distribution fits the expected distribution when the cell size is sufficient. When the cell size is not sufficient, Fisher's exact tests will be used. We will create a directed acyclic graph (DAG) to examine the relationships between the covariates and the exposure and outcome variables.
Multivariable Analysis
We will model the relationship between early pregnancy stress and hypertensive disorders of pregnancy using multivariable logistic regression to calculate ORs and 95% CIs.
Potential confounders will be evaluated by running all models with and without each covariate. Any covariate that changes the estimate for early pregnancy stress by 10% or greater will be retained in the model as a confounder.
Sensitivity Analysis to Address Potential Bias
We will compare characteristics of women missing delivery information to those with complete delivery information to determine whether there are any significant differences between those lost to follow-up versus those remaining for analysis.

Power and Sample Size

13

Power is a critical component of any grant proposal. In fact, failing to include power calculations for all or even some of your specific aims is often considered a **fatal flaw** by a grant review panel and is one of the most common reasons for reviewers to streamline (e.g., triage) a proposal (see Chapter 20, "Review Process").

This chapter is designed to give you an applied view of power for the most common study designs in epidemiology and preventive medicine: cohort studies, cross-sectional studies, and case-control studies. The chapter discusses the factors that influence power, the study design strategies that you can use to maximize your power, user-friendly approaches to calculating power, and how to best display your power calculations in a proposal. Throughout the chapter, I include annotated examples with strategies and tips.

Note that this chapter is not designed to take the place of a power and sample size chapter in a statistics textbook. In writing a grant proposal in epidemiology and preventive medicine, it is always best to consult with your collaborating statistician, a statistical consulting center, or data analysis core for your sections on power and sample size. This chapter will make you an informed participant in that conversation.

13.1 TIMELINE

As noted in Chapter 1, "Ten Top Tips for Successful Proposal Writing," after drafting your aims, the very next step in the proposal writing process is to calculate your statistical power to achieve these aims. This will help you to answer the question, "Will your sample size provide you with sufficient power to detect a difference between groups, if there is truly a difference?"

13.2 WHAT IS POWER?

Power is the probability of statistically detecting a difference between groups when a difference indeed exists. For the purposes of proposals in epidemiology and preventive medicine, power is typically the likelihood of observing a statistically significant difference in the occurrence of an **outcome** between **exposed** and **unexposed** groups, when there is indeed a difference. So, even the most beautifully designed proposal will be irrelevant if it can't detect what it is designed to detect.

In Figure 13.1, *reality* reflects what truly exists while *investigator's decision* reflects the decision that you as an investigator will make based on your observed findings.

The last column of Figure 13.1 demonstrates what happens when the groups are, in reality, truly different. We might conclude, in error, that the groups do not differ (*type II error*). Or we might conclude, correctly, that the groups differ (*power*). This probability, 1-beta, is the power of our study. In epidemiology and preventive medicine, power of 80% is generally considered acceptable. In other words, your

DOI: 10.1201/9781003155140-15

	Reality	
Investigator's decision	Groups are not different	Groups are different
Conclude that groups are not different	Correct decision	Type II error probability = beta
Conclude that groups are different	Type I error probability = alpha	Correct decision probability = 1– beta (power)

FIGURE 13.1 Possible study outcomes.

proposal should have **at least 80% power** to detect a difference between exposed and unexposed groups if a difference truly exists.

13.3 KEY CHARACTERISTICS OF POWER

There are several key principles to be cognizant of when calculating power.

- Key characteristic #1: The larger the sample size, the larger your power. In other words, simply due to the fact that you have more people in your study, and therefore greater precision to estimate an effect, you will be more likely to detect a difference between groups in a larger study when there is truly a difference. This does not mean, however, that the effect that you detect will be **clinically significant** but simply that, in a large study, you will be able to detect even small differences between groups.
- Key characteristic #2: The larger the true difference between groups, the easier it will be to have power to detect it. It is always easier to detect large differences between groups than small differences. Therefore, power increases as the expected true differences between groups get larger. In contrast, power decreases as the differences between groups get smaller. In other words, it is harder to find a needle in a haystack than to see an elephant in the room.

13.4 WHEN IS IT OK NOT TO INCLUDE A POWER OR SAMPLE SIZE CALCULATION?

The typical purpose of a feasibility study, or pilot study, is to generate rates on which you will base subsequent power calculations for the purposes of a larger proposal. For example, feasibility studies are critical in generating anticipated recruitment rates, eligibility rates, and retention rates—all necessary for subsequent power calculations. Therefore, including a statement in your proposal reminding the reviewers that you have not included power calculations because this is a pilot/feasibility study is usually sufficient.

A Feasibility Study for a Behavioral Intervention
Specific Aim #1: To assess process measures related to the administration of the intervention. These include the rates of recruitment and rates of follow-up.
Corresponding section on power: Findings from this pilot study will serve as the basis for power calculations to support a larger prospective cohort study designed to investigate the effects of iron levels on diabetes risk in older African Americans.

13.5 DO I NEED TO INCLUDE A POWER OR SAMPLE SIZE CALCULATION WHEN I AM PROPOSING A SECONDARY ANALYSIS OF AN EXISTING DATASET?

As an early-career investigator, your first grants may involve conducting a secondary data analysis of an **existing dataset** (e.g., the National Health and Nutrition Examination Survey [NHANES], the Behavioral Risk Factor Surveillance System [BRFSS]) as you may not have had the opportunity and funding to collect your own data. In these situations, it is still critical to include a Power and Sample Size section. This section will tell the reviewers, for the purposes of your analysis, whether you will be making additional exclusions to the dataset and how many participants will have complete data on your key variables of interest. Even more importantly, if recruitment in these preexisting studies is **ongoing**, your sample size will depend on the success of projected recruitment and retention rates. Therefore, your proposal should delineate these rates and demonstrate how they will yield in a sample size that is adequate for testing your hypotheses.

13.6 STEP #1: ESTIMATE YOUR SAMPLE SIZE

Your first step in calculating power is to estimate your sample size. This section should include your projected eligibility, recruitment, and retention rates as well as your final expected sample size for analysis. A corresponding table (e.g., see Table 13.1) can be included as well.

Your proposed sample size will be one of the primary factors influencing the costs of conducting your study as it is associated with so many aspects of study operations (e.g., number of participant incentives, number of assays to be run). Ask yourself whether it is feasible to actually recruit this number of participants. For example, if you are proposing to conduct a hospital-based study, find out if the hospital actually sees that number of patients per day/week/year. Are that many patients likely to be eligible *and* agree to participate?

If you are proposing to recruit participants de novo, you will likely not yet know all the figures in Table 13.1. However, for the purposes of ensuring feasibility, it will be critical to provide estimates. These estimates can be based on your own preliminary work, that of your coinvestigators, or that by other investigators at your proposed study site.

A **pilot study**, conducted at the same study site as your proposal, will be the best way to assure the reviewers that you have a well-grounded basis for your expected recruitment and retention rates and therefore the corresponding sample size. This highlights the need, as discussed in Chapter 1, "Ten Top Tips for Successful Proposal Writing," to conduct a pilot or feasibility study prior to proposing a larger grant.

However, if such pilot data are not available, then search for **prior similar studies** at the proposed study site conducted by your research team or others. Such prior studies, if they had similar eligibility criteria, can also provide evidence to support your proposed rates.

TABLE 13.1 To Estimate Your Sample Size, You Will Need to Project the Number of:

- Eligible participants
- Those who will agree to participate
- Participants who will remain at the end of follow-up (if a prospective study)
- Participants who will have complete data for analysis

Lastly, look to the prior literature. Base your recruitment and retention rates upon a published study at a site as similar as possible to your own in terms of sociodemographic status and other key variables. Clarify in the proposal how you expect the rates might change in your own setting.

---

eg
example

Imagine a proposal to assemble a prospective cohort of older African American patients. Proposed Sample Size: Taylor Health Clinic sees approximately 4040 patients per year, of which approximately 37% are older African Americans (>50 years of age). We expect 1495 (85.7%) of older African Americans to agree to participate, 1181 (79% of those who agree) to be eligible, 1075 (91% of eligible participants) to be followed through the end of the study, and valid questionnaires to be completed by 1000 (93% of the final sample). The above rates are based on (1) recruitment figures observed in prior studies conducted in this population at Taylor Hospital and (2) the rates reported by a prior study conducted in a similar setting.[1]

13.7 STEP #2: CHOOSE USER-FRIENDLY SOFTWARE TO CALCULATE POWER

There are several software packages commonly used by investigators in epidemiology and preventive medicine to calculate power, some of which are free and publically available.

Examples of free software packages include the following:

- ClinCalc Sample Size Calculator (https://clincalc.com/stats/samplesize.aspx)
- EpiInfo (www.cdc.gov/epiinfo/) has a *statcalc* function that includes power calculations for typical study designs in epidemiology and preventive medicine
- G*Power (www.psycho.uni-duesseldorf.de/aap/projects/gpower)
- PASS software (http://www.ncss.com/)
- nQuery Advisor (http://www.statistical-solutions-software.com/nquery-advisor-nterim/)
- Statistical analysis software such as SAS (www.SAS.com) can be used to calculate power

These software packages take the intimidation factor out of power calculations. With this software in hand, you will be empowered to experiment by entering a range of projected sample sizes and/or anticipated outcome rates. In real time, you can then observe the impact on your subsequent power. In this way, such software not only facilitates the calculation of your power but can provide vital information on the robustness of your intended inferences.

13.8 STEP #3: REMIND YOURSELF OF YOUR MEASURE OF ASSOCIATION

The type of test that you will use to calculate power will depend on the measure of association that you proposed to calculate in your Data Analysis section.

Below are two common measures of association in epidemiology and preventive medicine:

A. **Ratio measures of association**: Measures of association in which *relative* differences between exposed and unexposed groups are being compared. That is, if your outcome is **dichotomous**, then your measure of association will typically be a ratio such as a relative risk

(RR) (i.e., an odds ratio [OR], rate ratio, or risk ratio). In general, **dichotomous outcomes** tend to be the most common in epidemiology and preventive medicine as we are often comparing the incidence of disease diagnosis (e.g., diabetes diagnosis: yes or no) between exposed and unexposed groups.

B. **Difference measures of association**: Measures of association in which *absolute* differences between exposed and unexposed groups are being compared. That is, if your outcome is **continuous**, then your measure of association will typically be a difference in means between groups. **Continuous outcomes** are also fairly common particularly for early-career investigators as they typically necessitate a smaller sample size to achieve adequate power than dichotomous outcomes. Examples of continuous outcomes include fasting glucose levels, blood pressure, and cholesterol levels.

13.9 STEP #4: CALCULATE POWER FOR RATIO MEASURES OF ASSOCIATION (I.E., RELATIVE RISKS)

The following sections will focus on the data that you will need to gather to calculate power for relative risks (e.g., risk ratios, rate ratios, ORs).

A relative risk is a comparison of proportions between groups. To detect this difference in proportions between exposed and unexposed groups, power is typically based on a **chi-square test**.

The information that you need to enter into the software package will vary according to your proposed study design. The sections below are divided into **cohort study and cross-sectional study and unmatched case-control study**.

13.9.1 For Cohort and Cross-Sectional Studies

The data that you will need to gather and enter to calculate power for cohort and cross-sectional studies is described in Table 13.2.

1. **Confidence level**: For all study designs, the generally accepted confidence level is 95%.
2. **Sample size**: Enter the sample size that you anticipate will be feasible or available to you.
3. **Ratio of unexposed to exposed**: If you are using an existing dataset, you can calculate the *ratio of unexposed to exposed* directly from the dataset. If not, the best approach is to use data from a pilot study or find prior literature that evaluated your exposure of interest. Note that relevant studies only need to have described the distribution of your exposure of interest to be useful here—regardless of whether they evaluated your outcome of interest. In searching the prior literature, prioritize studies with a study population and setting most similar to your own.

TABLE 13.2 Data Needed for Power Calculations for Cohort and Cross-Sectional Studies with Relative Risks as the Measure of Association

1. Confidence level (95%)
2. Sample size
3. Ratio of unexposed to exposed
4. Frequency of disease in the unexposed
5. Risk ratio

Example Technique to Determine the *Ratio of Unexposed to Exposed* for a Power Calculation

Imagine a proposal to evaluate the association between iron levels measured via serum ferritin (i.e., your exposure of interest) and risk of type 2 diabetes (i.e., your outcome of interest) in older African Americans in New York State. You plan to categorize participants as having high or low ferritin levels according to a previously published cut point. To determine the anticipated ratio of exposed to unexposed, you search the prior literature for the distribution of iron levels among older African American adults in New York State. If you cannot find these specific studies, broaden your search step by step—only going as broad as you have to: ferritin levels in African American adults of similar socioeconomic status in other parts of the United States, ferritin levels in younger African American adults, or ferritin levels in older adults of any race, etc.

Tip for Success: Cite the sources upon which you are basing your exposure distribution. The closer these citations are to your proposed study population, the more relevant your ultimate power calculations will be. Reviewers will look for these citations to demonstrate your thoughtful, quantitative, literature-based approach to calculating power.

What if Your Exposure Is in Quintiles, Quartiles, or Tertiles?

If you plan to categorize your exposure variable into quintiles, quartiles, and tertiles, then your ratio of exposed to unexposed will be 1:1. In other words, by definition, each category will be of equal size and each of these categories will be compared to the referent category. Therefore, the ratio of exposed to unexposed (referent category) will always be 1:1.

Example Exposure Variable in Quartiles

Consider that you are proposing to evaluate a continuous exposure variable among 200 participants and plan to divide it into quartiles:

- Quartile 1: 50 participants (referent group)
- Quartile 2: 50 participants
- Quartile 3: 50 participants
- Quartile 4: 50 participants
- Total sample size = 200 participants

In the above example, comparing quartile 4 (n = 50) to quartile 1 (n = 50) results in a ratio of exposed to unexposed of 50:50 or 1:1. Just be certain to remember that your sample size needs to be large enough to populate all four quartiles for a total sample size of 200.

4. **Frequency of disease in the unexposed**: This is the disease frequency in those without your exposure of interest. In the example above, this is the percentage of type 2 diabetes in your study population of older African American adults who had low ferritin levels (unexposed). This information may be difficult to find unless you are using an existing dataset in which you can calculate it directly. If not, it is considered acceptable to use the overall frequency of disease (diabetes) in the entire study population (e.g., both exposed and unexposed). Again, prioritize studies with a study population and setting most similar to your own and **cite the source** of your disease frequency.

If you cannot find measures of disease frequency in a study population similar to your own, you may need to calculate a **weighted estimate of disease frequency**. Disease frequency will vary according to sociodemographic characteristics such as sex and age. Therefore, the calculation of a weighted disease frequency simply involves multiplying the percent of your study population with that characteristic by the disease frequency among people with that characteristic.

> Weighted disease incidence rate (IR) = (% sample with characteristic #1 * IR among those with characteristic #1) + (% sample with characteristic #2 * IR among those with characteristic #2) + etc.

Example Technique to Determine the *Frequency of Disease in the Unexposed* for a Power Calculation

We expect our study population to have the following distribution: 39% male and 61% female. We have calculated the expected percentage of those with diabetes using a weighted average of this distribution multiplied by the best available data on diabetes in African American older adults. These are 15% for men[1] and 10% for women.[2] This weighted disease frequency is therefore 12%.

- Weighted diabetes frequency = men [0.39 × 0.15] + women
- [0.61 × 0.10] = 0.12 or 12%

---

5. **Risk Ratio:** Your goal is to demonstrate that you will have adequate power (>80%) to detect risk ratios that have been observed by the prior literature and that are clinically significant. If you have not conducted a pilot study, search for prior literature that evaluated the relationship between your exposure and outcome of interest in a population as similar as possible to your own and note their observed risk ratios. Be sure to cite the source of these risk ratios. For example, "We have 80% power to detect a relative risk of 1.5; this relative risk is clinically significant[3] and is comparable to prior studies of ferritin levels and diabetes risk in which relative risks ranging from 1.3 to 1.8 have been observed."[4-6]

13.9.2 For *Unmatched* Case-Control Studies

Because case-control studies are designed to compare exposure odds in the cases to exposure odds in the controls, a different formula is used for power calculations. Therefore, there are some key differences in the data that you will need to gather and enter (Table 13.3).

TABLE 13.3 Data Needed for Power Calculations for Case-Control Studies with Odds Ratios (ORs) as the Measure of Association

---

1. Confidence level (95%)
2. Sample size
3. Ratio of controls to cases
4. Percent of controls exposed
5. Odds ratio

---

1. **Confidence level**: For all study designs, the generally accepted confidence level is 95%.
2. **Sample size**: Enter the sample size that you anticipate will be feasible or available to you.
3. **Ratio of controls to cases**: If you are using an existing dataset, you can calculate the *ratio of controls to cases* directly from the dataset. If not, the best approach is to use data from a pilot study or find prior literature that evaluated your disease of interest. Note that relevant studies

only need to have evaluated your disease of interest—regardless of whether they evaluated your exposure of interest. In searching the prior literature, prioritize studies with a study population and setting most similar to your own.

4. **Percent of controls exposed**: Enter the percent of controls who are exposed. This information may be difficult to find unless you are using an existing dataset in which you can calculate it directly. Instead, it is generally considered acceptable to present exposure rates among a population that is as similar to your own as possible (and not be concerned about whether or not they had your disease of interest because most diseases are fairly rare).

Example Technique to Determine the *Percent of Controls Who Are Exposed* for a Power Calculation

Consider a proposal to conduct a case-control study of ferritin levels (exposure) and type 2 diabetes (outcome) in older African American adults in New York State. Your cases have diabetes and your controls do not. To calculate the percent of controls who are exposed, ideally, you should identify the percent of those without type 2 diabetes (your controls) who have high levels of ferritin (your exposure). As you can imagine, it is unlikely that ferritin levels will be published only among adults without diabetes. Instead, you can use the percent of people with high ferritin levels in a population that is as similar to your own as possible (and not be concerned about whether or not they had diabetes, knowing that this percent is relatively low). **Cite the source** of these percentages.

5. **Odds ratio**: Lastly, determine the odds ratio that you wish to detect. Your goal is to demonstrate that you will have adequate power (>80%) to detect odds ratios that have been observed by the prior literature. If no prior studies have been published on your exposure–outcome relationship, it is also sufficient to choose a range of clinically meaningful odds ratios. Be sure to **cite the source** of these odds ratios.

13.10 STEP #5: CALCULATE POWER FOR DIFFERENCE MEASURES OF ASSOCIATION (I.E., CONTINUOUS OUTCOME VARIABLES)

Many proposals in epidemiology and preventive medicine will have continuous outcome variables (e.g., blood pressure, cholesterol levels, weight). If your proposal involves a **continuous outcome variable**, your measure of association will likely be differences in means of this outcome between exposed and unexposed groups. To detect these mean differences between exposed and unexposed groups, power is typically based on a **two-sample *t*-test** (Table 13.4).

TABLE 13.4 Data Needed for Power Calculations for a Cohort or Cross-Sectional Study to Detect Differences in Means

1. Confidence level (95%)
2. Standard deviation of the outcome variable
3. Mean difference in the outcome variable between the exposed and unexposed groups that you wish to detect
4. Number exposed
5. Number unexposed

Proposals to detect differences in mean values of an outcome of interest between exposed and unexposed groups typically require smaller sample sizes to achieve adequate power. Indeed, given the budgetary constraints for pilot/feasibility studies and early-career awards, selecting a continuous outcome can be a very **strategic study design decision**. Note that, by definition, continuous outcomes cannot be utilized if you are proposing to conduct a case-control study.

1. **Confidence level**: For all study designs, the generally accepted confidence level is 95%).
2. **Standard deviation of the outcome variable**: The best approach to finding the **standard deviation of your outcome variable** is to locate prior papers that evaluated your outcome in a study population as similar as possible to your own, regardless of whether they evaluated your exposure variable. Be sure to cite these sources.

Example Technique to Determine the *Standard Deviation of the Outcome Variable* for a Power Calculation

Consider a proposal to evaluate the association between ferritin levels (the exposure) and fasting glucose levels (a continuous outcome variable) in older African American adults in New York State. The best source of data on the standard deviation of fasting glucose levels would be from a pilot study in your study population. If not available, search for previous studies that evaluated the distribution of fasting glucose levels in older African American adults in New York State. If this is not available, then search for glucose data among older African Americans in the United States to serve as a proxy.

3. **Mean difference in the outcome variable** between exposed and unexposed groups that you wish to detect should be based on clinical significance. Clinical significance can be determined by consulting with your physician collaborators on the project or published papers in the field. The bottom line is to consider what magnitude of difference in your outcome variable will have an important impact on public health.
4. **Number exposed**: The number with your exposure of interest.
5. **Number unexposed**: The number without your exposure of interest.

Example Technique to Determine the *Mean Difference in the Outcome Variable* for a Power Calculation

Consider the same proposal to evaluate the association between ferritin levels (the exposure) and fasting glucose levels (a continuous outcome variable) in older African American adults in New York State. Consult with a physician-collaborator on what would constitute a clinically meaningful difference in fasting glucose levels. Therefore, differences in glucose levels that led to increased risk of disease would be clinically meaningful. Or, search for publications that evaluated the impact of differences in fasting glucose levels on risk of subsequent diabetes. Be sure to cite these sources.

13.11 HOW TO DISPLAY YOUR POWER IN THE PROPOSAL

13.11.1 Display Your Power for a Range of Relative Risks

When you have a **fixed sample size**, your proposal should include a table that displays the calculated power for a range of relative risks given your sample size (Table 13.5). Most importantly, this table should display where power falls below 80%.

TABLE 13.5   TEMPLATE TABLE Power for a range of Relative Risks for a Sample of N = xxx (Exposed = xxx, Unexposed = xxx) Assuming xx% Disease Frequency in Unexposed

RELATIVE RISKS	POWER (%)
xx	xx
xx	80
xx	xx
xx	xx

Choose a range of relative risks or odds ratios **observed by prior studies** that evaluated your association of interest. Provide citations for these studies. If your study has the power to detect relative risks comparable to those observed by other studies, this will be considered a study strength by reviewers. If, on the other hand, you don't have power to detect comparable relative risks, it will not be fruitful to try to hide this fact. Instead, reviewers will be looking for an explanation for why your study will still be worth conducting.

Therefore, **the text accompanying the table** should describe the implications of the table to the reviewer.

Items to mention in the text accompanying the power table:

- The name of the **statistical test** used to calculate the displayed power and its corresponding citation
- The **smallest relative risk** that you will have the power to detect with 80% power
- A comment upon the **degree of observed power** (e.g., adequate, insufficient, excellent) given your sample size
- A comment on the **clinical significance** of these power calculation findings

It is true that the reviewer may be able to deduce this information from the table, but you want to be kind to the reviewer and do this work for them. Remember that the smaller the relative risk that you can detect, the better.

Example Grant Section on Power for a Range of Relative Risks

Based on our pilot study,[1] we anticipate that 50% of our study population will have high ferritin levels and 50% will have low ferritin levels for a 1:1 ratio of the exposed to the unexposed groups. Based on state surveillance data, we chose 12% as the diabetes incidence rate among the unexposed.[2] Given our sample size of 1000 participants, a two-group chi-squared test with a 0.05 two-sided significance level will be able to detect a relative risk of as small as 1.5 with 80% power and 95% confidence (Table 13.6). This relative risk is clinically significant[3] and is comparable to prior studies of ferritin levels and diabetes risk in which relative risks ranging from 1.3 to 1.8 have been observed.[4–6]

TABLE 13.6   Power and Relative Risks (RR) for Total Study, N = 1000 (Exposed = 500, Unexposed = 500) Assuming 12% Disease Frequency in Unexposed

RR[a]	POWER (%)
1.6	88
1.5	80
1.4	58
1.3	38

a   Rounded to one decimal place.

Note that Table 13.6 shows that a larger power is needed to detect smaller relative risks.

13.11.2 Display Your Power for a Range of Exposure Distributions and Outcome Frequencies

Depending on the dataset you will be using, you may be unsure of the ratio of the unexposed to exposed group or the frequency of disease. In this situation, including a table that displays power for a **range of exposure and outcome frequencies** may be preferable, as in Table 13.7.

TABLE 13.7   Template Table: Power to Detect a Relative Risk of x.x for Outcome x with 95% Confidence based on a Sample Size of n = xxx for a Range of Exposure Prevalences

	EXPOSURE PREVALENCE		
OUTCOME PREVALENCE AMONG THE UNEXPOSED (%)	30%	40%	50%
10	xx%	xx%	xx%
12	xx%	xx%	xx%
15	xx%	xx%	xx%
20	xx%	xx%	xx%

Example Grant Section on Power for a Range of Exposure and Outcome Frequencies
Table 13.8 shows the power to detect a relative risk of 1.5 given a range of exposure and disease frequencies based on a two-group chi-squared test[2] with a 0.05 two-sided significance level and a fixed sample size of 1000. For example, given a diabetes prevalence of 15%, we will have 80% or greater power to detect a relative risk of 1.5 if the prevalence of high ferritin levels is 40% or above. Given a higher diabetes prevalence (20% or greater), we will have >80% power to detect a relative risk of 1.5 if the prevalence of high ferritin is 30% or greater (Table 13.8).

TABLE 13.8   Power to Detect a Relative Risk of 1.5 for Diabetes with 95% Confidence based on a Sample Size of n = 1000

	HIGH FERRITIN		
DIABETES PREVALENCE AMONG UNEXPOSED (%)	30%	40%	50%
10	56%	63%	67%
12	66%	73%	76%
15	77%	83%	86%
20	91%	94%	95%

13.11.3 Display Your Power for a Range of Sample Sizes

If you are proposing to conduct a new study, your **sample size may not be fixed** and still be flexible. In this situation, your proposal could have a table that displays the smallest relative risks that you would be able to detect at 80% power given a range of sample sizes (Table 13.9).

TABLE 13.9   Template Table: Relative Risks (RR) Detected at 80% Power Given a Range of Sample Sizes

RR	SAMPLE SIZE[a]
2.0	300
1.7	600
1.5	1000
1.3	3000

[a] Rounded to the closest hundred.

Example Grant Section on Power for a Range of Relative Risks and Sample Sizes
Based on an expected incidence rate of diabetes of 12% and a 1:1 ratio of exposed to unexposed group, a two-group chi-squared test[2] with a 0.05 two-sided significance level will have 80% power to detect the relative risks displayed in Table 13.6 given the following sample sizes. For example, with a sample size of n = 1000, we will have 80% power to detect a relative risk as small as 1.5 (Table 13.10).

TABLE 13.10   Relative Risks (RR) Detected at 80% Power Given a Range of Sample Sizes

RR	SAMPLE SIZE[A]
2.0	300
1.7	600
1.5	1000
1.3	3000

[a] Rounded to the closest hundred.

13.11.4 Display Your Power for a Continuous Outcome Variable

For a continuous outcome variable, your proposal could have a table that displays the power to detect a clinically significant mean difference in your outcome (Table 13.11).

TABLE 13.11   Template Table Power to Detect a Clinically Significant Mean Difference in a Continuous Outcome based on a Cohort of n = xxx

	FASTING GLUCOSE
Confidence level	95%
Standard deviation of outcome variable	xx
Clinically meaningful mean difference in outcome variable	xx
Number exposed	n
Number unexposed	n

Example Grant Section on Power for a Continuous Outcome Variable
Using a two-group t-test[1] with a 0.05 two-sided significance level and assuming a 7 mg/dL standard deviation in fasting glucose,[2] a sample size of 1000 has >99% power to detect a 9 mg/dL clinically meaningful mean difference[3] in fasting glucose (Table 13.12).

TABLE 13.12   Power to Detect a Clinically Significant Mean Difference in Fasting Glucose based on a Cohort of n = 1000

	FASTING GLUCOSE
Confidence level	95%
Standard deviation of fasting glucose	7 mg/dL[2]
Clinically meaningful mean difference in fasting glucose	9 mg/dL[3]
Number with high ferritin (exposed)	500
Number with low ferritin (unexposed)	500

13.12 WHAT IF YOUR POWER IS NOT ADEQUATE?

Now that you have calculated your expected power, it's time to consider whether your power is sufficient to achieve your specific aims. If not, before discarding your aims, consider the factors that influence power (i.e., sample size, disease frequency, exposure prevalence) and consider whether you can make any adjustments to these factors to increase your power.

The following are examples:

- Consider selecting a population that has a **higher disease incidence**—for example, a group at higher risk of disease. This can be done by selecting a new study site or by changing your inclusion criteria to limit participants to those at high risk of your disease.
- Consider selecting a population with a **higher prevalence of exposure**. This can be done by over-enrolling exposed participants and/or selecting a study site with a higher prevalence of exposure.
- Consider **extending the recruitment time** as a way to increase your sample size.
- Consider **adding study sites** (e.g., conducting a multisite study) in conjunction with other collaborators as a way to increase your sample size.

13.13 HOW TO ADJUST YOUR SAMPLE SIZE UPWARDS TO ACCOUNT FOR MISSING DATA

A well-written section on Power and Sample Size should anticipate missing data due to refusals to participate, exclusions, and loss to follow-up. Based on these anticipated rates, you can *a priori* adjust your sample size upwards. Reviewers will appreciate the thought that you put into these expected realities.

The following formula is useful to calculate the number of participants that you would need to recruit to compensate for anticipated refusals to participate, exclusions, and loss to follow-up:

> **FORMULA TO ADJUST SAMPLE SIZE UPWARDS TO**
> **ADDRESS ANTICIPATED MISSING DATA:**
>
> Sample size * (100% ÷ [100% − Total rate of missing usable response])

Example Adjustment of Sample Size to Address Anticipated Missing Data
Imagine that you conduct your power calculations and determine that you require a sample size of 200 participants to have adequate power to observe an effect. However, you estimate that 8% of subjects will refuse to participate, 5% will be excluded, 4% will be lost to follow-up, and 3% will have missing data on your exposure variable of interest.
Total rate of missing usable response: 8% + 5% + 4% + 3% = 20%
- 200 * (100% ÷ [100% - 20%])
- = 200 * (100% ÷ 80%)
- = 200 * 1.25
- = 250
Therefore, you need to recruit 250 participants to have a final usable sample size of 200.

13.14 OTHER FACTORS THAT INFLUENCE POWER

This chapter has covered the main factors that influence power for traditional study designs in epidemiology and preventive medicine. However, note that there are a variety of other study design and analysis issues that may also impact your power—these will be useful to discuss with a statistician:

- Adjusting for multiple covariates
- Clustering
- Less traditional study designs; for example, complex sampling designs that use sample weights to produce nationally representative data

13.15 FINAL PEP TALK

Overall, it's important to remember that power calculations are more of an art than a science. The estimates that go into the power and sample size calculations are at best well-considered estimates of what you expect will occur in your study. Life is unpredictable, and your recruitment and retention rates, as well as disease incidence and exposure prevalence rates, may all be different than what you expect.

13.16 EXAMPLE

Power for a grant proposal to evaluate the impact of a prenatal exercise intervention on postpartum mental health outcomes.

Specific Aim #1: To evaluate the impact of a 12-week individually targeted prenatal exercise intervention on postpartum mental health.

Hypothesis #1: Compared to subjects in the comparison health and wellness intervention, women in the individually targeted exercise intervention will have lower chronic physiological stress (measured via hair cortisol concentration), psychosocial stress, anxiety, depressive disorder, and anxiety disorder.

Power calculations for our continuous outcome variables (Table 1) are based on two-sample t-tests for independent means assuming equal variance and standard deviations observed in Proyecto Buena Salud (PBS) and the prior literature with a significance level of alpha = 5% (NCSS PASS 2020). Based on this data, our power ranges from 88% to 98% for exposure prevalence rates ranging from 18.1% to 31.4%.

For our dichotomous outcome variables, a two-group chi-squared test with a 0.05 two-sided significance level will be able to detect an odds ratio of at least 1.52 and greater for depressive and anxiety disorders based on rates of these disorders observed in prior studies among this study population[1] with 80% power and 95% confidence (EpiInfo).

TABLE 1   Power Calculations Corresponding to Specific Aim #1

Continuous Outcomes	Sample Size	SD	Clinically Meaningful Difference
Hair cortisol concentration (pg/mg)	276	13.50	4.05
Psychosocial stress	300	7.00	2.1
Anxiety	300	11.7	3.51
Dichotomous Outcomes	**Sample Size**		**Odds Ratio**
Depressive disorder	300		1.54
Anxiety disorder	300		1.52

Study Limitations to Consider

14

When writing a grant proposal, it is critical to try to identify as many of your study limitations as possible—before your reviewer does. Reviewers are selected because they are among the top experts in their fields. Therefore, it is not wise to *hide* potential limitations in a proposal by not mentioning them. In fact, if a reviewer discovers a limitation that you have not discussed, they might assume you are not aware of the limitation and attribute this to a lack of expertise on your part.

Remember that there is no perfect study. In addition, there exist true controversies in the field regarding the ideal study methods and designs. Indeed, often these controversies may be the rationale/driving force behind your proposed research. Therefore, this chapter provides a brief **review** of the **most common** sources of bias and confounding in epidemiology and preventive medicine studies. At the end of this chapter, you will find a section titled **Issues for Critical Reading**—this can assist you in identifying potential limitations associated with your proposed approach.

Please note that this chapter is not meant to be a substitute for an introductory epidemiology textbook—to which you can turn for a more comprehensive review of each of these topics.

Chapter 15, *"How to Present Limitations and Alternatives,"* follows up where this chapter leaves off, describing grantsmanship strategies for presenting study limitations with a focus on techniques to minimize their impact.

14.1 STUDY LIMITATIONS: CHANCE, BIAS, AND CONFOUNDING

The classic limitations faced by studies in epidemiology and preventive medicine are summarized in Table 14.1. These limitations can be divided into threats to **internal validity** and threats to **external validity**. Specifically, chance, bias, and confounding can all be considered as *alternate explanations* for a true relationship between your exposure and disease of interest.

TABLE 14.1 Threats to Validity

a. Threats to internal validity
    i. Chance
    ii. Bias
        1. Nondifferential
            a. Nondifferential misclassification of exposure
            b. Nondifferential misclassification of outcome
        2. Differential misclassification
            a. Selection bias
            b. Information bias
    iii. Confounding
b. Threats to external validity
    i. Generalizability

DOI: 10.1201/9781003155140-16

14.2 CHANCE

Studies in epidemiology and preventive medicine involve samples of the population about which we wish to make inferences. Therefore, chance may affect study results simply because of **random variability** from sample to sample.

At this point, it will be helpful to revisit the figure presented in Chapter 13, "*Power and Sample Size,*" and repeated here (Figure 14.1).

In the above figure, the subheading "Reality" reflects what truly exists while *Investigator's Decision* reflects the decision that you as an investigator will make.

Focusing on the first column of this table, you will see that there are two possibilities when the groups are in reality **not different**. We might conclude, correctly, that the groups are not different *(correct decision)*. Or we might conclude, in error, that the groups are different *(type I error or alpha)*. Our goal is to keep this alpha value low and, by convention, it is typically set to 5% (e.g., we will only make this error less than one out of 20 times).

$p < .05 =$ statistically significant
$p \geq .05 =$ **not** statistically significant

Therefore, a p-value can be defined as follows:

Assuming that there is no difference (e.g. the null hypothesis), the probability of observing your study results, or results even more different from the null hypothesis, by chance alone.

- Interpretation of a p-value of 0.05 in words:

There is a 5% chance of observing your study's results, or findings even further from the null hypothesis, if the null hypothesis were true.

Potential pitfalls to avoid   It is important to note that p-values that are not statistically significant do not mean that the null hypothesis is true. It just means that it is not unreasonable to conclude that sampling variability accounts for your study results even if the null hypothesis were true. On the flip side, a statistically significant p-value does not mean that the null hypothesis is not true; it simply means that it is very unlikely to have observed the evidence provided by your study if the null hypothesis were true. Therefore, statistical significance can never tell us definitively about the truth—just the likelihood.

Even if a p-value is statistically significant ($p < .05$)

- The null hypothesis may still be accurate (we can never know; we can only infer)
- Your results could still be due to bias or confounding
- Your results could lack biological importance or plausibility

Investigator's decision	Reality	
	Groups are not different	Groups are different
Conclude that groups are not different	Correct decision	Type II error probability = beta
Conclude that groups are different	Type I error probability = alpha	Correct decision probability = 1– beta (power)

FIGURE 14.1 Possible study outcomes.

- *p*-values give no indication of the direction or magnitude of the effect
- *p*-values give no information about the power of the study to detect a difference

So, even if your observed *p*-value is statistically significant, your proposal still needs to address the threats of bias and confounding.

14.3 BIAS

Bias is an integral aspect of study design and execution. Bias cannot generally be corrected by analytic methods and therefore it must be prevented by careful study design and execution. Bias encompasses both **nondifferential** and **differential** misclassification. As you will see from the descriptions below, in general, nondifferential misclassification is viewed as the lesser of these two potential threats.

14.4 NONDIFFERENTIAL MISCLASSIFICATION

Nondifferential misclassification addresses the question of whether your exposure or outcome is accurately measured. In any study, inaccuracies in the collection of data are inevitable. Nondifferential misclassification minimizes the differences between the two groups being compared, making them seem more similar than they actually are. Therefore, nondifferential misclassification typically results in an underestimate of any true association.

One should consider nondifferential misclassification in light of both the exposure of interest and the outcome of interest.

14.4.1 Nondifferential Misclassification of Exposure

Almost all forms of exposure assessment are subject to some degree of misclassification. Potential misclassification (error) includes inaccuracies in exposure measurement. These include reliance on proxy respondents, self-report, or recall. Even biomarkers can be subject to error. For example, samples of stored urine and blood can degrade over time. In addition, a biomarker may not be truly reflective of your exposure of interest—or may be influenced by other factors. For example, blood levels of vitamin D are influenced not only by diet but also by sunlight exposure. As you can see from Figure 14.2, nondifferential misclassification of exposure minimizes the differences between the exposed and unexposed groups, making them seem more similar in regard to their disease experience than they actually are. Therefore,

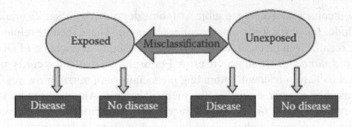

FIGURE 14.2 Nondifferential misclassification of exposure.

nondifferential misclassification typically results in an underestimate of any true association between exposure and disease.

---

e g
example

Example Nondifferential Misclassification of Exposure

Consider a proposal to conduct a cohort study to assess the impact of alcohol consumption on laryngeal cancer (Figure 14.3). Alcohol consumption will be measured via a food frequency questionnaire (FFQ). An FFQ may be subject to error simply due to the difficulty faced by all participants in accurately remembering and reporting their alcohol consumption. There may also be differences in reporting of alcohol consumption between drinkers and nondrinkers (e.g., drinkers may be more likely to underestimate their alcohol consumption). All these types of error would fall under the category of nondifferential misclassification. This misclassification mixes up the exposed (drinkers) and unexposed (nondrinkers) leading to more similar incidence rates of laryngeal cancer in these groups leading to a weaker association between alcohol and laryngeal cancer than is true or a *bias toward the null*. In other words, our study might conclude that alcohol does not have an adverse impact on laryngeal cancer when indeed it does.

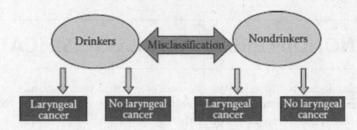

FIGURE 14.3   Nondifferential misclassification of exposure (drinkers vs. nondrinkers) in a cohort study of alcohol consumption and laryngeal cancer.

A pitfall to avoid: Regardless of the *direction* of the confusion between your exposed and unexposed groups, this source of error still falls under the category of "nondifferential misclassification." In other words, "nondifferential" means that these sources of error are not influenced by your outcome variable. That is, even if all your drinkers said that they were nondrinkers, this type of error would still be termed nondifferential. (Note that concerns about the influence of your outcome variable on your exposure categorization are a type of differential misclassification that will be discussed later in the chapter.)

14.4.2 Nondifferential Misclassification of Outcome

Almost all forms of outcome assessment are subject to some degree of misclassification. Potential misclassification (error) includes inaccuracies in outcome measurement. These include reliance on proxy respondents, self-report, or recall. Even medical records or International Classification of Diseases (ICD) codes, often considered a *gold standard,* are subject to error. For example, medical records may be completed by a variety of personnel including residents, attending physicians, and nurse midwives. In addition, *coders* assign ICD codes based on notes recorded in the medical record. Any of these personnel can make an error in recording key information in the medical record or in selecting the appropriate diagnostic code. There may also be error associated with the technique used to abstract data from the medical record.

As you can see from Figure 14.4, nondifferential misclassification of the outcome minimizes the differences between the diseased and nondiseased groups, making them seem more similar in regard to their

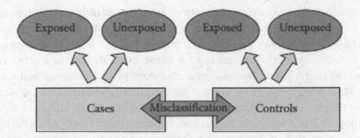

FIGURE 14.4 Nondifferential misclassification of outcome.

exposure history than they actually are. Therefore, nondifferential misclassification typically results in an underestimate of any true association between exposure and disease.

Example Nondifferential Misclassification of Exposure
Consider a proposal to conduct a case-control study of strenuous exercise and risk of miscarriage (Figure 14.5). Information on miscarriage will be self-reported by women. However, miscarriages that happen very early in pregnancy may be undetected (i.e., if a woman miscarried before she recognized that she was pregnant). Therefore, some of the controls (women reporting no miscarriages) may have been unaware that they miscarried and therefore actually may have been cases (women with miscarriages). Or, some of the controls may have terminated their pregnancies and did not want to report this. Such error would be termed nondifferential misclassification of outcome. It mixes up the cases and controls leading to more similar odds of exposure (exercise) between the two groups. This then leads to a weaker association between exercise and miscarriage than is true.

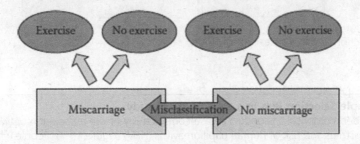

FIGURE 14.5 Nondifferential misclassification of outcome in a case-control study of exercise and miscarriage.

A pitfall to avoid: Regardless of the *direction* of the confusion between your cases and control groups, this source of error is still described as "nondifferential misclassification." In other words, "nondifferential" means that these sources of error are not influenced by your exposure variable. That is, even if all the women who thought they had no miscarriages actually had a miscarriage, this type of error would still be termed nondifferential. (Note that concerns about the influence of your exposure variable on your outcome categorization are a type of differential misclassification that will be discussed later in the chapter.)

14.5 SELECTION BIAS

Selection bias is bias in the **selection** of your study population. It can be viewed as a biased way in which participants come into your study. Selection bias is a **differential** bias and, unlike nondifferential misclassification, can lead to either an **overestimate** or an **underestimate** of the true association between your exposure and outcome of interest. Therefore, it is typically considered a more serious study limitation by reviewers. Once selection bias has occurred, no analysis techniques can alleviate it.

Selection bias is generally more of a concern for a case-control study or a cross-sectional study than for a prospective cohort study. Why? Because in a case-control and cross-sectional study, both the outcome and exposure have already occurred at the time the investigator initiates the study. Because of this timing, it is possible that having both the exposure and the disease can influence a person's decision to participate in the study. In other words, selection bias becomes more likely when being exposed differentially influences the participation of diseased and nondiseased people into the study.

14.5.1 Selection Bias in a Case-Control Study

As you can see in Figure 14.6, in a case-control study, selection bias occurs when **selection** of cases and controls is influenced by their exposure status.

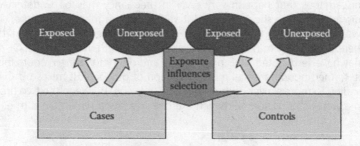

FIGURE 14.6 Selection bias in a case-control study.

Example Selection Bias in a Case Control Study

Consider a proposal to conduct a case-control study of the association between multiple sexual partners and risk of human papillomavirus (HPV) (Figure 14.7). People who have HPV (cases) **and** who have had multiple sexual partners (exposed) may be more motivated to participate because they are concerned that their HPV infection was caused by their having had multiple sexual partners. In other words, the cases' knowledge of their exposure influences their decision to participate in the study. This results in an overestimate of the number of cases with multiple partners, and therefore a stronger association between having multiple sexual partners and HPV than is true.

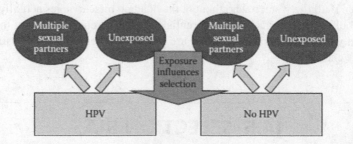

FIGURE 14.7 Selection bias in a case-control study of multiple sexual partners and HPV.

14.5.2 Selection Bias in a Cohort Study

Prospective cohort studies are less prone to selection bias because they enroll participants who do not have the disease of interest and follow them for disease incidence. Therefore, the disease (outcome) of interest is unknown at the beginning of the study (baseline) and should not influence selection of participants into exposed and unexposed groups.

However, instead, selection bias is possible in a prospective study through **differential loss to follow-up**. Just as participants who do not agree to participate will not be in your final dataset, participants who are lost to follow-up will also not be present in your final dataset. That is why loss to follow-up in a prospective cohort study can also be viewed as a type of **potential** selection bias. I use the term *potential* because not all loss to follow-up is differential and therefore not all loss to follow-up meets the criteria for selection bias.

Specifically, if those lost to follow-up were more likely to develop the disease of interest **and** be in our exposed group, this would constitute selection bias and bias our results toward the null. One way to assess this possibility is to compare characteristics of those lost to follow-up versus those not lost to follow-up.

14.6 INFORMATION BIAS

Information bias is bias in the collection of **information**. There are several subtypes of information bias (e.g., recall bias, interviewer bias, and surveillance bias). As noted in the Table 14.2, depending on your proposed study design, your proposal may be particularly susceptible to certain subtypes of information bias.

TABLE 14.2   Types of Information Bias

STUDY DESIGN	TYPE OF INFORMATION BIAS
Case-control or cross-sectional	Recall bias
	Interviewer (observer) bias
Cohort	Surveillance (detection) bias

14.6.1 Information Bias in a Case-Control or Cross-Sectional Study

Case-control and cross-sectional studies are particularly susceptible to recall bias and interviewer bias. Why? Because in these study designs, the outcome of interest has already occurred at the time that exposure information is collected. So, it is more likely that a participant's disease status will influence the collection of information on their exposure.

In a case-control study, information bias occurs when *collection of information* on exposure is performed differently among cases than controls, as shown in Figure 14.8.

Recall bias occurs when having the disease influences the way that information is *recalled*. Most typically, cases tend to remember or report exposures differently than controls. For example, those diagnosed with a disease may *overreport* their history of a particular exposure because they suspect that it may have caused their disease. Recall bias is even more likely when the hypothesis of a potential association between exposure and disease is well known.

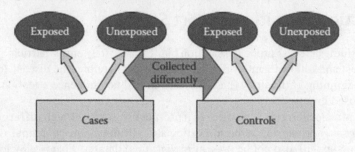

FIGURE 14.8   Information bias in a case-control study.

Example Information Bias (i.e., Recall Bias)
Consider a proposal to conduct a case-control study of the association between infant conjunctivitis and risk of infant mortality (Figure 14.9). Parents of cases (infants who died) may be more likely to recall information on conjunctivitis than parents of healthy children (controls). That is, due to the infant's death, case parents are likely to think back more carefully on every single exposure that occurred and therefore are more likely to recall and report conjunctivitis than parents of healthy children. This results in an overestimate of the frequency of conjunctivitis among the cases and therefore a stronger association between having conjunctivitis and infant mortality than is true.

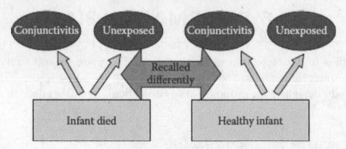

FIGURE 14.9   Recall bias in a case-control study of conjunctivitis and infant mortality.

Interviewer (observer) bias occurs when interviewers ascertain exposure information differently among the cases as compared to the controls. For example, if interviewers are aware of the study hypothesis, they may probe and prompt cases more for information on exposures than they do for controls.

Example Information Bias (i.e., Interviewer Bias)
Consider a proposal to conduct a case-control study of smoking during pregnancy on risk of preeclampsia (Figure 14.10). If the interviewers are aware of this study hypothesis, they may prompt women with preeclampsia (cases) more for smoking information than they do for controls. This would lead to an overestimate of the smoking rate among cases and the findings of a stronger effect of smoking on preeclampsia than is actually true.

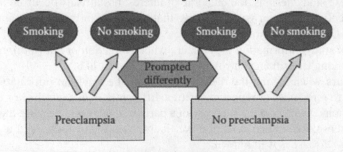

FIGURE 14.10   Interviewer bias in a case-control study of smoking and preeclampsia.

14.6.2 Information Bias in a Cohort Study

Recall bias and interviewer bias are less of a concern for prospective cohort studies. Why? Because in a prospective cohort study, the collection of information on exposure happens **before** the outcome (disease) has occurred. So, the disease, by definition, cannot influence collection of information on the exposure.

However, over the course of follow-up, exposed groups may be monitored more closely for disease than unexposed groups—this is called surveillance bias and is a particular concern for cohort studies.

Surveillance bias (detection bias) is a form of information bias typically faced by cohort studies. Most commonly, it occurs when information on the disease (outcome) of interest is collected differently among exposed participants than among unexposed participants. That is, if the person collecting information on the outcome is aware of the participant's exposure status and of the study hypothesis, they may be more motivated to search for incident disease. For example, a medical record abstractor may search the medical records of exposed participants more thoroughly for signs of the disease (outcome) than they do for unexposed participants (Figure 14.11).

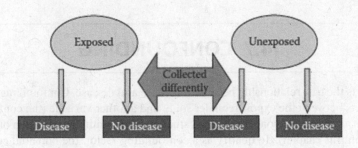

FIGURE 14.11   Surveillance bias (detection bias) in a cohort study.

 Example Information Bias (i.e., Surveillance Bias)
Consider a proposal to conduct a cohort study of oral contraceptives (OCs) and risk of venous thromboembolism (VTE) (Figure 14.12). OC users must attend regular medical appointments in order to have their prescriptions continued. In contrast, women not on OCs would likely not be attending doctors' visits in such a regular fashion. Therefore, VTEs are more likely to be detected among OC users because they are monitored more closely than nonusers of OCs who may have the same symptoms. This leads to a stronger association between OCs and VTE than is actually true.

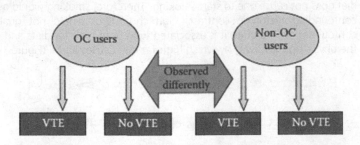

FIGURE 14.12   Surveillance bias (detection bias) in a cohort study of OCs and risk of VTE.

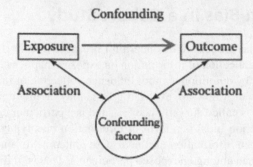

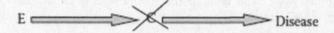

FIGURE 14.13   Diagram of confounding.

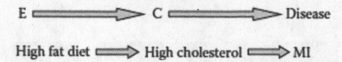

FIGURE 14.14   A confounder must not be in the causal pathway between the exposure and disease; E = exposure, C = confounder.

14.7 CONFOUNDING

Confounding distorts the true relationship between exposure and disease. Confounding can be considered a *confusion of effects* between the exposure under study and another variable (the confounder).

Confounding is an important concern for most study designs, with the exception of randomized trials (as discussed later in this chapter). To qualify as a confounding factor, the potential confounder must be independently associated with both the exposure and outcome (Figure 14.13):

- A confounder must be a risk factor for the disease of interest.
- A confounder must be associated with the exposure of interest.
- A confounder must *not* be in the causal pathway between the exposure and disease.

In other words, the confounder cannot be on the causal (e.g., physiologic or psychological) pathway for how the exposure potentially causes the disease (Figure 14.14).

Example Confounding

Consider a proposal to study the impact of a high-fat diet (exposure) on risk of myocardial infarction (MI). Those with a high-fat diet may be more likely to smoke, and smoking, in turn, is independently associated with MI. Smoking is also NOT on the causal pathway between a high-fat diet (exposure) and MI (outcome). In other words, having a high-fat diet does not *cause* one to start smoking. Therefore, smoking would qualify as a potential confounding factor. In contrast, high cholesterol would not qualify as a potential confounder even though it is associated with both high-fat diets and MI because it is on the physiologic pathway by which high-fat diet causes an MI (Figure 14.15).

$$E \Longrightarrow C \Longrightarrow Disease$$

$$\text{High fat diet} \Longrightarrow \text{High cholesterol} \Longrightarrow MI$$

FIGURE 14.15   Example causal pathway between high-fat diet and MI; E = exposure, C = confounder.

Example Confounding

Consider again a proposal to conduct a study of coffee drinking and risk of bladder cancer (Figure 14.16). You are concerned that cigarette smoking might be a confounding factor. Smoking is associated with both your exposure (coffee drinking) and with your disease (bladder cancer). In addition, smoking is not on the causal pathway between coffee drinking and bladder cancer. That is, coffee drinking doesn't *cause* smoking. Therefore, smoking does indeed qualify as a potential confounding factor for this study.

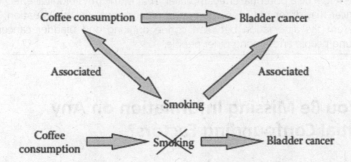

FIGURE 14.16 Smoking as a confounder of the relationship between coffee consumption and bladder cancer.

A pitfall to avoid: A common mistake is to forget that both the left and right sides of the above triangle in Figure 14.13 are necessary to qualify as a potential confounder. That is, in addition to being associated with exposure of interest, the confounder also needs to be associated with the outcome of interest. Consider the same study of coffee (exposure) and risk of bladder cancer (disease), but this time we are considering height as a confounder instead of smoking. While coffee drinkers differ from noncoffee drinkers in terms of their height, we know that height is *not* associated with bladder cancer example. Therefore, the right side of the triangle is missing and height cannot be a potential confounder of the association between coffee and bladder cancer.

14.7.1 Confounding in Randomized Trials

Typically, confounding is not a concern in a randomized trial. The use of randomization in a trial not only randomly distributes the exposure between study arms, but also both **known** and **unknown confounding factors**. The one caveat to this rule is the setting of a small trial. Depending on the sample size, randomization may not always be successful. Therefore, it is always wise to specify in the grant proposal that you will conduct analyses to check that baseline characteristics (potential confounding factors) do not significantly differ between the study arms. (More on techniques to address limitations can be found in Chapter 15, *"How to Present Limitations and Alternatives"*).

14.7.2 Difference between Confounding and Effect Modification

Unlike confounding, which is a nuisance effect that distorts the true relationship between an exposure and disease, effect modification is a characteristic of nature. Most simply, effect modification is a true physiological/psychological difference in the relationship between your exposure and outcome of interest within different subgroups (e.g., age groups, sex/gender groups).

While confounding can be controlled through careful study design and analysis, you do not want to control effect modification. Instead, you want to display effect modification; that is, the effect of your exposure on your outcome **within that particular subgroup**.

Example Effect Modification

Consider our prior example of coffee drinking and risk of bladder cancer. You hypothesize that age might be a potential effect modifier. That is, the physiological effect of coffee on bladder cancer may differ between young and older people. In this situation, you would want to present the association between coffee drinking and bladder cancer separately among young people and among older people.

14.7.3 Will You Be Missing Information on Any Potential Confounding Factors?

In writing a proposal, it is important to consider if there are any potential confounders that you will be unable to control for. This is a critical exercise, as reviewers will be looking for this as well. Be transparent about any potential uncontrolled confounders and then clarify how lack of control for these factors may influence your study findings.

Figure 14.17 and Tables 14.3 and 14.4 describe the potential impact of uncontrolled confounding on your exposure–outcome relationship.

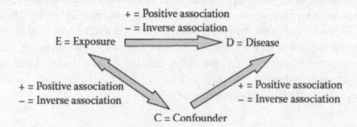

FIGURE 14.17   Schematic of potential confounding.

TABLE 14.3   Impact of Uncontrolled Confounding (C) on the Relative Risk Given a Hypothesized *Positive* Association between Exposure (E) and Disease (D) (Relative Risk >1)

E–C (+)	C–D (+)	Unadjusted RR is incorrectly overestimated. (e.g., unadjusted RR = 1.5; true RR = 1.2)
E–C (–)	C–D (–)	Unadjusted RR is incorrectly overestimated. (e.g., unadjusted RR = 1.5; true RR = 1.2)
E–C (+)	C–D (–)	Unadjusted RR is incorrectly underestimated. (e.g., unadjusted RR = 1.2; true RR = 1.5)
E–C (–)	C–D (+)	Unadjusted RR is incorrectly underestimated. (e.g., unadjusted RR = 1.2; true RR = 1.5)

E, exposure; C, confounder; D, disease; RR, relative risk.

The impact of confounding is always a bit more challenging to envision if you are hypothesizing an inverse or protective association between your exposure and disease.

TABLE 14.4 Impact of Uncontrolled Confounding (C) on the Relative Risk Given a Hypothesized *Inverse* Association between Exposure (E) and Disease (D) (Relative Risk <1)

E–C (+)	C–D (+)	Unadjusted RR is incorrectly underestimated (closer to the null value of 1.0). (e.g., unadjusted RR = 0.8; true RR = 0.5)
E–C (–)	C–D (–)	Unadjusted RR is incorrectly underestimated (closer to the null value of 1.0). (e.g., unadjusted RR = 0.8; true RR = 0.5)
E–C (+)	C–D (–)	Unadjusted RR is incorrectly overestimated (further away from the null value of 1.0). (e.g., unadjusted RR = 0.5; true RR = 0.8)
E–C (–)	C–D (+)	Unadjusted RR is incorrectly over estimated (further away from the null value of 1.0). (e.g., unadjusted RR = 0.5; true RR = 0.8)

Example Impact of Confounding in the Setting of a *Positive* Association between an Exposure and Outcome

Consider that you are hypothesizing a positive association between coffee and bladder cancer (i.e., that coffee consumption increases the risk of bladder cancer). Prior studies have found that coffee drinkers are more likely to smoke (E–C [+]) and that smoking increases risk of bladder cancer (C–D [+]). Therefore, failure to control for smoking would lead to an unadjusted RR that is incorrectly overestimated (Table 14.3, row 1).

Example Impact of Confounding in the Setting of an *Inverse* Association between an Exposure and Outcome

Consider a proposal to conduct a cohort study of fruit and vegetable intake and risk of lung cancer. Prior cross-sectional studies have found that individuals who eat five or more servings of fruits and vegetables have a 50% lower risk of developing lung cancer than those who eat fewer servings of fruits and vegetables. In addition, you know from the previous literature that individuals who consume five or more servings of fruits and vegetables are less likely to smoke than those who consume less of these foods (E–C [–]). Cigarette smoking is a known risk factor for lung cancer (C–D [+]). In this situation, you are hypothesizing that the unadjusted exposure–outcome (fruit/vegetable-lung cancer) relationship is inverse. If you fail to adjust for smoking (Table 14.4, last row), the inverse association will be artificially low (further away from the null value of 1.0). That is, some of the health benefit that you will be attributing to a healthy diet will actually be due to the fact that these people are less likely to smoke.

14.8 OTHER LIMITATIONS SPECIFIC TO CROSS-SECTIONAL AND CASE-CONTROL STUDIES

Survivor bias: Survivor bias is typically only a concern in cross-sectional and case-control studies. It can occur when high levels of your exposure lead to death from your outcome of interest or any similar inability to participate (e.g., due to illness from your outcome). Therefore, these people cannot be recruited into your study. Survivor bias will result in an underestimate of the impact of your exposure upon your outcome.

Example Survivor Bias

Consider a proposal to conduct a cross-sectional study of weight and risk of MI. Those who were of the heaviest weights (e.g., obese) may be more likely to die from an MI and therefore would not be available to participate in your study at the time of enrollment. This would result in an underestimate of the true association between weight and MI.

Temporal bias: Temporal bias is another concern typically faced by cross-sectional and case-control studies. Because both the exposure and outcome of interest have already occurred at the time the investigator launches the study, we cannot ensure the temporality of the association; that is whether the exposure led to the disease, or vice versa, the disease led to the exposure. Thus, temporal bias is often referred to as *reverse causality*.

Example Temporal Bias

Consider a proposal to conduct a case-control study of vitamin D deficiency and risk of cancer. You enroll cases of cancer and controls who are cancer-free and take blood samples to measure plasma vitamin D. Temporal bias is a concern because the cancer itself (the outcome) may have led to the vitamin D deficiency (the exposure), as opposed to the vitamin D deficiency (the exposure) leading to the cancer (the outcome).

14.9 GENERALIZABILITY

Generalizability is an issue of external validity. It should only be considered after thoroughly considering all the threats to internal validity discussed above (bias, confounding, misclassification). At this point, you want to suspend disbelief and assume that your study is internally valid.

In my experience, students and early-career faculty are often too conservative in generalizing their study findings. In contrast, the more that you can generalize your study findings to other populations, the greater **potential public health impact** and **potential for funding** your proposal will have.

The main questions to answer in determining generalizability are the following:

- **"Assuming causality**, to what larger population may the results of this study be generalized?" In other words, "Assuming that there is a true independent association between your exposure and outcome, will the **physiological or psychological mechanism** between exposure and outcome differ among groups not represented in the study?"

Therefore, in generalizing, we are assuming that our exposure causes our outcome. *The decision to generalize should be based primarily upon the physiologic or psychological mechanism.* If you do not generalize to certain groups, *the burden is on you* to justify why you are not generalizing and this justification must be based on a physiologic or psychological rationale. If you don't expect the physiologic impact of the exposure on the risk of disease to be any different in these groups, then you should definitely generalize.

Ask yourself each of these questions in a stepwise fashion:

1. Can you generalize to those of a different race/ethnicity than your study sample?
2. Can you generalize to those of different ages than your study sample?
3. Can you generalize to those of different sex/gender than your study sample?
4. Can you generalize to those of different geographical locations than your study sample?

To answer each of these above questions, ask yourself if the physiologic or psychological mechanism between your exposure and disease would differ in those groups.

Example of Generalizing

Consider a proposal to conduct a case-control study of cigarette smoking and lung cancer among white males in the United States. Based on the postulated physiologic mechanism between smoking and lung cancer, you must judge whether the findings can be generalized to (1) nonwhite males, (2) females, and (3) individuals in other countries. In this case, *you can indeed generalize to these groups because* being male and white and from the United States is irrelevant to the carcinogenic action that smoking has on lung tissue.

Example of Generalizing
Consider a proposal to conduct a study of hair dye and risk of breast cancer among a large cohort of female nurses in 25 states in the United States. Based on the postulated physiologic mechanism between hair dye and breast cancer, you must judge whether the findings can be generalized to (1) nurses in the other 25 states, (2) females in the United States who are not nurses, and (3) females in other countries. *If you presume that* being a nurse and being from the United States is irrelevant to the carcinogenic action that hair dye has on the breast, *then you can generalize your findings to each of these three groups.*

A pitfall to avoid   **Do not limit** the generalizability of your anticipated observed associations between exposure and outcome according to the **representativeness** of your study sample. Study populations should be selected to maximize internal validity and not to maximize representativeness. The issue of representativeness does not impact the generalizability of study findings. Instead, the generalizability of findings is based on the question of whether the physiologic or psychological mechanism between your exposure and outcome would be the same in other groups. In terms of our above example with the US nurses: *Even though the nurses* who volunteered to participate may not be representative of women who live in other parts of the country, and even if they are less likely to use hair dye, there is little basis for believing that the physiological relation between hair dye and breast cancer observed in this study population of nurses would be substantially different from that in most American women. Therefore, you can still generalize your findings of the association between hair dye and breast cancer to US women.

Example Generalizing When Your Sample Is Not Representative
Consider a proposal to conduct a study of eating disorders on risk of dental disease. You will recruit a convenience sample of volunteers. Adults who volunteer to participate may not be representative of adults who live in other parts of the country—they may have fewer eating disorders, be older, or be of different race/ethnic groups. *However, because there is little basis for believing that the physiological relation between eating disorders and dental disease would be different in adults of different sociodemographic groups, you can still generalize to all US adults.*

14.9.1 Reasons to Limit Generalizability

While the overall theme is to encourage generalizing, there are three situations in which you should limit generalizability.

Reason #1 (discussed above): Difference in expected physiologic association between your exposure and outcome in a different population.

Reason #2: Differences in the content or formulation of the exposure between your study population and the population to which you hope to generalize.

Example Limiting Generalizability Based on Different Content of Exposure
Consider a proposal to conduct a study of OCs and risk of breast cancer among women in the United States. One potential reason for not generalizing to European populations would be the difference in European formulations of OCs as compared to OCs used in the United States. In other words, because the OCs (the exposure) are not chemically the same, European OCs may have a different physiologic impact on the breast and therefore limit generalizability to the United States.

Reason #3: Nonoverlapping range of exposure between your study population and the population to which you hope to generalize.

Example Limiting Generalizability Based upon Different Range of Exposure
Consider a proposal to conduct a study of exercise on risk of preterm birth in a sample of non-Hispanic white female athletes. National figures show that Hispanic pregnant women engage in less activity than other racial/ethnic groups. Therefore, the range of exercise participation in this sample of athletes may not overlap with the range of exercise in a sample of sedentary Hispanic pregnant women. That is, your least active athlete may be more active than your most active Hispanic women. Therefore, you would not generalize your findings to a sedentary group of Hispanic pregnant women.

14.10 EXERCISES

1. In a case-control study of condom use and risk of human papillomavirus (HPV), you suspect that the cases were more likely to remember that they had used a spermicide-coated condom than were the control women. This is:
   a. Nondifferential misclassification of exposure
   b. Nondifferential misclassification of disease
   c. Information bias
   d. Selection bias
   e. Confounding

2. A study of alcohol intake and heart disease was performed among 80,000 male health professionals. The authors classified the men as regular drinkers (≥5 drinks/week) or nondrinkers (<5 drinks/week). Men were followed four years for development of heart disease.
   The investigators suspect that men may not tell the truth about their alcohol consumption. Some may say they do not drink when they actually do. This is:
   a. Nondifferential misclassification of exposure
   b. Nondifferential misclassification of disease
   c. Information bias
   d. Selection bias
   e. Confounding

3. A case-control study of exercise (regular vs. irregular) during pregnancy and preeclampsia reports a relative risk of 1.5. The investigators suspect that smoking is a confounder. In their sample, smoking is inversely associated with preeclampsia but not associated with exercise. Is smoking a confounder of the relationship between exercise and preeclampsia?
   a. Yes
   b. No

4. A prospective study of education level and risk of sexually transmitted infections was performed among active duty servicewomen deployed to Iraq and Afghanistan between 2014 and 2019. The authors classified the women as having obtained at least a high school diploma or not. Women were followed for one year for development of a sexually transmitted infection.
   The investigators suspect that active duty servicewomen may not feel comfortable sharing information about their sexually transmitted infections. This is:
   a. Nondifferential misclassification of exposure
   b. Nondifferential misclassification of disease
   c. Information bias
   d. Selection bias
   e. Confounding

5. In a case-control study of condom use and risk of urinary tract infection (UTI) in young women, the investigators reported a relative risk of 2.4 for the association between use of a spermicide-coated condom in the previous month and UTI.

You suspect that the case women were more likely to agree to participate in the study if they knew that they used spermicide-coated condoms. This is:
a. Nondifferential misclassification of exposure
b. Nondifferential misclassification of disease
c. Information bias
d. Selection bias
e. Confounding

Answers: 1c, 2a, 3b, 4b, 5d

14.11 ISSUES FOR CRITICAL READING

Below, issues for critical reading of cohort studies (Table 14.5), randomized trials (Table 14.6) and case–control and cross-sectional studies (Table 14.7) are listed.

TABLE 14.5 Issues for Critical Reading of Cohort Studies

POTENTIAL PROBLEM	IMPLICATION	SOURCE OF PROBLEM	EXAMPLE
Nondifferential misclassification of exposure	Results underestimated	Poor indicator/ inaccurate	Is your exposure measure subject to inaccuracies? For example, does it rely on proxy respondents, self-report, unstable urine levels, and recall?
Nondifferential misclassification of outcome	Results underestimated	Poor indicator/ inaccurate	Is your outcome measure subject to inaccuracies? For example, is there lack of clear diagnostic criteria for the disease such as ICD codes? Will self-report be used instead?
Selection bias	Results biased	Noncomparable selection	None if prospective cohort.
		Loss to follow-up	Will diseased people be lost to follow-up? If so, will they be more likely to be exposed?
Information bias	Results biased	Recall bias	None if prospective cohort.
		Surveillance bias	Will the disease be measured more carefully in the exposed group? For example, will the exposed group be screened for disease more often than the unexposed group? Or, will the exposed be more likely to visit the doctor?
Confounding	Results biased	Confounding	Are you missing information on any confounders? And, will you adjust for confounders on which you do have information? For example, other characteristics of the exposed people that may lead to their developing the disease.
Generalizability	Limited application	Restricted selection/ selective attrition	Who will the study be limited to? Who can you generalize to? For example, you can generalize to people in whom we could expect the same physiologic relationship between exposure and disease.

TABLE 14.6   Issues for Critical Reading of Randomized Trials

POTENTIAL PROBLEM	IMPLICATION	SOURCE OF PROBLEM	EXAMPLE
Nondifferential misclassification of exposure	Results underestimated	Poor indicator/ inaccurate	Will you use an inaccurate way to measure who receives the intervention? For example, will you rely on self-report?
Nondifferential misclassification of outcome	Results underestimated	Poor indicator/ inaccurate	Is your outcome measure subject to inaccuracies? For example, will there be clear diagnostic criteria for the disease such as ICD codes? Will self-report be used instead?
Selection bias	Results biased	Noncomparable selection	None.
		Loss to follow-up	Will diseased people be lost to follow-up?
Information bias	Results biased	Recall bias	None.
		Surveillance bias	Will the disease be measured more carefully in those that receive the intervention? For example, will the intervention group be screened for disease more often than the control group? Will the intervention group be more likely to receive medical care?
Confounding	Results biased	Confounding	Low, but need to demonstrate that all relevant variables were randomized (i.e., equally distributed between the intervention and control group).
Generalizability	Limited application	Restricted selection/ selective attrition	Who will the study be limited to? Who can you generalize to? For example, you can generalize to people in whom we could expect the same physiologic relationship between exposure and disease.

TABLE 14.7   Issues for Critical Reading of Case–Control and Cross-Sectional Studies

POTENTIAL PROBLEM	IMPLICATION	SOURCE OF PROBLEM	EXAMPLE
Nondifferential misclassification of exposure	Results underestimated	Poor indicator/ inaccurate	Is your exposure measure subject to inaccuracies? For example, will your rely on proxy respondents, self-report, unstable biomarkers, and recall?
Nondifferential misclassification of outcome	Results underestimated	Poor indicator/ inaccurate	Is your outcome measure subject to inaccuracies? For example, will there be clear diagnostic criteria for the cases such as ICD codes? Will self-report be used instead?
Selection bias	Results biased	Noncomparable selection	Will cases who have been exposed be more likely to participate?
		Loss to follow-up	None.

(Continued)

TABLE 14.7 (CONTINUED) Issues for Critical Reading of Case–Control and Cross-Sectional Studies

POTENTIAL PROBLEM	IMPLICATION	SOURCE OF PROBLEM	EXAMPLE
Information bias	Results biased	Recall bias	Will cases be more motivated to remember exposure than controls? Will the interviewers probe the cases more for exposure than the controls?
		Surveillance bias	None.
Confounding	Results biased	Confounding	Are you missing information on any confounders? And, will you adjust for confounders on which you do have information? For example, will the cases and controls differ in other characteristics that may lead to their developing the disease?
Generalizability	Limited application	Restricted selection	Who will the study be limited to? Who can you generalize to? For example, we can generalize to people in whom we could expect the same physiologic relationship between exposure and disease.

14.12 EXAMPLES

Note that each of these examples will be repeated in Chapter 15, "*How to Present Limitations and Alternatives,*" with the addition of techniques to minimize these threats to validity.

14.12.1 Example #1

A PROPOSAL TO CONDUCT A CASE-CONTROL STUDY OF MATERNAL HEAT EXPOSURE AND CONGENITAL HEART DEFECTS AMONG SOUTH ASIAN WOMEN

STUDY LIMITATIONS

Nondifferential Misclassification of Exposure

Parents of cases and controls will be asked to recall hours per week of heat exposure in the first trimester, but this will be on average five years after the delivery has occurred. While women's memory of their pregnancy might be better than for other life periods, inaccuracy is likely to result from the extended time lapse and difficulty in estimating average heat exposure over a several-month time period in the distant past.

Another possible source of nondifferential misclassification is in the definition of heat exposures, which requires some judgment by participants. No objective heat exposure measurements will be used in this study.

Nondifferential Misclassification of Outcome

Congenital cardiovascular malformations will be abstracted from the San Francisco birth defects registry. Inaccuracies in classifying birth defects as congenital cardiovascular malformations are possible, and such misclassification would bias our findings toward the null.

Selection Bias

In our pilot study, the response rate was 55.4% due to the difficulty in locating study subjects. Respondents were significantly different from nonrespondents with regard to age, race, ethnicity, and geographic location of residence. If these sociodemographic factors were associated with both our exposure (heat exposure) AND our outcome (congenital heart defects), this would raise the possibility of selection bias, leading to an under- or overestimate of our findings. In addition, if the hypothesis of an association between heat exposure and congenital heart defects was known, those who had been exposed to heat during pregnancy and had a child with a congenital heart defect might be more motivated to participate in our study as they suspected that their heat exposure caused the heart defect.

Information Bias: Recall Bias

In searching for possible causes for their children's heart defects, parents of cases may be more motivated to report heat exposures as compared to parents of controls. This recall bias would result in an overestimation of the association between heat exposure during pregnancy and congenital cardiovascular malformations.

Information Bias: Interviewer Bias

In this study, exposure information will be collected by an interviewer. If the interviewer is aware of our hypothesis of an association between heat exposure and congenital heart defects, it is possible that they will prompt case parents to recall heat exposures more than they do for control parents. This would result in an overestimate of the association between heat exposures and congenital cardiovascular malformations.

Confounding

The questionnaire will include information on all known risk factors for congenital cardiovascular malformations, including maternal chronic diabetes, fever during pregnancy, sex of the infant, and family history of congenital cardiovascular malformations. As with the main study exposures, information on these variables will be obtained through self-report. For information that was difficult to recall or associated with social stigma, such as drinking alcohol during pregnancy, some women's answers may be inaccurate. Failure to adequately control for these variables may lead to over- or underestimates of the association between heat exposures and congenital cardiovascular malformations. In addition, we are missing information on binge drinking during pregnancy. Prior studies have found that binge drinking during pregnancy is positively associated with heat exposure during pregnancy (e.g., sauna use). In addition, binge drinking during pregnancy is independently and positively associated with congenital cardiovascular malformations. Therefore, any failure to adjust for binge drinking may lead to an overestimate of the association between heat exposures and congenital cardiovascular malformations.

Generalizability

We do not expect the physiological association between pregnancy heat exposure and congenital cardiovascular malformations to differ according to race, ethnicity, or age. Therefore, in spite of the fact that study participants were limited to South Asian women, we will still be able to generalize our findings to pregnant women in the United States.

14.12.2 Example #2

A PROPOSAL TO CONDUCT A PROSPECTIVE COHORT STUDY OF STRESS AND RISK OF PREECLAMPSIA AMONG AFRICAN AMERICAN WOMEN

STUDY LIMITATIONS

Nondifferential Misclassification of Exposure

Trained, bilingual interviewers will administer the Perceived Stress Scale during a structured interview in early pregnancy (mean = 15 weeks gestational age). It is possible that women will over- or underreport their perceived stress. This may occur to the extent that perceived stress may be a sensitive issue. This type of misclassification would bias our results toward the null, thereby reducing our effect estimate for the relationship between perceived stress and preeclampsia. We expect this misclassification to be minor.

Nondifferential Misclassification of Outcome

Cases of preeclampsia will be ascertained through medical record abstraction, as well as through a review of ICD codes for preeclampsia. Nondifferential misclassification could occur if diagnoses are missed by physicians or via the data collection methods employed. This would result in a bias of our results to the null, but we expect the effect to be minimal.

Selection Bias: Differential Loss to Follow-Up

Due to the prospective nature of this study, selection bias is unlikely to occur as exposure status (stress) will be collected before the disease (preeclampsia) occurs. However, selection bias is possible in a prospective study through differential loss to follow-up. For example, if women lost to follow-up were more likely to be low-income and therefore in the high-stress group AND if low-income women were also more likely to have preeclampsia. This would mean a differential loss to follow-up among exposed (high-stress) women with disease (preeclampsia) and therefore would meet the definition of selection bias. This differential loss of exposed, disease participants would bias our results toward the null.

Information Bias: Surveillance (Detection) Bias

Surveillance bias will be unlikely in this study because women are not monitored differently for onset of preeclampsia according to their stress levels.

Confounding

We are not aware of any key confounders that are not available through our dataset. It is possible, however, that we measured one or more of these confounders inadequately. This residual confounding could result in a change in our effect estimate in either direction depending on the direction of the measurement error.

Generalizability

The results of this study may be generalized to all pregnant women as the physiological mechanisms through which stress may impact preeclampsia should not vary by race or ethnic origin.

How to Present Limitations and Alternatives

15

Now that you have identified the potential sources of bias and confounding in your proposal with the checklists at the end of Chapter 14, "Study Limitations to Consider," this chapter describes strategies for presenting study limitations with a focus on techniques to minimize their impact. The Approach section of your proposal should discuss these potential study limitations and alternative strategies.

Therefore, Part I of the chapter starts with a fourfold approach to strategically presenting limitations. Part II of the chapter applies this approach to a set of typical study limitations along with design and analytic techniques for minimizing these threats to validity.

15.1 PART I: HOW TO STRATEGICALLY PRESENT LIMITATIONS—A FOURFOLD APPROACH

The key principle in presenting limitations is **transparency**. As mentioned in Chapter 14, "Study Limitations to Consider," instead of trying to hide limitations in a grant proposal, you want to identify and present them. Be open about your thought process and describe the pros and cons of your study design decisions. Remember that there is no perfect study. All studies face limitations, and being humble and knowledgeable about these limitations will be more impressive to reviewers than hiding or ignoring them.

In a grant proposal, space is limited, therefore focus on the most important/major limitations of your proposal. This gives you the opportunity to address what you anticipate will be the most important threats to validity and to discuss the methods that you will use to minimize these concerns. A fourfold approach can be used when presenting limitations as outlined in Figure 15.1: (1) describe the potential limitation, (2) describe the potential impact of the limitation on your study findings, (3) discuss alternative strategies and why they were not selected, and (4) describe the methods that you will use to minimize the impact of this limitation. The advantage of this approach is that it ends on a positive note—always a good strategy when writing grant proposals!

Step 1: Identify the limitation
Step 2: Describe the impact on your findings
Step 3: Discuss alternatives
Step 4: Describe methods to minimize

FIGURE 15.1 A fourfold approach for presenting study limitations in a proposal.

DOI: 10.1201/9781003155140-17

15.1.1 Step #1: Describe the Potential Limitation

The most important key to success in writing a limitations section is to avoid the use of professional jargon. *Professional jargon* refers to the use of such terms as *selection bias*, *information bias*, *nondifferential misclassification*, and *confounding* without an accompanying lay person's explanation. Recall that not all of your reviewers will have training in epidemiology and preventive medicine; some will have expertise in other pertinent fields. Therefore, describing your study limitations in a direct manner using simple terms will show the reviewers that you have a clear grasp of these limitations.

For each limitation that you identify, specify the type. For example, is it nondifferential misclassification of exposure or outcome (e.g., error), or is it a more dangerous limitation—that is, a differential bias such as selection bias, information bias, or confounding? Or, perhaps the limitation is not related to internal validity, but is instead a matter of external validity such as limited generalizability of study findings.

As a starting point, consider limitations mentioned by the prior studies that evaluated the same association of interest that you will be evaluating. Even if you will not face the same limitations, you will want to highlight this fact as a study strength.

Example Layperson's Description of a Study Limitation
Consider a proposal to conduct a prospective study of menopausal hormone therapy (MHT) on risk of breast cancer
Original Version
"This proposal may face detection bias."
Improved Version
"One potential source of bias in our study is detection bias. In other words, users of MHT are more likely to have mammograms and thus more likely to be diagnosed with breast cancer than nonusers. This would lead to an overestimate of the association between MHT and breast cancer."

Note that the improved example still includes professional jargon (i.e., *detection bias*) but then goes on to define it.

15.1.2 Step #2: Describe the Potential Impact of the Limitation on Your Study Findings

For each limitation, it is important to try to state the:

- Likelihood
- Magnitude
- Direction of the limitation on your study findings

Remember, as discussed in Chapter 14, "Study Limitations to Consider," that some limitations are more likely to bias your findings toward the null value, while others are more likely to bias your findings away from the null. Other limitations may have an unpredictable impact on your findings.

In general, limitations that lead to a bias toward the null are considered less dangerous than limitations that cause a bias away from the null. These latter limitations lead you to conclude an association when there isn't one and therefore are often considered more dangerous. Such limitations will lead your reviewers to carefully scrutinize your methods, as well as the alternatives that you considered. The reviewers will assess whether you have minimized these limitations to the extent possible.

Example Description of the Impact of a Study Limitation
(Underlining for emphasis)
Consider a proposal to conduct a prospective study to assess the impact of coffee on bladder cancer. In this study, coffee consumption was measured via a food frequency questionnaire (FFQ).

It is possible that self-reported information on coffee intake will have error. This source of nondifferential misclassification would bias our findings toward the null resulting in an <u>underestimate</u> of the relationship between coffee intake on bladder cancer. However, because we collected coffee information every year as part of a validated FFQ, nondifferential misclassification is <u>unlikely</u>, and if it occurred, its impact would be <u>modest</u>. This is supported by the finding that validation studies have indicated that self-reported coffee intake correlates well with true intake.

Note that the example indicates the likelihood, direction, and magnitude of the study limitation—as indicated by the underlining.

A potential pitfall to avoid   Unlike a doctoral dissertation in which you are expected to show mastery of all potential study limitations, in a grant proposal you will only have space to comment on the most important limitations. See the checklists at the end of Chapter 14, "Study Limitations to Consider," for a critical reading guide for identifying limitations associated with standard study designs in epidemiology and preventive medicine. For example, let's say that you are proposing to conduct a prospective cohort study. Given this design, it is probably not necessary to dedicate space to a discussion of recall bias and selection bias. The robustness of your prospective study design against these potential biases could instead be highlighted.

15.1.3 Step #3: Discuss Alternatives

In any proposal, there will be alternative approaches that you could have, but chose not to, propose. Discuss these alternatives—both their pros and cons—and clearly explain to the reviewer why you chose the approach that you did. In writing this section, be up to date on approaches that prior studies in your field have used and the subsequent impact on their findings. Be sure to cite any review articles or convened panels that make particular recommendations—this can be persuasive evidence in support of the approach that you ultimately chose to take, or it can lead you to reconsider this decision.

Example Consideration of an Alternative Approach
Consider a proposal to conduct a prospective study to assess the impact of coffee on bladder cancer. In this study, coffee consumption was measured via a food frequency questionnaire (FFQ).

• "We selected a food frequency questionnaire (FFQ), as opposed to 24-hour dietary recalls, as FFQs are less prone to error due to the day-to-day variability in diet and have demonstrated relationships between dietary patterns and cancer incidence."[1]

A word of reassurance   Remember that for many study design and data analysis issues, there are true controversies in the field and even established investigators may disagree on the ideal strategy to take. Therefore, be transparent about your thinking as to why you chose one type of design or analysis, over and above other alternatives. In this manner, you will show that you have a grasp of the current state of the field and thoughtfully considered all the issues in making a final decision. While this decision may not be perfect, you are indicating to the reviewer that you are aware of the alternatives as well as the impact of your decision on the interpretation of your study findings.

15.1.4 Step #4: Describe Methods to Minimize the Limitation

In describing methods to minimize your study limitations, first consult prior published studies of your proposed association of interest. Did these studies use design or analysis techniques to minimize limitations that would be prudent for you to adopt as well?

Examples of Design Techniques to Minimize Study Limitations Include:
- Choosing a prospective study design over a case-control study design—to minimize such issues as recall bias and selection bias
- Blinding interviewers in a case-control study—to minimize interviewer bias
- Incorporating repeated administrations of questionnaires over the course of follow-up—to minimize nondifferential misclassification of exposure due to changes in behaviors over time
- Use of life events calendars—to boost the accuracy of recall thereby reducing nondifferential misclassification of exposure

---

Example Analysis Techniques to Minimize Study Limitations Include:
- Comparing baseline characteristics of the intervention and control arms in a clinical trial—to ensure that the randomization was successful
- Performing subgroup analyses among participants with and without missing data on key variables of interest—to address potential selection bias
- Conducting analyses among participants with asymptomatic disease—to address concerns regarding temporality, that is, that whether preclinical symptoms of disease may have influenced exposure

---

In Part II, I provide specific examples of design and analysis techniques to address each of the classic study limitations in epidemiology and preventive medicine proposals.

15.1.5 Conclusion to Fourfold Approach to Address Limitations: Putting It All Together

This fourfold approach of identifying the study limitation, describing its potential impact on study findings, discussing alternatives considered, and ending with methods to minimize limitations has a **key strategic benefit**. By ending with the steps that you are taking to minimize your limitations, you leave the reviewer with a **positive impression**. This leads us to the issue of where to place your study limitations in a grant proposal.

Example Fourfold Approach to Address Nondifferential Misclassification
Consider a proposal to conduct a prospective study to assess the impact of coffee on bladder cancer. In this study, coffee consumption was measured via a food frequency questionnaire (FFQ).
1. *Identify* the limitation: "Women may generally underreport their coffee consumption."
2. *Describe* the impact on your findings: "The effect of such misclassification, however, will be to underestimate any true association between coffee consumption and bladder cancer."
3. *Discuss* alternatives: "We selected a food frequency questionnaire (FFQ), as opposed to 24-hour dietary recalls, as FFQs are less prone to error due to the day-to-day variability in diet and have demonstrated relationships between dietary patterns and cancer incidence."[1]
4. *Methods* to minimize: "Because we collected dietary information every year as part of a validated FFQ, nondifferential misclassification is unlikely, and if it occurred, its impact would be modest. This is supported by the finding that validation studies have indicated that self-reported coffee intake correlates well with true intake."[2]
Note that, in your proposal, you would write this up as one complete paragraph without the subheadings.

15.2 WHERE TO PLACE YOUR STUDY LIMITATIONS IN A GRANT PROPOSAL

In general, there are two schools of thought on where to place your study limitations in a grant proposal. The first is to place your limitations section near or at the end of the Approach section. The second school is to intermingle your limitations within each relevant subsection of the Approach. Below, I discuss the advantages and disadvantages of each technique. Regardless of which technique you choose, the Study Limitations section(s) can be titled, *Limitations and Alternatives*. This is a key catch phrase that reviewers will search for—and will criticize proposals for failure to include.

15.2.1 Limitations Section at the End of the Approach Section

This technique involves writing **one section** with a subheading titled "Limitations and Alternatives" in which you discuss **all** the potential limitations of your proposal typically at or near the end of your proposal. For each limitation, you use the above fourfold approach—discussing the source of the limitation, the potential impact on the findings, the alternatives considered, and the methods that you will use to minimize this problem.

The advantage of this technique is that in one centralized section, you can carefully and thoroughly evaluate and discuss each potential limitation.

The first disadvantage of this technique is that, as the reviewer reads your proposal, they will be thinking of limitations in real time but will be forced to wait until the end of the Approach section to see if you have addressed their concerns. A careful reviewer will keep a list of these concerns as they arise in your application and will then have to cross-check this list with your limitations summary at the end. Therefore, this approach is less *kind* to reviewers.

The second disadvantage of this approach is that you are essentially ending the grant on a fairly negative note. Accumulating all study limitations in one section at the end of the Approach can inadvertently lead to a diminished enthusiasm for the proposal on the part of the reviewer—immediately before they need to assign their score. One way to modestly diminish this concern is to add a final section, immediately after the Limitations and Alternatives section, titled "Summary of Significance and Innovation," where you have a few lines rehighlighting the importance of the application. However, with strict page limitations on grant proposals, it is often difficult to have space for this final upbeat note.

15.2.2 Intermingled Limitations Sections

In contrast, the technique I prefer is to intersperse limitations—as they arise—throughout the Approach section. In this manner, you can address in real-time concerns that arise for the reviewer and don't leave them waiting and concerned until the end of the application. This approach is kinder to the reviewer—just as they are about to put pen to paper to note a concern, you immediately address it.

For example, when you are describing the study design, you intersperse a few lines discussing limitations of your study design and your rationale for choosing it. Further on, when you discuss participant recruitment, you insert another small limitation section discussing limitations and alternatives to your approach. In other words, each of these limitations sections is a micro-version of the fourfold approach presented above—dismissing each limitation individually, as it occurs. Each of these subsections can be titled *Limitations and Alternatives*.

An intermingled limitations section also works well if your methodology differs for each specific aim (e.g., in terms of the dataset used, sample size, and methodology). In this case you would insert your *Alternatives and Limitations* section within the individual methods sections corresponding to each specific aim.

15.3 PART II: METHODS TO MINIMIZE CLASSIC LIMITATIONS—DESIGN AND ANALYSIS TECHNIQUES

15.3.1 Methods to Minimize Nondifferential Misclassification

There are a number of different techniques that can be used to minimize nondifferential misclassification—both via study design and via data analysis.

15.3.1.1 Design Techniques to Minimize Nondifferential Misclassification

Design techniques to minimize nondifferential misclassification of your study *exposure* can include shorter recall periods, use of validated questionnaires, interviewer administration of questionnaires, use of calendars to assist participant recall, and many other techniques. Design techniques to minimize nondifferential misclassification of your study *outcome* include the use of clear diagnostic criteria to identify disease outcomes (e.g., based on published consensus guidelines).

Example Design Technique to Minimize Nondifferential Misclassification
Consider a proposal to evaluate physical activity and risk of breast cancer.
Design techniques: "Physical activity will be based upon self-report and therefore is subject to misclassification. Due to the prospective nature of the study, this misclassification should not be differential according to breast cancer diagnosis. However, to the extent that nondifferential misclassification occurs, our observed odds ratios will be biased toward the null. As prior studies have observed strong relationships between self-reported physical activity and diseases such as cancer and cardiovascular disease, this threat should not be substantial."

15.3.1.2 Analysis Techniques to Minimize Nondifferential Misclassification

One example of an analysis technique to minimize nondifferential misclassification would be to propose to use findings from a validation study to correct for measurement error. Such a validation study may be available from your preliminary studies or from the prior published literature. Measurement error techniques are discussed in detail in several excellent textbooks on the topic, and you could consult a statistician for assistance in this regard.

Example Analysis Technique to Minimize Nondifferential Misclassification
Consider a proposal to evaluate physical activity and risk of breast cancer.
Analysis technique: "We will use data from our physical activity questionnaire validation study to evaluate the extent of measurement error (see "Data Analysis" section)."

15.3.2 Methods to Minimize Selection Bias

The only way to avoid or minimize selection bias up-front is through study design techniques such as random selection into the study and ensuring that invited participants are unaware of the study hypothesis. Unlike nondifferential misclassification, selection bias cannot be removed by data analysis techniques after it has occurred, but data analysis techniques such as sensitivity analyses can be used to evaluate the *extent* of selection bias.

15.3.2.1 Study Design and Analysis Techniques to Minimize Selection Bias

Examples of study design approaches to minimize selection bias could include identifying participants via random sampling and ensuring that they are blinded to the proposed hypotheses. Analysis techniques to minimize selection bias include sensitivity analyses such as comparing the characteristics of participants with and without missing data in a cohort study; or comparing characteristics of cases and controls in a case–control study to see if they differ on sociodemographic and other medical history variables.

Example Design and Analysis Technique to Minimize Selection Bias

Consider a proposal to conduct a case-control study of the association between multiple sexual partners and human papillomavirus (HPV). People who have HPV (cases) **and** who have had multiple sexual partners (exposed) may be more motivated to participate because they are concerned that their HPV infection was caused by having multiple sexual partners.

Design techniques: "Participants will be identified via random sampling of medical records. In addition, we will ensure that participants are blinded to the proposed hypothesis when they are invited to participate."

Analysis techniques: "In addition, we will compare characteristics of cases and controls to see if they differ on sociodemographic and other medical history variables."

15.3.3 Methods to Minimize Information Bias

Remember from Chapter 14, "Study Limitations to Consider," that information bias includes recall bias, interviewer bias, and detection or surveillance bias. Just as with selection bias, information bias can only be prevented through study design approaches. Analysis techniques can be used to address the extent of information bias—but cannot remove information bias once it has already occurred.

15.3.3.1 Study Design Techniques to Minimize Information Bias

One of the best ways to reduce the threat of information bias is to blind the assessor to the participants' exposure (in a cohort study) or to the participants' case/control status in a case-control study. For example, in a prospective cohort study, if medical record abstractors are blinded to exposure status, information on exposure cannot influence the collection of information on the outcome.

Similarly, in a case-control study, if interviewers are blinded to case/control status, then information on case/control status cannot influence the collection of information on the exposure. In addition, bias is also reduced when the hypothesized association between the exposure and the outcome is not known to the assessor or to the participants.

Example Design Technique to Minimize Information Bias

Consider again our proposal to conduct a cross-sectional study of acid-lowering agents (ALA) and risk of vitamin B12 deficiency. Participants in this study will be asked to self-report their ALA during a home interview.

Design techniques: "It is possible that people with vitamin B12 deficiency will be more motivated to remember ALA use than people without vitamin B12 deficiency. Such a recall bias would result in an overestimate of the relationship between ALA use and vitamin B12 deficiency. However, the home interviews were conducted by trained interviewers and participants were blinded to the study hypothesis. Additionally, vitamin B12 deficiency was ascertained by serum concentration and results were not shared with participants until after exposure quantification; thus, they were unaware of their disease status at the time of the interview. Therefore, it is unlikely that information bias occurred in this study, and, if it occurred, we would expect its effect to be minor."

15.3.3.2 Analysis Techniques to Minimize Information Bias

Sensitivity analyses can be used to examine the extent of information bias. For example, if there are concerns about detection bias or surveillance bias in a cohort study, one analytic approach is to compare the number of medical visits or screenings between the exposed and unexposed groups. Another sensitivity analysis would be to repeat the analysis after excluding nonsymptomatic cases (i.e., *in situ* cases) as these cases would only tend to be detected during regular medical screening.

Example Analysis Technique to Minimize Information Bias
Consider a proposal to conduct a prospective study of menopausal hormone therapy (MHT) and risk of breast cancer.

Analysis techniques: "One potential source of bias in our study is the difference in the rates of mammographic screening between hormone users and nonusers. Those who are taking MHT are more likely to have a mammogram and thus more likely to be diagnosed with breast cancer than those women not taking MHT. This would lead to an overestimate of the association between MHT and breast cancer. We will address this problem in several ways. We will compare rates of mammography screening among MHT users as compared to nonusers. We will also exclude *in situ* breast cancers because they are more likely to be diagnosed through mammography."

Example Analysis Technique to Minimize Information Bias
Consider a proposal to conduct a prospective study of dietary factors and risk of diabetes.

Analytic technique: Bias could arise if those with early signs of diabetes, but not a formal diabetes diagnosis, started to change their diet in response to these early indicators. This bias would cause an overestimate of the association between diet and diabetes. To minimize this potential bias, we will perform a subanalysis only among participants without reported symptoms of diabetes. If we observe a comparable association between diet and diabetes in this subgroup as in the overall sample, this would reduce concerns about the impact of information bias.

15.3.4 Methods to Minimize Confounding

15.3.4.1 Study Design Techniques to Minimize Confounding

There are a number of study design techniques to minimize the threat of confounding—as summarized in Table 15.1.

TABLE 15.1   Study Design Techniques to Minimize Confounding

- Subject restrictions
- Collect information on confounders
- Matched design
- Randomization

1. *Subject restrictions*: Design approaches to minimize confounding include restricting subjects to particular characteristics. Specifically, you could propose to restrict subjects to particular strata of a confounding factor such that your exposed and unexposed groups will have this factor in common. Because most study designs have exclusion criteria, by definition, most

proposals are already taking a first step in limiting confounding. For example, if you are concerned about parity as a potential confounding factor, you could propose to restrict the study sample to nulliparous women (women who have not had prior children). In this way, parity cannot act as a potential confounder because all the women will have the same level of that potential confounding factor (i.e., no children).

Even if you cannot logistically rely on exclusion criteria to rule out all confounders, you can try to limit the range of a potential confounder. For example, if you were concerned about confounding by age, you could exclude extreme ages (e.g., children or the elderly). This will not remove the need to address potential confounding by age in your analysis, but will limit the potential extent of this confounding.

Example Design Technique to Minimize Confounding

Consider a proposal to evaluate the impact of vitamin D intake on cataract incidence. You will be using an existing dataset of dental hygienists.

"Although we collected information on many cataract risk factors, we did not have information on exposure to sunlight. Because sunlight is positively associated with vitamin D, and positively associated with cataract incidence, the lack of control for sunlight may lead to an overestimate of the association between vitamin D and cataract incidence. However, because the cohort is not occupationally exposed, variation in sunlight is not likely to be as large as in a general population sample."

Note that the example ends by minimizing the threat of confounding by pointing out that the study population does not vary significantly according to the level of sunlight. Remember, as described above, that if all participants do not differ according to the confounding factor (e.g., all one sex/gender, or all one age), then there cannot be confounding by this factor. That is, differences between participants in levels of this confounding factor will not be responsible for the observed association between vitamin D and cataract incidence. However, some residual confounding is likely to remain.

2. *Collect information on confounders*: The second approach to minimize confounding involves proposing to collect information on potential confounders. The variable table described in Chapter 11, "Study Design and Methods," is an excellent location to list these potential confounders. Carefully considering all potential confounding factors assures your reviewers that you are taking a thoughtful approach. As a first step, reviewing your summary table of the prior literature (described in Chapter 3, "Identifying a Topic and Conducting the Literature Search"). The construction of directed acyclic graphs (DAGs) (see Chapter 12, "Data Analysis Plan") is also a common approach. By having these data in hand, you will be able to adjust for these potential confounders once you get to the data analysis phase.

The flip side of this approach is the potential for heavy participant burden. That is, collecting information on each potential confounder (e.g., either through questionnaires or biomarkers) may take up an inordinate amount of participant time or require a high amount of biomarker assessment (e.g., multiple blood draws, biopsies).

It is also important to note that this approach does not remove the potential threat of **residual confounding**, but does minimize this concern. For example, if you are concerned that sleep is a potential confounder of the relationship between depression and preterm birth, you may choose to administer a sleep questionnaire to collect information on sleep. However, if this questionnaire has some error associated with it (e.g., reliance on self-report), adjusting for sleep in your analysis will only address a portion of the confounding by sleep and some residual confounding will remain.

3. *Matching*: The third design approach to minimize confounding is matching participants on potential confounders. Matching is a design technique typically used in case-control studies whereby cases are matched to controls on several key confounding factors (e.g., age, sex/

gender, study site). In this way, the cases and controls will not differ on these factors, and in turn, these factors cannot be responsible for the observed association between exposure and disease. However, it is typically not feasible to match on a multitude of factors because logistical concerns come into play. For example, it may become difficult to find a control that matches your case according to a long list of matching criteria.

4. *Randomization*: The fourth design approach to minimize confounding involves conducting a randomized trial. Randomized trials include clinical trials in which medical treatments are randomized. Randomized trials can also include behavioral interventions in which, for example, educational programs may be randomized. As long as the investigator is assigning the exposure in a random fashion, the study design qualifies as a randomized trial. Randomized trials are considered the gold standard design because the use of randomization not only randomly distributes *known* confounders, but just as importantly, randomly distributes *unknown* confounders between study arms.

15.3.4.2 Analysis Techniques to Minimize Confounding

There are a variety of analysis approaches to minimize confounding and the most common are listed in Table 15.2. For a more detailed discussion of these techniques, see Chapter 12, "Data Analysis Plan."

TABLE 15.2 Analysis Techniques to Minimize Confounding

- Stratification
- Matched analysis
- Multivariable regression

1. *Stratification*: Stratification involves analyzing the association between your exposure and outcome separately within individual strata of your confounding variables. In other words, if you are concerned about confounding by sex, you could conduct the analysis only among your female participants and then again among your male participants. Statistical techniques are available to derive a summary measure of association that pools the measure of association across each stratum (e.g., Mantel–Haenszel summary odds ratios).

2. *Matched analysis*: If you choose to use matching in the design of your study, then your analysis plan has to follow suit. Typically, for a matched case-control study, conditional logistic regression is used. However, there are other approaches to handling a matched study design that can be discussed with a statistician.

3. *Multivariable regression*: Lastly, the most common data analysis approach to address potential confounding is to propose to conduct multivariable analyses. Such analyses typically involve the construction of multivariable regression models that include your confounding factors. Chapter 10, "Data Analysis Plan," discusses techniques for incorporating confounding factors in multivariable models. Even if you have conducted a randomized trial, it will be important to assess whether the randomization actually worked. If there are any observed differences in covariate status between the treatment groups at baseline, you could propose to adjust for these in multivariable analyses. The smaller your study, the more likely that these baseline characteristics will differ in spite of the random assignment of treatment arm.

The example below uses several of the above approaches to minimize confounding. First, it uses two design approaches: subject restrictions and collecting information on confounders. Then, to further minimize the threat of confounding, it points out that specific subcomponents of the exposure (occupational and household physical activity) are less prone to confounding by "health status" because those aspects of physical activity are more fixed than voluntary sports and exercise.

Example Analysis Technique to Minimize Confounding
Consider a proposal to evaluate physical activity and risk of gestational diabetes.
"Women who are more active during or prior to pregnancy could be healthier in some overall way that decreases their risk of gestational diabetes. We will have information on a variety of confounding factors that reflect overall health and will include them in multivariable models. In addition, the study population has excluded women with more severe diseases such as existing diabetes, hypertension or heart disease, and chronic renal disease. In addition, while healthier women may be more likely to engage in sports and exercise, they may have little choice whether to undertake occupational or household activity. Our analyses will include an assessment of the independent contribution of occupational activity and household activity, as well as sports and exercise on gestational diabetes risk."

15.3.4.3 Techniques to Minimize Lack of Data on a Confounder

There are several ways that you can address anticipated lack of data on a potential confounding variable in your proposal.

First, you can propose to adjust for a **proxy variable** in place of the confounder of interest. In our cataract example earlier in the chapter, you could propose to adjust for geographic region (e.g., northern vs. southern latitude) as a proxy for adjusting for sunlight exposure, your confounder of interest. Or, if you are missing information on income level, you could consider adjusting for the highest level of education as a proxy. While a proxy will not be a perfect substitution, it will help to reduce confounding.

A second approach is to propose that you will perform a **sensitivity analysis**. For example, let's say you are conducting a study of exercise during pregnancy and risk of preterm birth but are missing information on history of preterm birth—an important confounder. In this situation, you could propose to repeat the analysis among women with no prior pregnancies (nulliparous women) who have never had the opportunity for a preterm birth. By comparing these findings to those among your entire sample of nulliparous and parous women, you can assess the extent of possible confounding by history of preterm birth.

15.3.5 Methods to Minimize Survivor Bias

As described in Chapter 12, "Study Limitations to Consider," survivor bias is a concern typically faced by cross-sectional and case-control studies. It can occur when those with high levels of your exposure may have died from your outcome or are no longer available to participate in your study. This concern can be addressed in several ways. First, you could discuss whether it's likely that high levels of your exposure would impact survival by your outcome. Secondly, you could propose a sensitivity analysis in which you compare survival rates among those with high vs. low levels of your exposure.

Example Analysis Technique to Minimize Survivor Bias
Consider again a proposal to evaluate acid-lowering agents (ALA) and risk of vitamin B12 deficiency. You propose a cross-sectional design in which you will recruit participants from an outpatient clinic. Given this design, participants involved in the study will have all, by definition, survived their vitamin B12 deficiency.
"If those with high levels of ALA use were more likely to die of vitamin B12 deficiency, they would not be available to be included in our study. This would constitute survival bias and findings would be biased toward null. However, this is not likely to be an important concern as the consequences of vitamin B12 deficiency are not usually life threatening. Therefore, we expect the possibility of survivor bias to be minor."

15.3.6 Methods to Minimize Temporal Bias

As discussed in Chapter 12, "Study Limitations to Consider," temporal bias is another typical concern faced by cross-sectional and case-control studies. Because both the exposure and outcome of interest have already occurred at the time the investigator launches the study, we cannot ensure that the exposure led to the outcome (disease) and not vice versa, that the outcome led to the exposure.

This concern is minimized if you are studying immutable exposures such as blood type and eye color. For these unmodifiable exposures, we can be sure that they definitely preceded the disease.

Example Technique to Minimize Temporal Bias
Consider a proposal to conduct a case-control study of blood type and risk of Asperger's syndrome. You enroll cases of Asperger's syndrome and controls that do not have Asperger's syndrome and abstract medical records for their blood type.
"Temporal bias is not a concern because Asperger's syndrome could not have led to the blood type of the patient. Instead, we can be sure that blood type preceded the diagnosis of Asperger's syndrome."

15.3.7 Methods to Minimize Lack of Generalizability

Generalizability was discussed in Chapter 12, "Study Limitations to Consider." The primary approach for minimizing reviewer concerns regarding the lack of generalizability involves clarifying the principles upon which generalizability is based. In other words, *the decision to generalize or not should be based primarily upon the physiologic or psychological mechanism.*

Example Technique to Minimize Lack of Generalizability
Consider a proposal to evaluate eating disorders and risk of weight loss. You are proposing to recruit a convenience sample of volunteers.
"Women who volunteer to participate may not be representative of women who live in other parts of the country. Perhaps those women who agree to participate in the study will have fewer eating disorders than those who decline to participate. **However, there is little basis for believing that the physiological relation between eating disorders and weight loss observed in this study will be substantially different in our population from that in most US women.**"

15.4 EXAMPLES OF METHODS TO MINIMIZE LIMITATIONS

Note that these examples extend the examples included in Chapter 12, "Study Limitations to Consider," by the adding **techniques to minimize the limitations in bold**.

15.4.1 Example #1

PROPOSAL TO CONDUCT A CASE-CONTROL STUDY OF MATERNAL HEAT EXPOSURE AND CONGENITAL HEART DEFECTS AMONG AFRICAN AMERICAN WOMEN

STUDY LIMITATIONS

Nondifferential Misclassification of Exposure

Parents of cases and controls will be asked to recall hours per week of heat exposure in the first trimester, but this will be on average five years after the delivery has occurred. While women's memory of their pregnancy might be better than for other life periods, inaccuracy is likely to result from the extended time lapse and difficulty in estimating average heat exposure over a several-month time period in the distant past. **To minimize the possibility for such misclassification, mothers were sent individualized, multicolored calendars of their pregnancy periods, which were used as visual aids during phone interviews.**

Another possible source of nondifferential misclassification is in the definition of heat exposures, which requires some judgment by participants. No objective heat exposure measurements will be used in this study. **However, misclassification resulting from poor participant recall is likely to be nondifferential (i.e., misclassification will not significantly differ between cases and controls), biasing results toward the null value.**

Nondifferential Misclassification of Outcome

Congenital cardiovascular malformations will be abstracted from the New York birth defects registry. Inaccuracies in classifying birth defects as congenital cardiovascular malformations are possible, and such misclassification would bias our findings toward the null. However, a validation study conducted by the New York birth defects registry in 2020 found reasonable validity for major congenital cardiovascular malformations with Spearman correlation coefficients ranging from 0.54 to 0.76 as compared to medical record abstraction.[1]

Selection Bias

In our pilot study, the response rate was 55.4% due to the difficulty in locating study subjects. Respondents were significantly different from nonrespondents with regard to age, race, ethnicity, and geographic location of residence within New York State. If these sociodemographic factors were associated with both our exposure (heat exposure) AND our outcome (congenital heart defects), this would raise the possibility of selection bias, leading to an under or overestimate of our findings. In addition, if the hypothesis of an association between heat exposure and congenital heart defects was known, those who had been exposed to heat during pregnancy and had a child with a congenital heart defect might be more motivated to participate in our study as they suspected that their heat exposure caused the heart defect. **However, we compared response rates and demographics between cases and controls and found no statistically significant differences, making the possibility of selection bias unlikely.**

Information Bias: Recall Bias

In searching for possible causes for their children's heart defects, parents of cases may be more motivated to report heat exposures as compared to parents of controls. This recall bias would result in an overestimation of the association between heat exposure during pregnancy and congenital cardiovascular malformations. **However, the hypotheses tested in this study are not well known to the public, and there is no reason to believe that mothers will particularly suspect these exposures as possible causes of their children's heart defects.**

Information Bias: Interviewer Bias

In this study, exposure information will be collected by an interviewer. If the interviewer is aware of our hypothesis of an association between heat exposure and congenital heart defects, it is possible that they will prompt case parents to recall heat exposures more than they do for control parents. This would result in an overestimate of the association between heat exposures and congenital cardiovascular malformations. However, interviewers will be blinded as to case/ control status of the subject until the end of the interviews. Their blinded status, in addition to the structured nature of the telephone questionnaire, will help to reduce the likelihood of such interviewer bias. In addition, the questions pertaining to our study exposures will represent a minor part of the overall study questionnaire, and it is possible that neither interviewer nor participant will have preconceived notions of the effects hypothesized for those exposures.

Confounding

The questionnaire will include information on all known risk factors for congenital cardiovascular malformations, including maternal chronic diabetes, fever during pregnancy, sex of the infant, and family history of congenital cardiovascular malformations. As with the main study exposures, information on these variables will be obtained through self-report. For information that was difficult to recall or associated with social stigma, such as drinking alcohol during pregnancy, some women's answers may be inaccurate. Failure to adequately control for these variables may lead to over- or underestimates of the association between heat exposures and congenital cardiovascular malformations. In addition, we are missing information on binge drinking during pregnancy. Prior studies have found that binge drinking during pregnancy is positively associated with heat exposure during pregnancy (e.g., sauna use). In addition, binge drinking during pregnancy is independently and positively associated with congenital cardiovascular malformations. Therefore, any failure to adjust for binge drinking may lead to an overestimate of the association between heat exposures and congenital cardiovascular malformations. **However, other important covariates in this study will be less likely to be misclassified by participants, such as whether they had chronic diabetes or whether an immediate family member had congenital heart disease.**

Generalizability

We do not expect the physiological association between pregnancy heat exposure and congenital cardiovascular malformations to differ according to race, ethnicity, or age. Therefore, in spite of the fact that study participants were limited to African American women, we will still be able to generalize our findings to pregnant women in the United States.

15.4.2 Example #2

PROPOSAL TO CONDUCT A PROSPECTIVE COHORT STUDY OF STRESS AND RISK OF PREECLAMPSIA AMONG AFRICAN AMERICAN WOMEN

STUDY LIMITATIONS

Nondifferential Misclassification of Exposure

Trained, bilingual interviewers will administer the Perceived Stress Scale during a structured interview in early pregnancy (mean = 15 weeks gestational age). It is possible that women will over- or underreport their perceived stress. This may occur to the extent that perceived stress may be a sensitive issue. This type of misclassification would bias our results toward the null, thereby reducing our effect estimate for the relationship between perceived stress and preeclampsia. We expect this misclassification to be minor. **However misclassification will be minimized through the use of a stress questionnaire that has been validated among African American women.[1] In addition, interviewers who are bilingual and/or native speakers of Spanish will assist women in completing the questionnaire.**

Nondifferential Misclassification of Outcome

Cases of preeclampsia will be ascertained through medical record abstraction, as well as through a review of International Classification of Disease (ICD) codes for preeclampsia. Nondifferential misclassification could occur if diagnoses are missed by physicians or via the data collection methods employed. This would result in a bias of our results to the null, but we expect the effect to be minimal. **The threat of nondifferential misclassification is minimized because all cases will be confirmed by the study obstetrician. Specifically, blood pressure measurements are obtained at every prenatal care visit as part of routine prenatal care, as well as regularly throughout labor and delivery. Therefore, it is unlikely that hypertension will be missed in any woman with complete delivery information. Additionally, women experiencing preeclampsia may have symptoms such as headache and visual disturbances, which would be recognized by the clinician as symptomatic of a hypertensive condition.**

Selection Bias: Differential Loss to Follow-Up

Due to the prospective nature of this study, selection bias is unlikely to occur as exposure status (stress) will be collected before the disease (preeclampsia) occurs. However, selection bias is possible in a prospective study through differential loss to follow-up. For example, if women lost to follow-up were more likely to be low-income and therefore in the high-stress group AND if low-income women were also more likely to have preeclampsia. This would mean a differential loss to follow-up among exposed (high-stress) women with disease (preeclampsia) and therefore would meet the definition of selection bias. This differential loss of exposed, disease participants would bias our results toward the null. **However, in our pilot study, women lost to follow-up were similar to those with complete delivery information, and therefore it is unlikely that selection bias will occur in this cohort.**

Information Bias: Surveillance (Detection) Bias

Surveillance bias will be unlikely in this study because women are not monitored differently for onset of preeclampsia according to their stress levels. **To reduce the threat of detection bias, the medical record abstractor will also be blinded to stress status.**

Confounding

We are not aware of any key confounders that are not available through our dataset. It is possible, however, that we measured one or more of these confounders inadequately. This residual confounding could result in a change in our effect estimate in either direction depending on the direction of the measurement error. **Given that we are not missing information on any factors that are strongly associated with both stress and hypertensive disorders, we do not expect that uncontrolled confounding will affect our results in a meaningful way.**

Generalizability

The results of this study may be generalized to pregnant women as the physiological mechanisms through which stress may impact preeclampsia should not vary by race or ethnic origin.

Project Summary/ Abstract

16

In the National Institutes of Health (NIH) grant review process, the abstract, referred to as the *project summary*, can be considered the most critical component of your proposal. The skill of learning to write a concise, persuasive Project Summary/Abstract will serve you well. Due to its short length and ability to encapsulate the crux of the study rationale and methods, the Project Summary/Abstract plays a powerful role in funding decisions. Importantly, it may be the only component of the proposal read by the entire review panel. Therefore, as noted in Chapter 1, "Ten Top Tips for Successful Proposal Writing," the bulk of your writing time should be spent refining your **Project Summary**/Abstract and specific aims.

The overall goal of the Project Summary/Abstract is to show how your proposed study will extend prior research in the area, briefly encapsulate the study methods (particularly any innovative methods), as well as provide the key public health and clinical significance of potential study findings. Keep in mind that your goal is to provide enough information for reviewer to make informed decisions on the rest of your proposal. The Project Summary/Abstract is the *teaser* or *appetizer*. If it doesn't grab the reader's attention, you may miss your window of opportunity.

Therefore, this chapter will provide tips and strategies for Project Summary/Abstract writing within the context of the strict space limitations typical of NIH as well as most funding agencies. In addition, guidelines and tips for how to **title** your grant proposal and for writing your **Project Narrative** will also be provided.

16.1 OUTLINE FOR PROJECT SUMMARY/ABSTRACT

In a grant proposal, a Project Summary/Abstract is usually the first scientific page of the proposal—coming immediately after the face pages (which contain contact data on the applicant and their institution). The Project Summary/Abstract for an NIH grant is limited to 30 lines of text with 0.5″ margins and does not include citations or references. It is meant to serve as a self-contained succinct and accurate description of the proposed work when separated from the application. It should be informative to others working in the same or related fields and insofar as possible understandable to a scientifically or technically literate lay reader.

Strategically, the Project Summary/Abstract is essentially a condensed version of your Specific Aims page and largely follows the same outline, but achieves these goals within 30 lines of text. For example, a well-written paragraph #1–2, *Significance and Innovation*, and paragraph #3, *Highlights of the Approach (Methodology)* from your Specific Aims page can serve as the basis of your abstract. Below, I provide strategies and techniques for this condensation and for **making every word count**.

Early-career faculty may be most familiar with journal article abstracts. The key difference between an abstract for a journal article and an abstract for a proposal is that the former will include study findings. In contrast, the Project Summary/Abstract for a proposal needs to convey the *potential importance of* **study findings**.

Table 16.1 provides a general outline for a proposal Project Summary/Abstract.

DOI: 10.1201/9781003155140-18

TABLE 16.1 Project Summary/Abstract Outline

I. Significance and Innovation
II. Highlights of the Approach (Methodology)
III. Overall Goal, Specific Aims, and Hypotheses
IV. Summary of the Significance and Innovation

Note again that this overall outline is the same as that for the Specific Aims page, but it is condensed into 30 lines of text.

16.2 STRATEGIES FOR MEETING THE WORD COUNT/LINE LIMITATIONS

As noted above, current NIH guidelines limit Project Summary/Abstracts to 30 lines with 0.5″ margins. Other funding agencies will have their own requirements but are not usually dissimilar.

Often, early-career faculty have difficulty fitting everything that they would **like** to say about their proposal within these strict word count or line limits. This difficulty is often due to insecurity or confusion as to which aspects of the proposal are most important to mention. By following the outline in Table 16.1 and the corresponding strategies below, you should be well on your way to fitting within these limits. Here is when you really want to follow the dicta that every word should count as described in Chapter 5, "Scientific Writing."

A *tactic* to try Before setting pen to paper, it is important to step back and try the following tactic. Pretend that you standing at the edge of a diving board. Immediately after you jump, someone yells out, "What is so important about your new proposal?" You quickly yell out the key factors before you hit the water. In my experience, this tactic is most productive when conducted **out loud** with a colleague (but not actually on a diving board!). It does not matter if this colleague is an expert in the field. To be successful, a proposal needs to be understandable by anyone with a scientific background. After answering this overall question, have the colleague hold a timer set to 15 s and ask you the following questions relating to each item in Table 16.1. You get 15 s to respond to each question:

- What **background** motivates your study?
- What are your key **aims**?
- What are the key aspects of your **methodology**?
- What is the **significance and innovation** of your proposed study?

I have used this verbal technique for years in my course on grant proposal writing. Students are always surprised how much easier it is to express themselves verbally when the identical questions, presented in writing, can cause them to freeze up or, even worse, use professional jargon.

16.3 WHEN TO FINALIZE THE PROJECT SUMMARY/ABSTRACT

It may be surprising to learn that the process of finalizing the Project Summary/Abstract ideally comes after the process of writing the entire proposal. This is also true when writing a journal article. Indeed, the chapters of this text were ordered purposefully to follow this recommendation. While you will start the Project Summary/Abstract along with your Specific Aims draft at the very beginning of your proposal writing process (see Chapter 2, "Setting Up a Time Frame"), it is not finalized until the very end.

The reason for this recommendation is efficiency. A well-written proposal will include within it the key sentences needed for a Project Summary/Abstract. Remember back in Chapter 8, "Significance and

TABLE 16.2 Correspondence between the Project Summary/Abstract with the Body of the Proposal and Corresponding Book Chapter

ABSTRACT OUTLINE	PROPOSAL SECTION	CHAPTER #
I. Significance and Innovation	Significance and Innovation	Chapter 8
II. Highlights of the Approach (Methodology)	Study Design and Methods	Chapter 11
III. Overall Goal, Specific Aims, and Hypotheses	Specific Aims/Hypotheses	Chapters 6 and 7
IV Summary of Significance and Innovation	Significance and Innovation	Chapter 8

Innovation," when I recommended setting in boldface key sentences in the Significance and Innovation section. Here, you are allowed to plagiarize from yourself! Simply start out by copying and pasting, with a modicum of tweaking, these key sentences into your Project Summary/Abstract. Continue on through the proposal choosing key sentences from your methods section. This repetitive use of key sentences (i.e., both in the Project Summary/Abstract and then again in the body of the proposal) makes it easier for the reviewer. It usually takes seeing these items at least twice, before the reviewer really *gets* the key aspects of your proposal (Table 16.2).

Excerpt the Key Sentences from Your Proposal That Relate to Each Component of the Project Summary/Abstract Outline

It is important to note here that this process serves a dual purpose. If you find that you are unable to find key sentences in the body of your proposal—this raises a red flag about your writing style (see Chapter 5, "Scientific Writing," for more advice on adding/highlighting key sentences).

16.4 NIH REVIEW OF A PROJECT SUMMARY/ABSTRACT

As discussed in more detail in Chapter 20, "Review Process," NIH grant reviews are conducted by study sections—panels of anywhere from 20 to 30 members. Prior to this meeting, your grant application will have been read in its entirety by one primary reviewer and two to three secondary and tertiary reviewers. The remainder of the grant review panel will likely have never seen your application prior to this meeting.

Some study sections will start the grant review process by asking the entire grant review panel to take two to three minutes to silently read over the Project Summary/Abstract and specific aims of the application under review. Others will not even allow this time before the discussion starts. Therefore, the majority of reviewers on the panel will only have time to read your Project Summary/Abstract. The remainder of the discussion typically lasts 10–20 minutes—not enough time for these members to read the body of your proposal. Therefore, the Project Summary/Abstract may be the first and only exposure to your grant for the majority of the review panel.

Because every review panel member's vote counts equally on your application— regardless of whether they are a primary/secondary/tertiary reviewer or a committee member—it is vital that your Project Summary/Abstract encapsulates the key significance and innovation of your proposal.

16.5 EXAMPLES OF FUNDED ABSTRACTS

An excellent resource in writing your Project Summary/Abstract is the NIH Reporter (http://projectreporter.nih.gov/reporter.cfm). This site provides the Project Summary/Abstracts for successfully funded grants. These Project Summary/Abstracts can serve as examples—in terms of both writing style and scope and depth.

You can limit your search of the NIH Reporter to key terms as well as particular grant mechanisms (e.g., early-career awards, smaller grant mechanisms, and larger grant mechanisms). In addition to listing the Project Summary/Abstract, the website will also provide the name of the review panel and the NIH institute that funded the proposal. Therefore, you can also limit your search to the specific NIH institute that you are targeting and see which applications were successfully funded by that institute.

The Project Summary/Abstracts that your search reveals can help you answer the questions:

"How did the writer convey the significance and innovation of the project? How many aims did the authors include? What was their sample size? How did they concisely summarize their study methods? How did they express the significance and innovation of their study?"

For general familiarity with Project Summary/Abstract writing style in your field, it is also advisable to read through the top journals in your area. For example, a perusal through the abstracts in *American Journal of Epidemiology* or *American Journal of Preventive Medicine* also provides excellent examples of concise Project Summary/Abstract writing.

16.6 ABSTRACT: STEP BY STEP

Table 16.3 provides a detailed outline for the Project Summary/Abstract.

TABLE 16.3   Detailed Project Summary/Abstract Outline

ABSTRACT SUBSECTION	# SENTENCES
I. Significance and Innovation	3–5
A. Importance of the topic	
i. Public health impact of the outcome	
ii. Physiology of the exposure–outcome relationship	
iii. Epidemiology of the exposure–outcome relationship	
B. How previous research is limited (Research Gap)	1–2
C. The overall goal of your proposal and how it will fill this research gap	1–2
II.Highlights of the Approach (Methodology)	4–5
A. Study design	
B. Sample size	
C. Measurement tools	
D. Preliminary study findings (if applicable)	
III.Overall Goal, Specific Aims, and Hypotheses	1–2
IV. Summary of the Significance and Innovation	1–2

16.7 I. SIGNIFICANCE AND INNOVATION

A pitfall to avoid   It is important to note that while this section is key, a common pitfall is to spend too much time on this section before getting to the aims and methods. Remember that there is an informal adage among reviewers that the longer your Significance (Background) section, the less likely your application will receive a good score. Remember that you will have a chance to expand in detail on the Significance in the body of the proposal. Your goal here is to concisely justify the need for your study—touching on the major points in the outline below but then immediately moving on to the highlights of the methodology.

16.7.1 A. Importance of the Topic

16.7.1.1 i. Public Health Impact of the Outcome (Disease)

Recall that Section I of the *Significance and Innovation* section of your proposal already specified the public health impact of your outcome. This is typically done by citing the prevalence and/or incidence rates of your outcome. Remember that if you have multiple outcomes of interest, then this information needs to be presented for all of them.

Excerpt the key sentences from your *Significance and Innovation* section from your Specific Aims page and insert them at the beginning of your Project Summary/Abstract. The example below demonstrates this process. Note again that Project Summary/Abstracts typically **do not allow citations or references**.

Example Public Health Importance of the Outcome
Example #1—Alzheimer's disease outcome: In the United States, 5% of women over age 60 years, 12% of those over 75 years, and as many as 28% of women over 85 years suffer from Alzheimer's disease. This is critical in light of the growing population of women in this age group.
Example #2—Low Birth Weight Outcome: Epidemiological evidence suggests that approximately 1 in 12 infants (approximately 8%) are born with low birth weight. Black infants are about two times as likely as white infants to be born low birthweight.

16.7.1.2 ii. Physiology of the Exposure–Outcome Relationship

The Project Summary/Abstract can also include a justification for the physiologic mechanism between your exposure and your outcome. You have already written a section on physiology as part of your Significance and Innovation section. Excerpt the key sentences from that subsection and insert them into your abstract.

Example Physiology of the Exposure–Outcome Relationship
Consider a proposal to conduct a study of prenatal physical activity and risk of low birth weight: Chronic exposure to aerobic exercise before and during pregnancy is associated with numerous maternal and neonatal adaptations which may have short- and long-term benefits to maternal and child health. Specifically, the chronic physiologic effects of moderate-to-vigorous exercise during pregnancy are increased maternal plasma volume, blood volume, cardiac output, vascular compliance, and placental volume.[1]

Remember that it is important to avoid focusing on simply the physiology of your outcome, or your exposure, in isolation. Instead, choose a sentence for the Project Summary/Abstract that focuses on the physiologic *link* between your exposure and your outcome; that is, in this case the mechanism by which physical activity could **impact** birth weight).

16.7.1.3 iii. Epidemiology of the Exposure–Outcome Relationship

Next, the Project Summary/Abstract should summarize the prior epidemiologic literature. Recall that when you wrote this section for the Significance and Innovation section of your proposal, you opened with a paragraph that gave the reader an overview of the number and designs of the prior epidemiologic studies that evaluated your exposure–outcome association of interest. The goal of this overview was to quickly give the reader a synopsis of the state of the research in this area. For example, is this a well-studied area? Or are prior studies sparse?

Although this overview will likely be too long for the Project Summary/Abstract, it can be readily condensed as demonstrated in the example below.

Example Epidemiology of the Exposure–Outcome Relationship
Consider a proposal to conduct a study of prenatal physical activity and risk of low birth weight.
Original sentences in the Significance and Innovation Section
Prior studies of physical activity and low birth weight have been contradictory.[1-21] Fifteen of the 21 published studies observed decreased risk of low birth weight for women who were physically active compared with inactive women.[1-15] No overall association between physical activity and low birth weight was found in four studies.[16-19] Increased risk of low birth weight was associated with higher levels of physical activity in the Springfield cohort study[20] and the Finnish case-control study.[21]
Corresponding sentence for the Project Summary/Abstract
Prior studies of physical activity and low birth weight have been contradictory with 15 observing a decreased risk for active women, 4 failing to find an association, and 2 observing an increased risk.

16.7.2 B. How Previous Research Is Limited (Research Gap)

Next, the Project Summary/Abstract should highlight the research gap that you discovered as part of reviewing the literature in Chapter 3, "Identifying a Topic and Conducting the Literature Search," and described in Chapter 8, "Significance and Innovation."

Example Research Gap
Consider again a proposal to conduct a study of prenatal physical activity and risk of low birth weight.
Original Sentences in the Significance and Innovation Section
A total of 15 epidemiologic studies have evaluated the relationship between physical activity and birth weight.[1-15] These studies, however, have assessed women's occupational activities only,[1-5] recreational activities only,[6-11] or a combination of occupational and household activities.[12,13] Only two studies have measured total activity (recreational, occupational, and household).[14,15]
Corresponding Sentence for the Project Summary/Abstract
The majority of prior studies that evaluated the relationship between physical activity and birth weight have failed to measure total activity (recreational, occupational, and household).

16.7.3 C. The Overall Goal of Your Proposal and How It Will Fill This Research Gap

Next, state the application's <u>broad, long-term objectives and specific aims</u>, making reference to the health relatedness of the project (i.e., relevance to the mission of the NIH institute that you are targeting; see Chapter 4, "Choosing the Right Funding Source"). You already wrote your Specific Aims and Hypotheses in Chapter 6, "Specific Aims." Here, in the Project Summary/Abstract you will insert a condensed version.

Example Specific Aims/Hypotheses for a Project Summary/Abstract
Consider again a proposal to conduct a study of prenatal physical activity and risk of low birth weight.
Original Specific Aims
Specific Aim #1: To prospectively evaluate the relationship between intensity of physical activity and low birth weight.

> Hypothesis #1a: Women who participate in activities of moderate and vigorous physical activity during pregnancy will have a reduced risk of low birth weight as compared to women who participate in activities of low intensity.

Specific Aim #2: To prospectively evaluate the relationship between type of physical activity and preterm birth.

> Hypothesis #2a: Increasing levels of housework/caregiving, occupational, and sports/exercise activity will be inversely associated with risk of low birth weight.

Corresponding Sentence for the Project Summary/Abstract
Our overall goal is to prospectively evaluate the relationship between total physical activity (according to type and intensity) and risk of low birth weight.

16.8 II. HIGHLIGHTS OF THE APPROACH (METHODOLOGY)

Next, describe the research design and methods for achieving your stated goals. The Project Summary/ Abstract should specify the study design, sample size, and the tools that you propose to use to measure your key exposure and outcome variables. Note that elements that make your research **innovative** deserve more emphasis (e.g., if you will be using a novel measurement tool or study design feature).

Key features of the methods to include in the Project Summary/Abstract:

- Study design
- Sample size
- Measurement tools (and any methodological innovations)
- Any preliminary studies

A pitfall to avoid   One common pitfall in Project Summary/Abstract writing is the failure to mention your sample size. Abstracts that do not include this number can be misinterpreted as trying to *hide* a study limitation—that is, a small sample size. The example methodology section of a Project Summary/Abstract below omits several items that would be useful for the reviewer and are study strengths, which if included could increase your chances of funding.

Example Project Summary/Abstract Methods
Original Version Needs Improvement
The investigation will be a supplementary study to an existing dataset of 8000 older adults based in New Mexico. We will conduct tests of cognitive function. Baseline data from this testing will serve as the initiation of a study of predictors of cognitive decline. Second interviews will be given to the same adults after a 2-year interval and again at 4 years. Multivariable logistic regression will be used to model the association between diet and risk of cognitive decline controlling for confounding factors.

Improved Version
(Underlining for emphasis)
The investigation will be a supplementary study to the Lincoln Health Study, an existing cohort study of 8000 older adults based in New Mexico. We will conduct tests of cognitive function using an instrument validated for use in this population. Baseline data from this testing will serve as the initiation of a prospective cohort study of predictors of cognitive decline. Second interviews will be given to the same adults after a two-year interval and again at four years. Multivariable logistic regression will be used to model the association between diet and risk of cognitive decline controlling for confounding factors.

The example Project Summary/Abstract above was improved by also stating the type of study design (e.g., prospective cohort study, case-control study, cross-sectional study), the name of the tool used to measure cognitive function and whether it has been validated, and the name of the existing database/study.

Remember that you want to be kind to the reviewer. You do not want to leave it to them to deduce your study design. In addition, if a study is particularly well known (e.g., NHANES) and has generated many published findings, it definitely adds to the value of the Project Summary/Abstract to mention it by name.

A pitfall to avoid Many grant proposals involve the use of existing datasets (i.e., secondary data from cohorts that are already established). While the use of these rich datasets can be viewed as a study advantage, it can be risky to emphasize **cost efficiency** as the reason for choosing to use such a dataset in the abstract. Instead, it is always best to provide a scientific rationale for your proposed methods. Then, as a secondary advantage, you could mention efficiency by stating that, for example, "the study capitalizes upon the existence of previously collected data" which implies, but does not overtly state, the cost savings.

Example Project Summary/Abstract Methods
Original Version Needs Improvement
The Lincoln Health Study provides a highly cost-efficient setting in which to investigate these issues.
Improved Version
The proposed secondary study capitalizes upon the comprehensive data on diet collected by the Lincoln Health Study as well as objective measures of key potential confounding factors such as cigarette smoking and physical activity. Retention rates to date have been excellent.

16.8.1 What if You Plan to Use Substantively Different Methods to Achieve Individual Specific Aims

Note that if your methodology differs *substantively* for each specific aim (e.g., in terms of the dataset used, sample size, and methodology), then an alternative approach for the Project Summary/Abstract is to intersperse your methods below each specific aim (Table 16.4). Be consistent with the approach you chose to take in the Approach section of your application.

TABLE 16.4   More Detailed Project Summary/Abstract Outline with Methods Interspersed within Each Specific Aim

Abstract Subsection	# Sentences
I. Significance and Innovation	3–5
~~II. Highlights of the Approach (Methodology)~~	~~4–5~~
III. Overall Goal, Specific Aims, and Hypotheses	
A. Aim #1	2–3
i. Highlights of the Approach for Aim #1	
B. Aim #2	2–3
i. Highlights of the Approach for Aim #2	
C. Aim #3	2–3
i. Highlights of the Approach for Aim #3	
IV. Summary of the Significance and Innovation	1–2

16.9 III. OVERALL GOAL, SPECIFIC AIMS, AND HYPOTHESES

The Project Summary/Abstract should convey the **overall goal** of the proposal and, if space permits, a concise version of your **specific aims**. Remember that you will have the entire Specific Aims page to expand upon the aims; therefore, they do not need to be included verbatim in their entirety here.

Below is an example that shows how to **condense** your Specific Aims page into a concise excerpt for the Project Summary/Abstract.

Example Specific Aims
Original Specific Aims
Specific Aim #1: Evaluate the impact of a 12-week individually targeted exercise intervention on risk of gestational diabetes.
 Hypothesis #1: Compared to subjects in the comparison health and wellness intervention, women in the individually targeted exercise intervention will have a lower risk of gestational diabetes.
Specific Aim #2: Evaluate the impact of a 12-week individually targeted exercise intervention on biochemical factors associated with insulin resistance M.
 Hypothesis #2: Compared to subjects in the comparison health and wellness intervention, women in the individually targeted exercise intervention will have lower fasting concentrations of glucose, insulin, leptin, TNF-α, and CRP and higher concentrations of adiponectin.
Specific Aim #3: Evaluate the impact of a 12-week individually targeted exercise intervention on the adoption and maintenance of physical activity during pregnancy.
 Hypothesis #3: Compared to subjects in the comparison health and wellness intervention, women in the individually targeted exercise intervention will participate in more physical activity in mid and late pregnancy.
Condensed Version of Specific Aims for the Project Summary/Abstract
Our overall goal is to evaluate the impact of an exercise intervention on risk of gestational diabetes mellitus (GDM). The specific aims of the proposal are to investigate the effects of a motivationally tailored, individually targeted 12-week physical activity intervention on (1) the risk of gestational diabetes, (2) serum biomarkers associated with insulin resistance, and (3) the adoption and maintenance of exercise during pregnancy.

16.10 IV. SUMMARY OF THE SIGNIFICANCE AND INNOVATION

When reading your Project Summary/Abstract, reviewers will be asking, "Why would it be worthwhile to conduct your study?" and "What is the demonstrated need for this new study?" Therefore, the Project Summary/Abstract ends with a summary of the significance and innovation of the *potential* findings. The **key principle** in summarizing the significance and innovation of the proposal is to highlight the research gap that your proposal will be filling and how it extends the prior research in your area. The more the research gaps that you can point out that you will be filling, the better. In other words, at least one is necessary but more are value-added.

Remember the example research gaps originally presented in Chapter 8, "Significance and Innovation," and repeated again in Table 16.5.

TABLE 16.5   Example Research Gaps

PRIOR LITERATURE IS ...
Limited to particular study designs
Limited to particular methodology
Limited sample size
Conflicting findings
Limited control for confounding factors
Limited to particular study populations
Limited number of prior studies

Excerpt the key sentences from your summary of the Significance and Innovation section on the Specific Aims page and insert them at the end of your Project Summary/Abstract. Recall that significance and innovation are both key drivers of the *overall impact* score on the NIH reviewer critique sheet. Don't rely upon the reviewer to figure it out for you—be kind to your reviewer! Lastly, the Summary of the Significance and Innovation sentences can also cite relevance of the project to the mission of the NIH institute to which you are targeting your submission as demonstrated in the example below.

Example Summary of Significance and Innovation:
Consider, again, a proposal to conduct a study of prenatal exercise and low birth weight:
Prior studies of prenatal exercise and low birth weight were limited by small sample sizes, limited generalizability, and failure to use tools validated for pregnancy and to adjust for important confounding factors. In contrast, our proposal is <u>innovative</u> by evaluating this association in a large, well-characterized prospective cohort of minority women using validated tools to assess physical activity. The <u>significance</u> of the proposal is reflected in the high rates of low birth weight in this understudied population. This proposal fits within Theme 3 of NICHD's 2020 Strategic Plan, "Setting the Foundation for Healthy Pregnancies and Lifelong Wellness".

As always, throughout this process, if you cannot identify the significance and innovation of your proposal, then it may be time to go back and rethink your specific aims and hypotheses. Remember that proposal writing is an iterative process, and it is always acceptable to go back and tweak or even entirely scrap your original aims.

Example Summary of Significance and Innovation for the Project Summary/Abstract:
Very little is known about ways to reduce Alzheimer's disease. Most prior investigations have been cross-sectional. In addition, while genetic aspects of Alzheimer's disease are increasingly being appreciated, virtually no studies have explored interactions between environmental and genetic factors. Therefore, the proposed study is <u>innovative</u> in prospectively evaluating genetic risk factors for Alzheimer's disease. The results of the proposed study are <u>significant</u> in that they will help to elucidate the etiology of Alzheimer's disease.

16.11 HOW TO WRITE A TITLE FOR YOUR PROPOSAL

There are several strategies to consider in writing the title for your proposal. Most importantly, the title should be **concise**, yet as informative as possible, while complying with the guidelines of NIH or the funding agency you are targeting. NIH requires that the title be limited to 200 characters, including spaces and punctuation. However, note that a 200-character title runs the risk of being too lengthy and often gets truncated in some of the reviewer's online spreadsheets. Just as emphasized in Chapter 5, "Scientific Writing," every word should count.

Example Title:
Original Version Needs Improvement
The Measurement of Physical Activity in Free-Living Humans and the Effect of Seasonal and Short-Term Changes in Physical Activity on Cardiovascular Disease Risk Factors
Improved Version
Seasonal Changes in Physical Activity and Cardiovascular Disease Risk Factors

The revised version in the example above is more concise while retaining the primary focus of the proposal (e.g., the key exposure and outcome variables)

16.11.1 Tip #1: Use Agency-Friendly Keywords

Using terms in the title that correspond to the names of review panels at the granting agency will help ensure that officials direct your proposal to the correct scientific review group at NIH (study section). The overall goal in crafting the title for an NIH grant proposal is to ensure that your proposal gets **routed to the correct review panel** and institute within NIH. While you can request what you feel is the appropriate review panel in the PHS Assignment Request form, your title will help to further ensure that your suggestion is followed. This issue is discussed in more detail in Chapter 17, "Submission of the Grant Proposal." The tips below not only help to correctly route your application but also reflect good practices in titling.

Using agency-friendly keywords to help support your requested study section and institute in the *assignment request form*. For example, for grant proposals in epidemiology and preventive medicine, using the term *epidemiology* in the title will help confirm the relevance of the application to an epidemiology review panel. It is one of the key ways to indicate that the study is population-based. In contrast, removing this term might lead the same application to be misdirected to more of a *bench science* review panel. Such groups may not be comfortable with the use of self-reported assessments or other techniques considered acceptable in large studies in preventive research. Including study design terms that are characteristic of grants in epidemiology or preventive medicine will also be helpful, such as *A Case-Control Study of …* or *A Prospective Study of …* Including your disease outcome of interest in your title can confirm relevance to the requested NIH institute.

Example Title:
Original Version Needs Improvement
Stress and Gestational Diabetes
First Improved Version
The Epidemiology of Stress and Gestational Diabetes
Second Improved Version
A Prospective Cohort Study of Stress and Gestational Diabetes

16.11.2 Tip #2: Titles Should Include the Key Variables Being Evaluated

A proposal title should list your key **exposure** and **outcome** variables. If there are too many exposure and outcome variables to fit concisely in the title, then the corresponding umbrella terms should be used. For example, if your outcome variables are risk factors for cardiovascular disease such as HDL, LDL, and triglycerides, it is more efficient to simply use the umbrella term *cardiovascular disease risk factors*. Similarly, if your exposures involve lifestyle behaviors such as diet, exercise, and weight management, use the term *lifestyle behaviors*. Additional examples include *nutritional factors*, *risk-taking behaviors*, or other terms that summarize groups of variables.

This tip has a second benefit. If you find that you are having trouble coming up with a concise title, this could be an indicator that your topic is overly ambitious and that you are taking on a dissertation/proposal topic that is too broad.

Example Title:
Original Version Needs Improvement
The Relationship between Blood Lead and HDL, LDL, and Triglycerides among Adult Women
Improved Version
The Relationship between Blood Lead and Cardiovascular Risk Profile among Adult Women

16.11.3 Tip #3: The Title Should Not State the Expected Results of the Proposed Study

Stating the expected or hypothesized outcome of your study in your title is considered inappropriate for several reasons. First, this is the title for a proposal and not a publication on your findings. That is, your proposal includes hypotheses to be tested that are not yet answered. Secondly, even if prior studies have observed an association between your exposure and outcome, causality has likely not been established. Indeed, the merits of your proposal rely upon your assertion that there is a research gap and that your association of interest is not fully known.

Example Title:
Example #1: Original Version Needs Improvement
Emphasis on Patient Care Delivery and Collegial Interaction Lead to Successful Recruitment of Physicians in Health Maintenance Organizations.
Improved Version
Critical Factors in Recruiting Health Maintenance Organization Physicians
Example #2: Original Version Needs Improvement
Chocolate Increases the Risk of Heart Disease
Improved Version
The Association between Chocolate and Heart Disease

16.11.4 Tip #4: Titles Should Mention the Study Design If a Strength

Including the study design in your title is important if the design is a particular strength of your proposal and a means by which you are extending prior research. For example, if you are conducting a large prospective study, or a randomized clinical trial, or using data from a national survey—these are strengths to highlight by including them in your title. On the other hand, conducting a cross-sectional study or a qualitative study may be an appropriate study design but likely not worth highlighting in your title.

Example Title:
(Underlining for emphasis)
Example #1
The Role of Alcoholism in Posttraumatic Stress Disorder: <u>A Prospective Study</u>
Example #2
Kindergarten Teachers' Definitions of Attention Deficit Disorder: <u>A National Survey</u>

16.11.5 Tip #5: The Title Should Mention the Study Population When Important

Including the study population in a title is important when one of the key strengths of your proposal is the study population. In other words, if your choice of study population is a means by which you are extending the prior literature, then mention this population in the title. Examples include proposals using large population-based cohorts or surveillance studies (e.g., the Behavioral Risk Factor Surveillance System [BRFSS]) or using data from well-established cohorts such as the Nurses' Health Study. Similarly, if your study population will be focused on an understudied racial or ethnic group, a specific age group, or to some other population subgroup (e.g., participants with overweight and obesity), try to mention your study population in the title.

To summarize, potential reasons to mention the study population in your title include:

- A new study population
- A large national database
- An established cohort
- A specific racial/ethnic group
- An at-risk study population with a particular disease or disability
- A particular age group

Example Title:
(Underlining for emphasis)
Example #1
Age and Automobile Crash Risk in a <u>Community Population</u> of Older Persons
Example #2
Relationship of Drug Therapy with Mortality in the <u>National Health Interview Survey</u>
Example #3
The Association between Vitamin D and Depression in <u>African American Men</u>

16.11.6 Tip #6: Titles Should Mention Any Other Unique Features of the Study

In addition to mentioning the study population and study design, titles should also mention any other unique features of the proposal. For example, if you will be conducting the first long-term follow-up study in your area, or using a novel measurement tool, point this out in your title—if space allows. The bottom line is to be sure that the title (or at least the Project Summary/Abstract) touches upon those aspects of your proposal that you believe will be pivotal in its funding success.

Example Title:
(Underlining for emphasis)
Example #1
The <u>Long-Term</u> Effects of Tetracycline on Tooth Enamel Erosion
Example #2
<u>Objective Measurement</u> of Physical Activity and Risk of Respiratory Disease

16.11.7 Tip #7: The Title Should Be Consistent with the Overall Study Goal

This may seem like a straightforward tip, but caution should be taken to draw your title from your overall goal and specific aims. It may be easy to get distracted by some of the above tips and emphasize the study methods to the exclusion of your overall exposure and outcome variables. In other words, be sure not to miss the forest for the trees.

Example Title:
Example #1 Specific Aim
The purpose of this study is to investigate whether those who experience sexual harassment have a higher rate of suicide ideation than those who do not experience sexual harassment.
Corresponding Title
The Relationship between Sexual Harassment and Suicide Ideation
Example #2 Specific Aim
To examine the association between alcohol consumption and cataract extraction in a prospective cohort of older adults.
Corresponding Title
A Prospective Study of Alcohol Consumption and Cataract Extraction among Older Adults

16.11.8 Stylistic Tip #1: Avoid Clever Titles

Dissertation proposals in the humanities often include a catchy phrase or subtitle to capture the attention of the audience. It is best to avoid the use of such clever titles for proposals in epidemiology and preventive medicine. Such titles are more appropriate for the popular press (i.e., material written for the general public as opposed to scholarly material written for an academic or research audience). If your topic is timely and important, it will speak for itself.

Example Title:
Original Versions Need Improvement
The Smoking Gun: The Association between Cigarette Use and Oral Cancer
Doctors without Borders: Health Care Utilization Patterns and HIV Risk in Developing Countries

16.11.9 Stylistic Tip #2: Avoid Writing Titles as Questions

While a title written in the format of a question might at first appear intriguing, the use of a question as a title is considered more appropriate for the popular press. It is not a generally acceptable approach for a scientific proposal.

Example Title:
Original Version Needs Improvement
Does a Mediterranean Diet Reduce Risk of Heart Disease?
Improved Version
The Mediterranean Diet and Risk of Heart Disease

16.12 HOW TO WRITE A PROJECT NARRATIVE FOR YOUR PROPOSAL

The NIH guidelines require that you write a project narrative that describes the relevance of your proposed research to public health in, at most, three sentences. Save this task for the very end of your grant writing process and choose the most persuasive sentences from your Project Summary/Abstract. Typically, these would be a combination of (1) your overall goal and (2) the summary of your Significance and Innovation. Remember that reviewers need to be reminded, repeatedly, of the overall goals and importance of your project as they are balancing multiple reviews.

In this section, it is important to be succinct and use plain language that can be understood by a general lay audience because, if the application is funded, this public health relevance statement will be combined with the Project Summary/Abstract and will become public information.

Note that the example below is limited to three sentences as per the NIH guidelines.

Example Project Narrative

Consider a proposal to conduct a prospective cohort study in postpartum Hispanic women:
The proposed research is relevant to public health because understanding how physical health during pregnancy can help predict cardiovascular disease in later adulthood is essential to women's health. The specific objective of the proposed research is to examine the association of pregnancy complications with subsequent cardiometabolic disorders among Hispanics of Puerto Rican heritage living in the continental United States, the Hispanic subgroup with the highest prevalence of diabetes, obesity, and major cardiometabolic risk factors. Study outcomes will inform culturally sensitive prenatal interventions for early life prevention of future chronic disorders in an understudied and particularly vulnerable population.

Example Project Narrative

Consider a proposal to conduct a randomized lifestyle intervention in Black women:
The Black population has grown by more than ten million since 2000 which represents a 29% increase over almost two decades, a population growth rate larger than that of the White population over the same time span (13%). Black women are more likely to begin their pregnancies overweight or obese as compared to white women. This randomized controlled trial of a culturally modified, individually tailored lifestyle intervention in Black pregnant women aims to reduce excessive gestational weight gain, postpartum weight retention, and subsequent obesity using a high-reach, low-cost strategy, which has great potential for adoption on a larger scale and reducing health disparities in the United States.

16.13 EXAMPLES

16.13.1 Example #1a: Needs Improvement

A PROPOSAL TO EXAMINE THE IMPACT OF DANCE PROGRAMS ON PHYSICAL ACTIVITY LEVELS OF AFRICAN AMERICAN GIRLS

ABSTRACT

African American girls suffer disproportionately from obesity and type 2 diabetes mellitus compared to their age matched non-Hispanic white counterparts. One factor associated with the development of obesity and type 2 diabetes disparities in children is a decrease in their physical activity (PA) levels. Reductions in PA are more prevalent in African American girls; therefore, effective PA interventions that result in behavior change and ultimately improvements in their PA levels are needed. For a PA intervention message to be effective among African American girls, the program must resonate among them and they must enjoy participating in the intervention activity (e.g., Afrocentric dance). Afrocentric dance has a strong cultural and historical significance in the African American community and can provide girls with sustained bouts of moderate-to-vigorous physical activity (MVPA). One study in African American girls has shown that Afrocentric dance can result in improvements of self-reported measures of PA but not objectively measured PA; it is possible that the participation in the dance program did not have any impact on girls' home PA environment due to lack of parental participation. It has been speculated that one way to increase children's PA level is to increase parental PA level, as there is a strong positive correlation between parental and children PA levels. In the African American culture, maternal health behaviors have a strong influence on children's health behaviors, making studies exploring methods to enhance maternal and child health behaviors critical. There are sparse data, mostly in non-Hispanic white families, suggesting that parent–child interventions could have a beneficial impact on children's PA. In one of the few family-based interventions in African American girls, Beech et al. examined the effects of a family-based behavioral intervention in the prevention of weight gain and found a 12% nonsignificant increase in girls' self-reported levels of MVPA compared to the control group. The lack of significant differences could potentially be attributed to the lack of impact on girls' home PA environment. **Currently, there are no studies examining the effects of a daughter–mother Afrocentric dance program on the PA levels of African American girls.** Therefore, we propose to examine the feasibility of a 12-week randomized control daughter–mother afterschool Afrocentric dance PA

COMMENTS

- Too much space is dedicated to background before transitioning to the research gap and the proposed study methods. Remember that there is an informal adage among reviewers that the more time spent on the significance (background) section of the abstract, the less likely your application will receive a good score.
- While the abstract points out that prior studies were limited by a lack of objective measures, it is not clear if the proposed study will use objective measures.
- Key features of the methods (as outlined earlier in the chapter) are not included. These include sample size, measurement tools (and any methodological innovations), and any preliminary studies.
- The terms "significance" and "innovation" are not used. Remember that reviewers will search for these terms and they are key aspects in your final score.

16.13.2 Example #1b: Improved Project Summary/Abstract

A PROPOSAL TO EXAMINE THE IMPACT OF DANCE PROGRAMS ON PHYSICAL ACTIVITY LEVELS OF AFRICAN AMERICAN GIRLS

ABSTRACT

African American girls suffer disproportionately from obesity and type 2 diabetes mellitus compared to their age matched non-Hispanic white counterparts. Physical activity (PA) reduces the risk of these disorders; however, African American girls participate in low levels of PA. Afrocentric dance has a strong cultural and historical significance in the African American community and can provide girls with sustained bouts of moderate-to-vigorous physical activity (MVPA) only. Only one vanguard study was conducted and found that Afrocentric dance resulted in positive impact on self-reported PA study in African American girls but not on objectively measured PA and was limited by lack of parental participation, an important correlate of child PA. Parent–child interventions among non-Hispanic white populations indicate that family-based interventions may have a beneficial impact on children's PA but are sparse. **Currently, there are no studies examining the effects of a mother–daughter Afrocentric dance program on the PA levels of African American girls.** Our overall goal is to examine the efficacy of a 12-week randomized control daughter–mother afterschool Afrocentric dance intervention among 50 mother–daughter pairs. Pairs will be randomly assigned to the dance intervention (n = 50) or to a comparison of health and wellness (control) intervention (n = 50). The intervention will utilize exercise intervention materials culturally adapted for and shown to be efficacious in our previous controlled trials in this ethnic group (R21 xxx; PI: Dr. Smith). Targets of the intervention are to meet US guidelines for physical activity among youth. The intervention draws from social cognitive theory and the transtheoretical model and includes strategies for family support to address the specific social, cultural, and economic challenges faced by this study population. The measures of compliance will include actigraphs. The proposed project builds upon the expertise of the investigative team in conducting randomized controlled trials of exercise interventions among African American girls and can readily be translated into practice in underserved and minority population. This proposal is **significant** in light of the growing rates of obesity and diabetes among African American youth and **innovative** in being the first, to our knowledge, to test a culturally modified intervention to increase physical activity among African American girls.

PART III

Submission and Resubmission

Submission of the Grant Proposal

17

The submission of a grant includes not only *scientific* sections such as the *Research Strategy* and human subjects protection but also *nonscientific* sections such as the biosketch, budget, and facilities. Because the National Institutes of Health (NIH) is the most typical funding source for epidemiology and preventive medicine, particularly for larger awards, this chapter uses NIH submission criteria as the primary example.

The NIH website instructions are extensive and tend to require considerable time to read and navigate; therefore, this chapter is designed to walk you step by step through the key required *scientific* and *nonscientific* components for the submission of your grant proposal to a funding agency and provides strategic tips for these forms.

In this spirit, I recommend exploring the All About Grants podcast in which the NIH Office of Extramural Research (OER) talks to NIH staff members about the ins and outs of NIH funding (https://grants.nih.gov/news/virtual-learning/podcasts.htm#3). Designed for investigators, fellows, students, and research administrators interested in the application and award process, the podcast provides additional insights on a wide range of NIH grant topics.

17.1 COMPONENTS OF THE GRANT PROPOSAL SUBMISSION

The NIH grant application instructions are described in great detail on their website in a document titled "General Instructions for NIH and Other Public Health Service (PHS) Agencies SF424 (R&R)": https://grants.nih.gov/grants/how-to-apply-application-guide/forms-f/general-forms-f.pdf. This document contains specific application instructions and links for: Research (R), Career Development (K), Training (T), and Fellowship (F) applications, among others. Be sure to check the website to see if there have been changes in policy since the publication of this text.

Table 17.1 highlights the **key** required components for the most typical NIH submissions. Note that Table 17.1 is divided into three sections. Section I includes the scientific component of the submission. Section II includes the nonscientific forms required of you. Sections II, IV, and V list the forms required from your collaborators. The table is not meant to be an exhaustive list of the forms, but instead focuses on key forms that you, as an investigator, can have a strategic hand in.

17.2 OVERALL FORMATTING GUIDELINES

NIH recommends the following fonts, although other fonts (both serif and non-serif) are acceptable if they meet the requirements below.

TABLE 17.1 Outline of the Scientific and Nonscientific Components of a Research Grant Submission

GRANT SUBMISSION COMPONENT	CHAPTER NUMBER
I. Scientific component	
a. Title	Chapter 16
b. Project Summary/Abstract	Chapter 16
c. Project Narrative	Chapter 16
d. Introduction to Application (for resubmission and revision applications)	Chapter 21
e. Specific Aims	Chapter 6
f. Research Strategy	Chapters 8–15
g. Training Information for Fellowship Grants (F series)	Chapter 18
h. Candidate Information for Career Development Grants (K series)	Chapter 19
i. PHS Human Subjects and Clinical Trials Information	**Current chapter**
j. Bibliography and References Cited	
II. Nonscientific Forms	
a. SF 424 (R&R) Form and other forms	
b. Facilities and other resources	
c. Equipment	
d. Biosketch	
e. Budget and budget justification	
f. Multiple PD/PI Leadership Plan	**Current chapter**
g. Resource Sharing Plan	
h. Authentication of Key Biological and/or Chemical Resources	
i. Appendix	
j. PHS Assignment Request Form	
III. Items Needed from Co-investigators at Your Institution	
a. Biosketches	**Current chapter**
b. Letters of Support	
IV. Items Needed from Subcontractors (at Other Institutions)	
a. Consortium/contractual arrangements	
b. Scope of work	
c. Budget and budget justification	
d. Biosketches	**Current chapter**
e. Facilities and other resources	
f. Equipment	
g. Letters of support	
V. Items Needed from Consultants	**Current chapter**
a. Biosketches	
b. Letters of support	

- Arial
- Georgia
- Helvetica
- Palatino Linotype

The **font size** must be 11 points or larger. Note that some PDF conversion software reduces font size; therefore, it is important to confirm that the final PDF document complies with the font requirements.

Smaller text in figures, graphs, diagrams, and charts is acceptable, as long as it is legible when the page is viewed at 100%. **Type density** must be no more than 15 characters per linear inch (including characters and spaces). **Line spacing** must be no more than six lines per vertical inch. Finally, there is no restriction on text color. However, note that black or other high-contrast text colors are recommended since they print well and are legible to the largest audience. Some reviewers who prefer to read hard copies of their assigned grant submissions may not have color printers.

17.2.1 Tips for Success

Tip #1: Strive for consistency in content. Even if your institution has a grants manager who assists you with these forms, as a Principal Investigator it is advantageous that you oversee and read all these components for consistency with the scientific component. For example, check for consistency between the research methods section, the biosketch personal statements, the budget justification, facilities statement, and the letters of support. Check for consistency in the delineated roles of your co-investigators between forms. Reviewers become concerned when they see internal inconsistencies.

Tip #2: Strive for consistency in tone. It is common for particular sections of the research strategy (e.g., the data analysis section) to be written by one of your co-investigators—such as a statistician. Read over and edit this section so that the writing style and content is consistent with the rest of the research strategy. Avoid the pitfall of simply cutting and pasting sections written by co-investigators into your research strategy without checking for errors.

Tip #3: Do not circumvent the strict formatting requirements (e.g., font size, margin size, and line spacing details). These requirements are designed to ensure equity across applicants in terms of proposal length. They are also designed to make the review easier on the reviewers— such that the proposal is readable and not densely packed. It is critical to follow these guidelines to the letter as failure to comply can be rationale for the grant not to be reviewed.

Chapter 5, "Scientific Writing," provides detailed strategies for scientific writing style, which will help you comply with these strict NIH page limitations. Several key tips from that chapter include:

- Use active voice
- Use figures and tables
- Be sure that every word is necessary
- Proofread

Remember that it takes longer to write a shorter research application. Only by reading and rereading your application will you have adequate time to make sure that every word counts.

17.3 SECTION I: SELECTED SCIENTIFIC FORMS

17.3.1 PHS Human Subjects and Clinical Trials Information Form

NIH has a helpful Decision Tool on their website titled "Am I Doing Human Subjects Research?" (https://grants.nih.gov/policy/humansubjects/research.htm), which is useful in determining whether your project involves non-exempt or exempt human subjects research. For example, Exemption 4 will be relevant for you if your proposed **research involves** the collection or study of existing data, or specimens, if the sources are publicly available or the information is recorded so subjects cannot be identified.

Most grant applications in epidemiology and preventive medicine involve human subjects, therefore you will be required to complete the **PHS Human Subjects and Clinical Trials Information Form**. Note that completion of sections of this form is required **whether or not** your study is proposing a clinical trial. The **PHS Human Subjects and Clinical Trials Information Form** is used to collect basic information along with study population characteristics, protection and monitoring plans, and a protocol synopsis (for clinical trials).

Table 17.2 provides an outline of the **PHS Human Subjects and Clinical Trials Information Form**, and key items are described in detail in the following sections of the chapter. Note that you will have already described many, if not all, of these aspects in the Study Design and Methods section of your Research Strategy (see Chapter 11, "Study Design and Methods"). Therefore, copying and pasting from your Research Strategy into this clinical trials form is recommended—in this way, you are killing two birds with one stone and ensuring consistency across the application.

TABLE 17.2   Outline of the PHS Human Subjects and Clinical Trials Information Form

Section 1—Basic information (**required for all studies involving human subjects**)
   1.1 Study title
   1.2 Is this study exempt from federal regulations?
   1.3 Exemption number
   1.4 Clinical trial questionnaire
   1.5 ClinicalTrials.gov identifier, if applicable.
Section 2—Study population characteristics (required for all studies involving human subjects unless Exemption 4)
   2.1 Conditions or focus of the study
   2.2 Eligibility criteria
   2.3 Age limits
  2.3.a Inclusion of individuals across the lifespan
   2.4 Inclusion of women and minorities
   2.5 Recruitment and retention plan
   2.6 Recruitment status
   2.7 Study timeline
   2.8 Enrollment of first participant
   2.9 Inclusion enrollment report
Section 3—Protection and monitoring plans (**required for all studies involving human subjects**)
   3.1 Protection of human subjects
   3.2 Is this a multi-site study that will use the same protocol to conduct non-exempt human subjects research at more than one domestic site?
   3.3 Data and safety monitoring plan
   3.4 Will a Data and Safety Monitoring Board be appointed for this study?
   3.5 Overall structure of the study team
Section 4—Protocol synopsis (**required for clinical trials only**)
   4.1 Study design
   4.2 Outcome measures
   4.3 Statistical design and power
   4.4 Subject participation duration
   4.5 Will the study use an FDA-regulated intervention?
   4.6 Is this an applicable clinical trial under FDAAA?
   4.7 Dissemination plan
Section 5—Other clinical trial-related attachments (**required for clinical trials only**)
   5.1 Other clinical trial-related attachments

Pitfall to Avoid   Although NIH instructions suggest that you can refer to relevant information in the **PHS Human Subjects and Clinical Trials Information Form** in writing your Research Strategy, in my experience, reviewers prefer that you mention these key aspects (e.g., recruitment and retention, statistical power) in **both** your *Research Strategy* **and** in the **PHS Human Subjects and Clinical Trials Information Form**. If reviewers sense that you are trying to circumvent the page length guidelines with these strategies, this can lead to an unhappy reviewer and a lower score to have your research strategy include these items.

17.3.1.1 Section 2: 2.3a Inclusion of Individuals across the Lifespan

The Inclusion of Individuals across the Lifespan requires that you justify the exclusion of any specific age or age range group (e.g., children or older adults). Individuals of all ages are expected to be included in all NIH-defined clinical research unless there are scientific or ethical reasons not to include them. For the purposes of NIH, a child is defined as an individual under the age of 18 years. This does not mean that your proposal must include such groups but that there needs to be a scientific rationale for their lack of inclusion. This can be straightforward. For example, a proposal to evaluate risk of Alzheimer's disease would likely not include children as they are not at risk for this disease.

Example Inclusion of Individuals Across the Lifespan
(Underlining for emphasis)
A proposal to conduct a lifestyle intervention in high-risk pregnant Hispanic women to prevent postpartum weight retention and risk of diabetes.
The population under study includes 300 pregnant and postpartum women between the ages of 18 and 45 years at Taylor Hospital. The study is designed to test a lifestyle intervention to control gestational weight gain and positively influence maternal metabolic profile; therefore, all subjects are women. <u>Mothers between the ages of 18 and 21 will be included.</u> <u>Mothers younger than 18 will not be included as modifiable determinants of gestational weight gain may differ substantively among pregnant women under age 18 therefore precluding direct applicability of hypotheses to this age group.</u> Hispanics have, overall, been underrepresented in prior research.

17.3.1.2 Section 2: 2.4 Inclusion of Women and Minorities

The section on Inclusion of Women and Minorities asks you to describe the planned distribution of subjects by sex/gender, race, and ethnicity in terms of the scientific objectives and proposed study design, and to describe proposed outreach programs for recruiting these groups. If you are limiting inclusion of any group by sex/gender, race, and/or ethnicity, as do many studies in epidemiology and preventive medicine, you are asked to provide a reason for limiting inclusion. This can be straightforward but needs to rely upon a scientific rationale. Avoid using logistics of cost as a reason not to recruiting certain groups.

Example Inclusion of Women and Minorities
(<u>Underlining for emphasis</u>)
Consider a proposal to conduct a lifestyle intervention in high-risk pregnant Hispanic women to prevent postpartum weight retention and risk of diabetes.
The population under study includes 300 pregnant and postpartum women between the ages of 18 and 45 years at Taylor Hospital. The study is designed to test a lifestyle intervention to control gestational weight gain and positively influence maternal metabolic profile; <u>therefore, all subjects are women.</u> <u>All subjects are Hispanic.</u> Hispanic women are the fastest-growing minority group in the United States and have the highest rates of sedentary behavior as well as elevated rates of prepregnancy overweight and obesity. Hispanics have, overall, been underrepresented in prior research.

17.3.1.3 Section 2: 2.5 Recruitment and Retention Plan

The **Recruitment and Retention Plan** form asks you to describe both planned recruitment activities and proposed engagement strategies for retention. Luckily, you will already have done this work in the Research Strategy section of the grant (see Chapter 11, "Study Design and Methods"). It is typical to simply copy and paste (and perhaps condense) the relevant section from the Research Strategy into this section. Take care not to use this section to save space in your Research Strategy as reviewers will be looking for your recruitment and retention efforts in the body of the grant.

17.3.1.4 Section 2: 2.7 Study Timeline

The Study Timeline is required if you answered "Yes" to all the questions in the "Clinical Trial Questionnaire" (i.e., your study is a clinical trial). It asks you to provide a description or diagram describing the study timeline. However, note that whether or not your study is a clinical trial, **including a timeline can strengthen your application**.

The timeline should be general (e.g., Year 1, first quarter, Year 2) and not refer to specific years and months (e.g., January 2024–April 2024). Be sure to include time for study start-up, participant assessments, subsequent data analysis, and final manuscript writing. Some overlap of phases of each activity is expected. For example, you may start collecting data for Aim 2 while you are working on manuscript writing for Aim 1. Similarly, if you are following participants over time, some preliminary data cleaning and analyses can occur during the follow-up time period.

Don't underestimate the time for data collection. Try to point to prior data when projecting the time it will take to recruit and adequate number of participants. And, most importantly, avoid the pitfall of continuing participant assessments to the very end of the study and not leaving time for data cleaning and data analysis.

The following example shows the timeline from the same proposal to evaluate the efficacy/impact of a pregnancy physical activity intervention on risk of gestational diabetes (Table 17.3).

17.3.1.5 Section 2: 2.9 Inclusion/Enrollment Report

An Inclusion/Enrollment Report is required for all human subjects studies unless your proposal falls under Exemption 4 (i.e., your proposed research involves the collection or study of existing data or specimens, if the sources are publicly available, or the information is recorded so subjects cannot be identified). Again, see the NIH Decision Tool (https://grants.nih.gov/policy/humansubjects/research.htm) to determine whether your project involves non-exempt or exempt human subjects research. Note that the majority of research in epidemiology and preventive medicine is **not** exempt. That is, at some point there will be an intervention or interaction with subjects for the collection of biospecimens or data (including health or clinical data, surveys, focus groups, or observation of behavior). Or, private information or identifiable biospecimens will be obtained, used, studied, analyzed, or generated for the purpose of this study. On the other hand, a proposal involving the use of a secondary dataset that is deidentified may qualify as exempt. In this situation, if the specimens or data were not collected specifically for your study and no one on your study team has access to the subject identifiers linked to the specimens or data, your study is not considered human subjects research. In your NIH application, you would indicate "No" to Human Subjects.

However, it is always wise to contact relevant NIH personnel first and, when in doubt, to include the complete section on protection of human subjects.

The Inclusion/Enrollment Report asks you to describe the planned enrollment at the study site(s) according to race/ethnicity and sex/gender categories. Planned enrollment generally means that individuals will be recruited into the study and/or that individuals have already been recruited and continue to be part of the study.

17.3.1.6 Section 3: 3.1 Protection of Human Subjects

For research that involves human subjects and is not considered exempt, you will need to include this section on **Protection of Human Subjects**. This section requires a justification for the involvement of human subjects

TABLE 17.3 Example Study Timeline

MONTH	YEAR 1						YEAR 2						YEAR 3						YEAR 4						YEAR 5					
	2	4	6	8	10	12	2	4	6	8	10	12	2	4	6	8	10	12	2	4	6	8	10	12	2	4	6	8	10	12
Training/protocol development	×	×	×																											
Recruitment				×	×		×	×	×	×	×	×	×	×	×	×	×	×	×	×	×	×	×							
Baseline assessment				×	×		×	×	×	×	×	×	×	×	×	×	×	×	×	×	×	×	×	×						
Intervention				×			×	×	×	×			×	×	×	×			×	×	×	×			×					
Follow-up assessment									×	×	×	×	×	×	×	×	×	×	×	×	×	×	×	×	×					
Diabetes screening						×						×						×			×			×	×					
Medical record review							×	×	×	×	×	×	×	×	×	×	×	×	×	×	×	×	×	×	×	×	×	×		
Analysis and manuscript writing																			×	×	×	×	×	×	×	×	×	×	×	×

TABLE 17.4   Outline of the Protection of Human Subjects Component of the Grant Submission

---

   i. **PHS Human Subjects and Clinical Trials Information Form**
     3.1   **Protection of human subjects**
         1.   Risks to human subjects
            a.   Human subjects involvement, characteristics, and design
            b.   Study procedures, materials, and potential risks
         2.   Adequacy of protection against risks
            a.   Informed consent and assent
            b.   Protections against risk
            c.   Vulnerable subjects, if relevant to your study
         3.   Potential benefits of the proposed research to research participants and others
         4.   Importance of the knowledge to be gained

---

and the proposed protections from research risk according to four criteria (see Table 17.4). Reviewers consider carefully issues in conducting research on humans in their overall *score* of your application.

17.3.1.7 *Data and Safety Monitoring Plan*

For any proposed clinical trial, NIH requires a data and safety monitoring plan (DSMP) that is commensurate with the risks of the trial, its size, and its complexity. The DSMP should describe the following:

- How many people and what type of entity will provide the monitoring (e.g., Principal Investigator, Independent Safety Monitor/Designated Medical Monitor, Independent Monitoring Committee, Data and Safety Monitoring Board [DSMB])
- What information will be monitored
- The frequency of monitoring including any plans for interim analysis and stopping rules
- The process by which adverse events will be managed and reported

NIH requires the establishment of Data and Safety Monitoring Board (DSMBs) for multi-site clinical trials involving interventions that entail potential risk to the participants; and generally, for all Phase III clinical trials, although Phase I and Phase II clinical trials may also need DSMBs. DSMBs are a formal independent board of experts including investigators and biostatisticians.

Example Data and Safety Monitoring Plan
This trial will be monitored in compliance with an independent Data and Safety Monitoring Board (DSMB) written in concordance with the guidelines from the National Institutes of Health. The DSMB will (1) review the research protocol and plans for data safety and monitoring; (2) evaluate the progress of the trial with biannual assessments of data quality and timeliness, participant recruitment, accrual and retention, participant risk versus benefit, and reports from related studies; and (3) make recommendations to the IRB and investigators concerning continuation or conclusion of the trial. The DSMB will consist of three members including a physician who will serve as Chair, a statistician, and an outside researcher at the University of Springfield all of whom will be knowledgeable about the study's content but not directly involved in the study nor in a supervisory role to study personnel. The DSMB will meet biannually. Prior to each meeting, the Principal Investigator will submit a report to the DSMB, which will include (1) safety of the protocol participants, specifically if any adverse events have occurred; (2) validity and integrity of the data; (3) enrollment rate relative to expectation; (4) retention of participants; (5) data completeness; and (6) preliminary data analysis. The Principal Investigator will receive a written response regarding the DSMB's approval or suspension of the study. The report will be forwarded to the Institutional Review Board. Monitoring activities by the Principal Investigator and the DSMB will continue until all participants have completed the study and are beyond the time point at which study-related adverse events would presumably be encountered.

17.3.2 Bibliography and References Cited

The NIH guidelines require a bibliography of all references cited in the research plan component and in the **Human Subjects and Clinical Trials Information** Form. Any standard scholarly format for citations is acceptable, but the references should be limited to relevant and current literature. While there is no page limitation for the bibliography, it is important to be concise and to select only those references pertinent to the proposed research.

One important tip is to not insert your references by hand, but instead use a reference manager such as Mendeley, EndNote, and RefWorks. Once you have the reference manager generate your reference list, be sure to double check that list corresponds to the correct articles and did not leave out important information such as volume and page numbers. And, finally, as noted earlier in Chapter 5, "Scientific Writing," use superscripted references to save space.

When you are citing articles that fall under the public access policy, were authored or coauthored by yourself, and arose from NIH support, provide *the NIH Manuscript Submission reference number* (e.g., NIHMS97531) or the *PubMed Central (PMC) reference number* (e.g., PMCID234567) for each article. If the PMCID is not yet available because the journal submits articles directly to PMC on behalf of their authors, indicate *PMC Journal—In Process*. NIH maintains a list of these journals is https://publicaccess .nih.gov/submit_process_journals.htm.

Citations that are not covered by the public access policy but are publicly available in a free online format may include URLs or PubMed ID (PMID) numbers along with the full reference.

You are also allowed to cite interim research products, but note that interim research products have specific citation requirements. See related Frequently Asked Questions for more information: https:// grants.nih.gov/faqs#/interim-research-product.htm.

17.4 SECTION II: NONSCIENTIFIC FORMS

17.4.1 SF 424 (R&R) Form and Other Forms

The **SF 424 (R&R) Form** is used in all grant applications. This form collects information including type of submission, applicant information, type of applicant, and proposed project dates. There are a number of other administrative pages required for an NIH grant submission (e.g., **Cover page supplement, R&R Other Project Information, Project/Performance Site Locations, R&R Senior/Key Person Profile Form**). Try to enlist a grants manager or office of grants and contracts to assist you in their completion.

17.4.2 Facilities and Other Resources

On the **Facilities and Other Resources** page, you are asked to describe how the scientific environment in which the research will be done contributes to the probability of success. This includes institutional support, physical resources (e.g., laboratory, animal, computer, office, and clinical), and intellectual rapport. For example, discuss the ways in which your proposed study will benefit from unique features of the scientific environment or from unique subject populations available to you or how you will employ useful collaborative arrangements. If there are multiple performance sites, describe the resources available at each site.

For early-stage investigators (ESIs), describe the institutional investment in your success. Your application will be strengthened by including the following elements if relevant:

- Resources for classes, travel, or training
- Collegial support, such as career enrichment programs, assistance and guidance in the supervision of trainees involved with your project, and availability of organized peer groups
- Logistical support, such as administrative management and oversight and best practices training
- Financial support, such as protected time for research with salary support

Tip for Success   Read over all the facilities statements including those sent to you by any off-site co-investigators) and be sure that the content and writing style is consistent with the remainder of your proposal. For example, if you state that you will assess participants in a sleep lab in your Research Strategy but the sleep lab is not included in the Facilities and Other Resource plan, this will raise a red flag among reviewers.

17.4.3 Equipment

List the major items of equipment already available for your project and, if appropriate, identify their location and pertinent capabilities. Again, watch for consistency with the remainder of your proposal.

17.4.4 Biosketch

The NIH provides a template for your **Biosketch**, which is divided into four subsections: sections A, B, C, and D, as described below. Note that the biosketch cannot exceed five pages.

A. *Personal statement*: This section asks you to briefly describe why you are well suited for your role(s) in this project. Relevant factors may include aspects of your training; your previous research on this specific topic or related topics; your technical expertise; your collaborators or scientific environment; and/or your past performance in this or related fields, including ongoing and completed research projects from the past three years that you want to draw attention to (previously captured under Section D of earlier versions of the biosketch).

It is recommended that you cite up to four publications or research products that highlight your experience and qualifications for this project. Research products can include conference proceedings such as meeting abstracts, posters, or other presentations; patents; data and research materials; databases; educational aids or curricula; software or netware; and others. Note that the use of hyperlinks and URLs to cite these items is not allowed. You are also allowed to cite interim research products. See related Frequently Asked Questions for more information: https://grants.nih.gov/faqs#/interim-research-product.htm. Note that figures, tables, or graphics are not allowed.

Tips for Success

Tip #1: Demonstrate relationships with your co-investigators. The personal statement should be used to describe established/ongoing relationships with your co-investigators, a critical factor in the review. Follow this up by including publications in Section C below that you have coauthored with your co-investigators, if available.

Tip #2: Adverse events. The personal statement is a good place to explain factors that adversely affected your past productivity, if relevant, such as family care responsibilities, illness, disability, or military service. In this section, you can also indicate whether you have published or created research products under another name.

Example Personal Statement (Section A) on an NIH Biosketch
I am an assistant professor of epidemiology in the Division of Epidemiology at the Jones School of Public Health. I am a reproductive epidemiologist with a focus on physical activity during pregnancy. The proposed project will build upon a history of collaboration among our investigative team in conducting culturally modified, motivationally targeted, individually tailored interventions among Hispanic women. I led the development and evaluation of the feasibility of the proposed lifestyle intervention in collaboration with Dr. Branson and Dr. Smith (co-investigators on the proposed study) in our pilot study, "Estudio Vida" (ASPH/CDC1234). My research experience has lent me an appreciation of both the importance and difficulties associated with study design, measurement, quality data management, and analyses that will be instrumental in conducting the proposed study.
Ongoing and recently completed projects that I would like to highlight include:
R01 DA942367
Branson (PI); Role: co-investigator
09/01/16-08/31/21
Health trajectories and behavioral interventions among older substance abusers

ASPH/CDC1234
Jones (PI)
09/01/20-08/31/21
Estudio Vida; a pilot feasibility study of a lifestyle intervention among Hispanic women.

B. *Positions, scientific appointments, and honors*: This section asks you to list in reverse chronological order all positions and scientific appointments. This includes titled academic, professional, or institutional appointments regardless whether or not remuneration is received, or whether full time, part time, or voluntary (including adjunct, visiting, or honorary). Students, postdoctorates, and early-career faculty should include scholarships, traineeships, fellowships, and development awards, as applicable.

C. *Contributions to science*: This section asks you to briefly describe up to five of your most significant contributions to science. The description of each contribution should be no longer than one half page, including citations. Graduate students and postdoctoral fellows may wish to consider highlighting two or three they consider most significant.

For each contribution to science, you are asked to describe the following:
- The historical background that frames the scientific problem
- The central finding(s)
- The influence of the finding(s) on the progress of science or the application of those finding(s) to health or technology
- Your specific role in the described work

Under each contribution description, you may cite up to four relevant publications. You should also provide a URL to a full list of your published work. This URL must be to a Federal Government website (a .gov suffix). NIH recommends using *My Bibliography*.

Potential pitfall to avoid   Co-investigators may send you versions of their biosketches that they've used on other grant applications. Therefore, check over their *personal statement* and make sure that their role is consistent with (1) the role that you delineated in the Research Strategy section, and (2) the budget justification section. Ensure that their selected list of publications includes those on which you've served as a coauthor and/or those that most directly relate to your study aims. Publications demonstrate the seniority of the co-investigator are also a plus (e.g., on which the co-investigator is the first or senior author, or those in top-ranked journals). For example, it would almost never make sense to leave out a *New England Journal of Medicine* paper.

Example Contribution to Science (Section C) on an NIH Biosketch

C. **Contributions to Science**

1. My early publications directly addressed the fact that substance abuse is often overlooked in older adults. However, because many older adults were raised during an era of increased drug and alcohol use, there are reasons to believe that this will become an increasing issue as the population ages. These publications found that older adults appear in a variety of primary care settings or seek mental health providers to deal with emerging addiction problems. These publications document this emerging problem and guide primary care providers and geriatric mental health providers to recognize symptoms, assess the nature of the problem and apply the necessary interventions. By providing evidence and simple clinical approaches, this body of work has changed the standards of care for addicted older adults and will continue to provide assistance in relevant medical settings well into the future. I served as the primary investigator or co-investigator in all of these studies.

   a. Gryczynski, J., Shaft, B.M., Merryle, R., & **Hunt, M.C.** (2013). Community based participatory research with late-life addicts. *American Journal of Alcohol and Drug Abuse*, 15(3), 222–238.

   b. Shaft, B.M., **Hunt, M.C.**, Merryle, R., & Venturi, R. (2014). Policy implications of genetic transmission of alcohol and drug abuse in female nonusers. *International Journal of Drug Policy*, 30(5), 46–58.

   c. **Hunt, M.C.**, Marks, A.E., Shaft, B.M., Merryle, R., & Jensen, J.L. (2015). Early-life family and community characteristics and late-life substance abuse. *Journal of Applied Gerontology*, 28(2), 26–37.

   d. **Hunt, M.C.**, Marks, A.E., Venturi, R., Crenshaw, W. & Ratonian, A. (2018). Community-based intervention strategies for reducing alcohol and drug abuse in the elderly. *Addiction*, 104(9), 1436–1606. PMCID: PMC1111000

17.4.5 Budget and Budget Justification

If available to you, engage the assistance of your office of grants and contracts to assist you with the budget and the budget justification section—a narrative in which you justify all your proposed costs, including personnel costs. Start this process early so that you can sketch out a draft budget.

Before such a meeting, be sure to calculate your power and sample size so that you have an approximate sense of the number of participants or samples that you will be analyzing. Think about the broad cost areas that you will include in the budget. Typical cost areas for grants in epidemiology and preventive medicine include

- Personnel
  - Professional (e.g., yourself and your co-investigators)
  - Staff (e.g., research assistants, health interviewers, health educators, laboratory personnel, data analysts)
  - Consultants
- Materials and supplies (e.g., computer supplies, participant monitors such as physical activity and sleep monitors)
- Other direct costs (e.g., computer lab charges, laboratory assays, travel, express mail, participant incentives)

There are two primary types of budget forms: the detailed **R&R Budget Form** and the PHS 398 **Modular Budget Form**. Generally, you will use the **R&R Budget Form** if you are applying for more than $250,000 per budget period in direct costs, and you will use the **Modular Budget Form** if you are applying for less than $250,000. The smaller research grants most typical of early-career investigators (e.g., R21s and R03s) require modular budgets. These budgets are simplified and do not require detailed categorical information. However, one caveat is that your institution may still require you to submit a detailed internal budget. Finally, some grant mechanisms or programs (e.g., training grants) may require other budget forms to be used.

Tips for the Budget Justification

Tip #1: Demonstrate established relationships with your co-investigators in the budget section. The budget justification section is an excellent place to describe the means by which you will communicate with your co-investigators. Recall that your co-investigators do not have to be at your institution as long as you have a clear plan for communication. Any remote/virtual relationship can be further bolstered by indicating that it has worked successfully in the past.

Example Personnel Section of a Budget Justification Demonstrating Established Relationships

Dr. Jones PhD, **Principal Investigator** (2.70 academic months and 0.90 summer months, years 1–5) assistant professor of epidemiology in the Division of Epidemiology at the School of Public Health. Dr. Jones will be responsible for the scientific conduct of the study and oversee all aspects of the project. These will include patient recruitment and follow-up, patient interviews, patient interventions, laboratory analysis, medical record review, data analysis and interpretation, and manuscript preparation. As in our pilot study, Dr. Jones will oversee quality control procedures ensuring that stage of change and social cognitive constructs are consistently represented in both the physical activity and dietary interventions. Dr. Jones will meet face to face with (1) the project manager weekly, (2) the statistician monthly, (3) the co-investigators at the recruitment sites monthly (Dr. Branson, Dr. Jones, and Dr. Smith), and (4) the intervention team via videoconference calls monthly (Dr. Smith, Dr. Francis, and Dr. Goldman). All the co-investigators and consultants will meet quarterly via videoconference calls as well as yearly in a face-to-face meeting.

Dr. Branson, PhD, **co-investigator** (0.45 academic months and 0.15 summer months in Years 1–5) is an associate professor of kinesiology at the School of Public Health whose research focuses on understanding how exercise, diet, and/or pharmacological agents interact to mediate insulin resistance and the risk for type 2 diabetes. Dr. Branson will provide expertise in the assessment and interpretation of the biomarker measures. He will participate, along with the other study investigators, in discussions of study design and in conducting analyses and disseminating study findings.

Tip #2: Check for consistency in the delineated roles of your co-investigators between forms. It is critical to check for consistency between the Research Strategy, the biosketch personal statements, the budget justification, and the letters of support. Similarly, reviewers will check that contributions delineated in letters of support match those mentioned in the Research Strategy and vice versa.

Tip #3: Ensure consistency between the budget justification section and the remainder of the proposal. Care should be taken that your budget justification section is consistent with your methods section. Inconsistencies can be viewed as a serious flaw in an application. For example, costs per participant listed in the budget justification should match the total number of projected participants outlined in your sample size calculations. Similarly, if you will use gift cards as a recruitment incentive, be sure to include the cost for these in the budget justification.

17.4.6 Multiple Principal Investigator Leadership Plan

The multi-Principal Investigator option presents an important opportunity for investigators seeking support for projects or activities that require a team science approach. NIH notes that the overarching goal of this option is to maximize the potential of team science efforts in order to be responsive to the challenges and opportunities of the 21st century.

If you are using this option, you will be asked to complete a Multiple Principal Investigator Leadership Plans which asks you to address the following administrative processes and Principal Investigator responsibilities:

- Roles/areas of responsibility of the Principal Investigators
- Fiscal and management coordination
- Process for making decisions on scientific direction and allocation of resources
- Data sharing and communication among investigators
- Policies for publication and intellectual property (if needed)
- Procedures for resolving conflicts

NIH provides examples of these plans: https://grants.nih.gov/grants/multi_pi/sample_leadership _plans.pdf

Tips for Success

Tip #1: If you are a new investigator, consider the appropriateness of the multiple Principal Investigator option. If you are a new investigator, it will be important to balance the benefits versus the potential downsides of choosing the multiple Principal Investigator option. Including an established Principal Investigator as a Co-principal Investigator may serve to reassure the reviewers of the feasibility of project and your ability to achieve your specific aims. However, it is important to note that the application will no longer be eligible for the new investigator payline (see Chapter 20, "Review Process"). Therefore, consider whether a career development award (K-series) might be more appropriate at this earlier point in your career. This type of application is described in Chapter 19, "Career Development Award", and will involve a mentor instead of another Principal Investigator

Tip #2. Consider your rationale for choosing a multiple Principal Investigator approach.
Reviewers like to see a solid, scientifically based answer to this question. Since the multiple Principal Investigator option is for collaborative, multidisciplinary research, be clear as to why your proposed research requires Principal Investigators with distinct and complementary expertise. For instance, describe why the Specific Aims of the project could not be accomplished without the combined leadership and expertise of all the Principal Investigators.

Pitfalls to avoid:　Weaker Leadership Plans tend to have poor organization, lack of specifics on roles and responsibilities, omit critical information such as plans for deciding scientific direction or resolving conflicts. Avoid the temptation to use additional Principal Investigators solely because they are prominent in your field as reviewers will become concerned if they don't have a truly distinct and independent role in the project. Another pitfall is stating that all Principal Investigators will take joint responsibility for all grant components (e.g., fiscal, compliance). Reviewers know that even with the closest collaborations, there will be times when Principal Investigators do not agree. Therefore, reviewers will look for a reasonable division of responsibilities to avoid a frequently implemented conflict resolution procedure.

Example Multiple Principal Investigator Leadership Plan
Principal Investigator #1 and Principal Investigator #2 will provide oversight of the entire program and development and implementation of all policies, procedures, and processes. In these roles, Principal Investigator #1 and Principal Investigator #2 will be responsible for the implementation of the scientific agenda, the Leadership Plan, and the specific aims and ensure that systems are in place to guarantee institutional compliance with US laws, DHHS, and NIH policies including biosafety, human and animal research, data, and facilities. Specifically, Principal Investigator #1 will oversee Aim 1. Principal Investigator #2 is responsible for Aims 2, 3, and 4 including the implementation of all human subjects research and approvals. Principal Investigator #1 will serve as contact Principal Investigator and will assume fiscal and administrative management including maintaining communication among Principal Investigators and key personnel through monthly meetings. She will be responsible for communication with NIH and submission of annual reports. The responsibilities of the contact Principal Investigator will be rotated to Principal Investigator #2 in even years of the grant award. Publication authorship will be based on the relative scientific contributions of the Principal Investigators and key personnel.

Intellectual Property: The Technology Transfer Offices at Institutions A and B will be responsible for preparing and negotiating an agreement for the conduct of the research, including any intellectual property. An Intellectual Property Committee composed of representatives from each institution that is part of the grant award will be formed to work together to ensure that the intellectual property developed by the Principal Investigators is protected according to the policies established in the agreement.

Conflict Resolution: If a potential conflict develops, the Principal Investigators shall meet and attempt to resolve the dispute. If they fail to resolve the dispute, the disagreement shall be referred to an arbitration committee consisting of one impartial senior executive from each Principal Investigator's institution and a third impartial senior executive mutually agreed upon by both Principal Investigators. No members of the arbitration committee will be directly involved in the research grant or disagreement.

Change in Principal Investigator Location: If a Principal Investigator moves to a new institution, attempts will be made to transfer the relevant portion of the grant to the new institution. In the event that a Principal Investigator cannot carry out his/her duties, a new Principal Investigator will be recruited as a replacement at one of the participating institutions.

17.4.7 Resource Sharing Plan

NIH considers the sharing of unique research resources developed through NIH-sponsored research an important means to further the advancement of research. Therefore, the **Resource Sharing Plan** includes plans for (1) data sharing, (2) sharing model organisms, and (3) genome wide association studies. The data sharing plan is unlikely to be relevant to early-career faculty or postdoctoral fellows as it is typically only required of very large projects. Specifically, investigators seeking $500,000 or more in direct costs in any year are expected to include a brief one-paragraph description of how final research data will be shared or explain why data sharing is not possible.

On the other hand, note that some specific Funding Opportunity Announcements (FOAs) may require that all applications include this information regardless of the dollar level. Therefore, it is important to read the specific FOA carefully. If so, in writing this section, discuss how raw data or other resources will be made available. Although a generic statement can be made, a more specific statement is preferred. Consider where data (particularly large file sizes) may be stored—both on-campus repositories to public access archives such as Dataverse or re3data.org.

Example Resource Sharing Plan

Research resources generated with funds from this grant will be freely distributed, as available, to qualified academic investigators for non-commercial research. Our institution (University of Springfield) will adhere to the NIH Sharing Policies and Related Guidance on NIH-Funded Research Resources including the NIH Research Tools Policy (Principles and Guidelines for Recipients of NIH Research Grants and Contracts on Obtaining and Disseminating Biomedical Research Resources). Should any intellectual property arise which requires a patent, we would ensure that the technology remains widely available to the research community in accordance with NIH Principles and Guidelines document.

Example General Data Sharing Plan

Final data will be shared primarily through the vehicle of peer-reviewed publication. Raw data will be considered for sharing under the following rules: Raw datasets to be released for sharing will not contain identifiers. Data and associated documentation will be made available to users only under a signed and properly executed data sharing agreement that provides for specific criteria under which the data will be used, including but not limited to (1) a commitment to using the data only for research purposes and not to identify any individual participant; (2) a commitment to securing the data using appropriate computer technology; and (3) a commitment to destroying or returning the data after analyses are completed.

17.4.8 Authentication of Key Biological and/ or Chemical Resources

This section asks you, if applicable to the proposed science, to briefly describe methods to ensure the identity and validity of key biological and/or chemical resources used in the proposed studies. A maximum of one page is suggested. This subsection relates to the rigor and reproducibility of the application (see Chapter 11, "Study Design and Methods"), which what reviewers look for as they evaluate the application for scientific merit. Key biological and/or chemical resources include, but are not limited to, cell lines, specialty chemicals, antibodies, and other biologics. Key biological and/or chemical resources may or may not have been generated with NIH funds and:

- May differ from laboratory to laboratory or over time
- May have qualities and/or qualifications that could influence the research data
- Are integral to the proposed research

NIH notes that the quality of resources used to conduct research is critical to the ability to reproduce the results. Each investigator will have to determine which resources used in their research fit these criteria and are therefore key to the proposed research.

17.4.9 Appendix

Read over the NIH guidelines for **Appendix** materials carefully and be sure to comply with them. A common pitfall is to try to use the Appendix as a way to circumvent the strict page limitations of the *Research Strategy* section. Reviewers are sensitive to this strategy and are not required to read appendices, although most try to do so. Refer to the FOA to determine whether there are any special **Appendix** instructions for your application.

Materials allowed in the Appendix:

- **Blank** data collection forms, blank survey forms, and blank questionnaire forms. Take care that these do **not** include data, data compilations, lists of variables or acronyms, data analyses, publications, manuals, instructions, descriptions, or drawings/figures/diagrams of data collection methods or machines/devices
- Simple lists of interview questions

- Blank informed consent/assent forms
- Other items *only if* they are specified in the FOA as allowable appendix materials

I can't emphasize enough to take care when including an Appendix. Simply relocating disallowed materials to other parts of the application will result in a noncompliant application. In other words, your application will be withdrawn and not reviewed if it does not follow the appendix requirements in these instructions or in your FOA.

17.4.10 PHS Assignment Request Form

The **PHS Assignment Request Form** requests the assignment of your application to up to three NIH institutes (termed "awarding components") and up to three NIH Scientific Review Groups (study sections). This form is optional but highly recommended in assisting NIH staff in correctly assigning your grant application as NIH receives thousands of applications per cycle.

See Chapter 4, "Choosing the Right Funding Source," for tips on findings the most relevant institutes for your application and Chapter 20, "Review Process," for tips on finding the most relevant study section.

In brief, each NIH institute provides information about its scientific mission and priorities on their websites. Similarly, the NIH Center for Scientific Review (CSR) website includes a description of each study section, their overall goals/objectives, and a list of the types of applications that they review. Take care that your proposed topic of interest fits within the goals/areas of the institute. For example, a grant focused on preventing postpartum depression as an outcome may or may not fit under the goals of the National Institute of Child Health and Human Development (NICHD) which tends to fund pregnancy research but instead may fit within the mission of National Institute of mental Health (NIMH) depending on their current listed priorities.

Quote key points from these descriptions in the **PHS Assignment Request Form** section on rationale (i.e., why you think the assignment is appropriate).

The NIH RePORTER website can also be useful in identifying institutes and study sections. Search on grants with similar topics and funding mechanisms, and the search output will provide the name of the NIH institute and study section which reviewed the application. A tool in NIH RePORTER, called "Matchmaker," allows you to paste your abstract/specific aims in a query box and get information about which NIH institutes/centers may have funded similar work in the past https://grants.nih.gov/grants/phs _assignment_information.htm#AwardingComponents.

Note that requested assignments are not guaranteed. However, if your application was inadvertently assigned to what you feel is an inappropriate study section or institute, you can contact the scientific research administrator (SRA) assigned to the application to clarify the fit of your application and to request reassignment if appropriate.

A pitfall to avoid   One caveat in terms of requesting an institute is if your application is in response to a Program Announcement (PA) or Request for Application (RFA). In this case, the list of institutes sponsoring these funding mechanisms will be prespecified, and you will need to choose one on this list. If multiple institutes are listed, you can specify which institute is your primary choice and also provide a second and third choice.

17.5 SECTIONS III, IV, V: ITEMS NEEDED FROM COLLABORATORS

17.5.1 Biosketches

Your collaborators (i.e., co-investigators, consultants) will be added to use the same **NIH biosketch** template. As noted above, be sure to assist them in modifying their biosketches to demonstrate your relationships with them. First, in the personal statement (Section A), describe your ongoing relationships with your co-investigators. Second, include publications (Section C), if available, that include your co-investigators as coauthors.

17.5.2 Letters of Support from Co-investigators and Consultants

If you have co-investigators and consultants on your project, the grant application is strengthened by including a signed letter from each collaborator that lists the contribution they intend to make and their enthusiasm for the proposal. Consultants will also need to state their rate for consulting services. These letters provide proof of principal for the reviewers and speak to the feasibility of the proposed project. Note that letters of support are not the same as letters of reference (also known as reference letters) which are required for some Career Development (K-series) applications as discussed in Chapter 19, "Career Development Grants."

As an early-career investigator, you will often find yourself in the position of soliciting collaborations with more senior faculty. Given their busy schedules, if they are willing to serve on your grant application, it is considered a courtesy for you to draft their letter of collaboration. They can certainly edit it as they see fit, but taking that first step of drafting the letter ensures timely receipt of this form and that the correct title and grant number (if a resubmission) will be referenced.

Recommended items to include in a letter of collaboration include:

- The title of the application
- The grant number (if a resubmission)
- Your prior history of collaboration if relevant (e.g., other grant funded research, publications, presentations)
- The importance of the topic of the grant proposal
- The role that the investigator will be playing

Finally, check for consistency in the delineated roles of your co-investigators between the letters of support and the Research Strategy, the biosketch personal statements, and the budget justification. Similarly, reviewers will check that contributions delineated in letters of support match those mentioned in the Research Strategy and vice versa.

Example Letter of Support for a Proposal of Physical Activity and Gestational Diabetes
[on letterhead]
Dear x [your name]:
I very much look forward to building on our previous work in connection with your proposed study, "Study Title." This proposal builds on our previous work [can insert grant numbers and titles here] and has the potential to advance our understanding of modifiable risk factors for gestational diabetes. It will provide an invaluable opportunity to comprehensively assess the frequency, intensity, and duration of physical activity during pregnancy: the first step toward critically examining the relationship between activity during pregnancy and gestational diabetes.
As we have discussed, I will be responsible, along with the other study investigators, for the analysis and dissemination of findings related to physical activity as well as weight gain and body fat distribution. I very much look forward to working with you on this important research.
Sincerely,
Dr. Smith
Co-investigator

17.5.3 Items Needed from Subcontractors (at Other Institutions)

If you have co-investigators from other institutions, they are considered subcontractors. Your institution's office of grants and contracts will communicate with theirs to complete the required forms. These consortium/contractual arrangements will include:

1. A scope of work
2. Detailed budget and budget justification
3. Biosketches
4. Facilities and other resources
5. Equipment

Tip for success While your grant officers communicate, you can work with your subcontractor Principal Investigator to help them draft their forms to ensure consistency with the Research Strategy. For example, be sure to carefully look over their scope of work, their biosketches, budget justification, and facilities document to ensure that everything is consistent, and where possible, that you demonstrate a track record of collaboration.

17.6 SETTING UP A TIME FRAME

NIH submission due dates are three times per year and termed cycle I, cycle II, and cycle III), typically corresponding to winter, spring and fall time periods https://grants.nih.gov/grants/how-to-apply-application-guide/due-dates-and-submission-policies/due-dates.htm. As noted in Chapter 2, "Setting up a Time Frame," it's ideal to start a grant application four months prior to the submission deadline. Table 2.1 in that chapter provides you with a step-by-step timeline.

Fellowship Grants* 18

This chapter focuses on fellowship grants (F-series awards), specifically Predoctoral and Postdoctoral Fellowships, which are a type of National Research Service Award (NRSA), https://researchtraining.nih.gov/programs/fellowships. The NRSA awards are named for Dr. Ruth L. Kirschstein, an accomplished scientist in polio vaccine development, who became the first female director of an NIH institute. She was a champion of research training and a strong advocate for the inclusion of underrepresented individuals in the scientific workforce.

The purpose of the fellowship award is to provide support to promising applicants with the potential to become productive, independent investigators in scientific health-related research fields relevant to the missions of participating NIH Institutes and Centers. It is essential to note that the fellowship awards are **primarily training awards** and not research awards. As such, they span the graduate school years as well as a postdoctoral period and largely fund the trainee's stipend but not research costs.

The NIH website instructions for Fellowship Grants are extensive and tend to require considerable time to read and navigate https://grants.nih.gov/grants/how-to-apply-application-guide/forms-e/fellowship-forms-e.pdf. Therefore, this chapter provides tips for success, pitfalls to avoid, and examples of reviewer comments.

A note: This textbook does not review the submission of Training Grants (T series) Ruth L. Kirschstein NRSA applications. These Institutional Training Programs are awarded to universities and are under the direction of a senior investigator who implements the program. Ask your department chair or mentor if your institution has such a training grant (e.g., T32 series for predoctoral students and/or postdoc trainees). You would then apply internally at your institution.

18.1 ARE YOU A GOOD CANDIDATE FOR A FELLOWSHIP GRANT?

Successful receipt of a fellowship grant reflects an investment in you and your potential for a career as an NIH-funded scientist. Therefore, consider your long-term goals when deciding whether you are a good candidate for a fellowship grant. Successful candidates for an F30 are interested in a career as a physician-scientist or other clinician-scientist. Successful candidates for an F31 have an excellent academic record, plan to subsequently become a postdoctoral fellow, and ultimately plan to obtain a faculty position in which they are doing independent research. Lastly, successful candidates for both the F31 and F32 have the strong potential to develop into productive, independent researchers.

Major considerations in the review are your potential for a productive career, your **need for the proposed training**, and the degree to which the research training proposal, the sponsor, and the environment will satisfy those needs. The **ideal fellowship application** is submitted by a candidate with high career potential, a strong mentorship team, and who proposes a research plan that is well balanced between originality and feasibility. (Note that the proposed research cannot involve leading an independent clinical trial, but can be within a clinical trial led by a sponsor or co-sponsor.)

---

* The author would like to acknowledge the expert contributions of Dr. Rebecca Spencer to this chapter.

DOI: 10.1201/9781003155140-21

TABLE 18.1 Overview of Characteristics of F-Series Grants for Predoctoral Students and Postdoctoral Fellows

PROGRAM	TARGET GROUP	YEARS OF SUPPORT	TIME OF APPLICATION
F30 Individual Predoctoral MD/PhD or other Dual-Doctoral Degree Fellowship Award	Mentored doctoral students enrolled in a Dual-Doctoral Degree program (e.g., MD/PhD, DDS/PhD, DVM/PhD, AuD/PhD, DO/PhD)	Up to six years of support during which at least 50% of the award period must be devoted to graduate research training	Typically in Year 4 and no later
F31 Predoctoral Fellowship Award	Mentored doctoral students performing dissertation research	Up to five years (typically two to three years) of support; the award period must be devoted to full-time research training (40 hours/week)	Typically in Year 3 and after an approved dissertation proposal (admitted to candidacy)
F31 Fellowship to Promote Diversity in Health-Related Research	Mentored doctoral students, performing dissertation research, from diverse backgrounds/including those from groups that are underrepresented in the biomedical, behavioral, or clinical research workforce	Up to five years (typically two to three years) of support; the award period must be devoted to full-time research training (40 hours/week)	Typically in Year 3 and after an approved dissertation proposal (admitted to candidacy)
F32 Postdoctoral Fellowship	Mentored postdoctoral training under the guidance of a faculty sponsor	Up to three years; the award period must be devoted to full-time research training (normally 40 hours/week)	Typically in Year 1 or 2 of a postdoc fellowship

In addition to the options above, also note that the **F99/K00 Predoctoral to Postdoctoral Fellow Transition Award** spans both the fellowship and career development phases. Specifically, the first phase (F99) supports up to two years of research training for individuals in PhD or dual-degree clinician-scientist programs. The second phase (K00) provides up to three years of mentored postdoctoral research career development support.

Table 18.1 provides an overview of characteristics of each of the fellowship grants for Predoctoral Students and Postdoctoral Fellows: the target group, years of support, and typical time of application within your training program. The decision to apply should not be taken lightly as the full application for a fellowship grant, with all its required forms, can be more than 60 pages. In other words, the application requires a large-time investment and significant advance planning (see the timeline at the end of the chapter). Some universities have fellowship grant writing programs or "clubs" to provide support during this process.

18.1.1 Consider if You Have a Strong Mentorship Team at Hand

Fellowship grants do not fund the research project and instead fund the mentorship/training plan. Therefore, they require a primary sponsor. A co-sponsor or mentoring team is also highly recommended. Most typically, the Principal Investigator of the lab in which you are conducting your research, or your dissertation committee chair, would serve as your **primary sponsor**. They should be able to mentor you in the content area and in career trajectory that you have selected and should have a key role in helping you to prepare the application.

That being said, it is critical to note that *either* your **primary sponsor** or the **co-sponsor** be a senior investigator (i.e., Full or Associate Professor) with a track record of NIH funding (specifically R01 or equivalent research funding) and a strong publication record. You can check out their funding record yourself on NIH RePORTER (select all awards, not just active awards) and their publication record (e.g., on PubMed). Just as importantly, either your primary sponsor or the co-sponsor should have a successful track record of mentoring including, ideally, other fellowship grant awardees.

A **co-sponsor** is not required but can be strategically selected to fill any gaps. Specifically, the co-sponsor can provide additional training and mentoring to complement the primary sponsor's strengths or weaknesses. For example, if your primary sponsor is an assistant professor, reviewers may consider that they are too early in their career to have the mentorship experience you require. In this case, a co-sponsor that is a full professor would be key. If your primary sponsor has not had recent research funding, a co-sponsor with active NIH funding will strengthen your application. Other gaps may be more around the research area. For example, if your primary sponsor does not have expertise in all the aspects of your proposed research plan—particularly if your research will combine two or more areas of expertise—a co-sponsor can fill this gap. For grants in epidemiology and preventive medicine, reviewers will also look for a statistical sponsor on the team.

If you choose to involve a co-sponsor, a **track record of collaboration** between your primary sponsor and your co-sponsor(s) will be considered a strength. Collaboration can include co-mentored trainees, co-authored publications and presentations, as well as collaboration on funded grants.

Similarly, **consultants**, **collaborators**, and/or **advisory committee members** are not required but can be strategically selected to fill any gaps. The key point to consider is that every person included should have a unique role. Note that while collaborators always play an active role in the grant, consultants typically help fill in smaller gaps by, for example, supplying software, providing technical assistance or training, or setting up equipment (however, they may also play a more active role as well).

Tips for Success in Choosing Your Mentorship Team

> **Tip #1:** Keep your team of investigators (i.e., sponsors, consultants, collaborators) small (e.g., three to five members) so that reviewers don't become concerned that there are "too many cooks in the kitchen." At the same time, if you are a doctoral student applying for an F31 grant, a mentoring committee is considered a plus.
>
> **Tip #2:** Avoid selecting a sponsor and co-sponsor who are **both** early-career faculty members as this raises a gap of mentoring experience that neither role can fill.
>
> **Tip #3:** Avoid selecting highly overcommitted sponsors (e.g., with too many mentees) or off-site sponsors as this may raise a red flag for reviewers. This is true even if the sponsor is internationally acclaimed; reviewers may be concerned that they are overcommitted and will not have adequate time to dedicate to your project.

18.1.2 Consider Your Experience Thus Far

In practice, approximately half of successful applicants for the F30 and F31 grantees have at least one first author publication (some reviewers look for at least three) and more than half of successful F32 grantees have three or more first author publications (some reviewers look for five to ten). Expectations will also vary depending on the year that you are in your program. For example, an application for a predoctoral F31 training grant who is in their second year of training will not be expected to have as many publications as an F31 applicant in their fourth year of training.

On a related note, consider the timing of your application. Some reviewers consider the date by which the funds would be received (see https://grants.nih.gov/grants/how-to-apply-application-guide/due

-dates-and-submission-policies/due-dates.htm) and compare this to the time remaining in your training program. If the remaining time is short, a reviewer may conclude that you will be nearing the end of your training and that you will no longer require funding to complete this process. At the same time, they may expect more publications due to the elapsed time in your program.

18.1.3 Eligibility

At the time of the award, candidates must be citizen or non-citizen nationals of the United States or permanent resident. Individuals on temporary or student visas are not eligible. Applicants to F30 and F31 Fellowship Grants must be enrolled in a program in the biomedical, behavioral, health services, or clinical sciences. F32 applicants must have a research or clinical doctoral degree from an accredited US or foreign institution. All applicants must show evidence of both high academic performance in the sciences and commitment to a career as an independent research scientist.

18.1.4 Consider the Benefits of a Fellowship Grant

The receipt of a Fellowship Grant is associated with a number of benefits. Because it is a competitive award, it will provide strong evidence of your success with grantsmanship, and position you well to compete for future grants. If you are a doctoral student, successful receipt of an F31 will position you well to obtain a subsequent F32 grants, and if you are a postdoctoral fellow, receipt of an F32 will position you well to compete for a subsequent Career Development Award (K series) (see Chapter 19, "Career Development Awards"). Therefore, consider applying for a Fellowship Grant even if you are already fully funded in your program.

If you are a doctoral student, the F31 grant application can serve as your dissertation proposal, and therefore will "kill two birds with one stone" by providing you with grant writing experience and a completed dissertation proposal at the same time. If awarded, the F31 would enable you to work on your dissertation full time. On the flip side, as noted earlier in the chapter, the application process includes a number of other required forms aside from the content of your dissertation proposal. Therefore, the application process and the additional courses that you may take as part of your proposed training plan, could slow down your dissertation progress.

Other benefits of Fellowship Grants include a stipend and monies toward tuition and fees. The applicant can request an institutional allowance to help defray the cost of fellowship expenses such as health insurance, research supplies, equipment, books, and travel to scientific meetings.

18.1.5 Before You Make a Final Decision

As with other funding mechanisms, it is particularly helpful to view examples of successfully funded fellowship applications to get a good sense of their depth and scope and whether they are appropriate for you. Search on NIH RePORTER http://projectreporter.nih.gov/reporter.cfm and limit your search to F-series projects, the institutes where your research will fall, and your key terms. The National Institute of Allergy and Infectious Diseases (NIAID) also posts examples of successfully funded fellowship applications on their website https://www.niaid.nih.gov/grants-contracts/three-new-f31-sample-applications. While these applications may not be in your area of expertise, they will give you an excellent sense of the components required.

You can also look up award success rates for F-series awards on the NIH website: https://report.nih.gov/funding/nih-budget-and-spending-data-past-fiscal-years/success-rates. The pay line is set for each fiscal year depending on the budget approved by congress and the number of applications received.

18.2 OUTLINE OF A FELLOWSHIP GRANT APPLICATION

Table 18.2 provides an outline of the key components required for the Fellowship Grant submission. Also included are the components of a standard research grant application which were described in Chapters 8–15. Therefore, the remainder of this chapter focuses on the *new sections required* (e.g., Applicant's Background and Goals for Fellowship Training) highlighted in **bold** in Table 18.2 but also provides strategic tips for the standard sections of a grant submission.

TABLE 18.2 Outline of the Key Components of the Fellowship Grant Submission

GRANT SUBMISSION COMPONENT	CHAPTER NUMBER
I. Scientific component	
a. Title	Chapter 16
b. Project summary/abstract	Chapter 16
c. Project narrative	Chapter 16
d. Introduction to application (for resubmission applications)	Chapter 21
e. **Applicant's background and goals for fellowship training**	**Current chapter**
f. **Specific aims**	**Current chapter**
g. **Research strategy**	**Current chapter**
h. **Training information for fellowship grants (F series)**	
i. **Respective contributions**	
ii. **Selection of sponsor and institute**	
iii. **Training in the responsible conduct of research**	**Current chapter**
iv. **Sponsor and co-sponsor statements**	
v. **Letters of support from collaborators, contributors, and consultants**	
vi. **Institutional environment and commitment to training**	
i. PHS human subjects and clinical trials information	Chapter 17
j. Bibliography and references cited	Chapter 17
II. Nonscientific forms (selected items)	
a. SF 424 (R&R) form and other forms	Chapter 17
b. **Facilities and other resources**	**Current chapter**
c. **Biosketch**	**Current chapter**
d. **Budget**	**Current chapter**

18.3 PROJECT SUMMARY/ABSTRACT

The Project Summary/Abstract for a fellowship grant is limited to 30 lines of text but, in addition to summarizing the research project to be conducted under the fellowship award, the Project Summary/Abstract for a fellowship grant also describes the Fellowship Training Plan and the environment in which the training will take place. Table 18.3 provides an outline for the Project Summary/Abstract for a fellowship grant, highlighting in bold the differences between this outline and the Project Summary/Abstract outline for a Research award (R series) as described in Chapter 16.

TABLE 18.3   Project Summary/Abstract Outline for a Fellowship Application

> I. Significance and innovation
> II. **Fellowship specific sentences**
>   A. **Long-term career goal**
>   B. **Training goals for this fellowship**
>   C. **Summary of training activities**
> III. Highlights of the approach (methodology)
> IV. Specific aims and hypotheses
> V. Summary of the significance and innovation

Note that the key differences between this fellowship outline and the outline for a research award are the insertion of sentences on your long-term career goal and training goals and activities to meet this career goal. The following *fill-in-the-blank exercise* is a helpful first step. Engage your mentor in this task.

1. Long-term career goal: _____
2. Training Goals to meet the above long-term career goal: (1) _____,
   (2) _____, (3) _____
3. Training Activities to reach the above training goals: _____

See Section 18.4 for more help on clarifying your training goals and activities.

In order to meet the 30 line limit for the Abstract with these new insertions, Sections I, III, IV, and V are somewhat condensed. Searching on NIH RePORTER for F-series projects will provide you with examples of fellowship grant abstracts.

Example Project Summary/Abstract for a Fellowship Application (Fellowship application-specific sentences are underlined):
<u>The goal of the proposed fellowship is to prepare the applicant, Jane Doe, a doctoral student in Epidemiology at Spring University, for an independent research career focused on informing approaches to reduce risk of Alzheimer's disease through the understanding of modifiable sensory and social risk factors. The applicant will be supported by a strong mentorship team with expertise in cognitive aging, social isolation, and statistical and epidemiologic methods. The Research Training Plan will help Ms. Doe (a) learn and apply rigorous methods for analysis of longitudinal data; (b) strengthen content expertise in social and cognitive Alzheimer's disease risk factors; and (c) effectively disseminate her findings and strengthen skills in teaching and leadership. Therefore, the proposed fellowship consists of two complementary components: (1) a research project that aims to assess the impact of social isolation on risk for Alzheimer's disease; and (2) a training plan composed of mentored research, didactic and informal training, and professional development.</u> In the absence of effective treatments, interventions to reduce Alzheimer's disease risk are critical. There is scientific premise to suggest social isolation is a strong risk factor for Alzheimer's disease, yet there is gap in the research in this area. In addition to conferring Alzheimer's disease risk, social isolation can impact efficacy of current Alzheimer's disease interventions yet is rarely considered in intervention design and implementation. To fill these gaps, this project proposes to use longitudinal data from the senior randomized controlled trial to investigate (1) the associations between social isolation and nine-year cognitive change and incident dementia; (2) socioeconomic status as a moderator of the social isolation—cognitive change and incident dementia associations; and (3) social isolation as a moderator of cognitive training intervention effects on ten-year cognitive change and incident dementia. The proposed research directly addresses high priority areas for NIA. The 2020-2025 NIA Strategic Directions for Research on Aging calls for more research to support "interventions for treating, preventing, or mitigating the impact of age-related diseases and conditions" (Goal 1.2). Findings from the proposed study may support inclusion of social isolation mitigation in multi-domain Alzheimer's disease interventions that promote health in older adults.

18.4 APPLICANT'S BACKGROUND AND GOALS FOR FELLOWSHIP TRAINING

Although each of these sections is crucial to success, most reviewers would agree that the Fellowship Training Plan sets the tone. A well-organized and carefully designed "Applicant's Background and Goals for Fellowship Training" section reflects a candidate who has clearly identified the training skills that are critical for their eventual success as an independent investigator. And, at the same time, it communicates to a reviewer that the mentor has been very actively involved in designing the grant. The Fellowship Training Plan is often the first section that is closely read by a reviewer, first impressions matter. This section is limited to six pages and should include the following subsections outlined in Table 18.4.

TABLE 18.4 Outline for Applicant's Background and Goals Section of a Fellowship Application

A. Doctoral dissertation and research experience	1–2 pages
B. Training goals and objectives	1–2 pages
C. Activities planned under this award	2–3 pages
1. Training plan	
a. Training activities for Goal # 1	
b. Training activities for Goal # 2	
c. Training activities for Goal # 3	
d. Training activities for Goal # 4	
2. Table of training activities for each training goal	
3. Monitoring applicant's progress	

The key concept to consider here is that, unlike a Research award (e.g., an R-series award such as an R21 R03, or an R01), the fellowship grant is intended to fund you, the candidate, as opposed to your research. Therefore, fellowship grants can (and should) be written in the first person (e.g., use "I/my" instead of "we/our"). In this section, your goal is to emphasize what makes you **unique**.

18.4.1 A. Doctoral Dissertation and Research Experience

Write this section chronologically starting with any undergraduate research experience and continue on to your graduate research experiences including your doctoral dissertation work. If you have had no research experience, describe other scientific experiences. The key is to describe how all of these experiences ultimately relate to the proposed fellowship. For example, will the fellowship build directly on your previous research experiences, results, and/or conclusions? Or have your past research experiences to led you to apply for a fellowship in a new or different area of research? Both these narratives are equally acceptable. Be sure to explain this to the reader. Note that coursework should **not** be listed in this section, however, if you had **poor academic grades** in the past or faced other challenges, you can address this up-front here. For example, you could describe how once you found your research niche, then you started to succeed. Your sponsor letter can also support this assertion as well.

This is a key section where you can talk about how long you've been interested in and working to achieve your proposed goals. Ideally this section will provide evidence of your commitment to a productive independent scientific research career in a health-related field—a major consideration in the overall impact score that reviewers give your application.

18.4.2 B. Training Goals and Objectives

Start this section by describing your overall long-term career goals and how the fellowship will enable the attainment of these goals. Then, specify your training goals (see the fill-in-the-blank exercise in Section 18.3). Training goals should be in two or three distinct areas in which you need training, that are outside of your current PhD or postdoctoral program, that will *facilitate your transition to the next career stage*, and ultimately achieve your long-term goal.

Determining your **long-term career goal**, beyond your doctoral degree should be made in conversation with your mentor. Most typically, reviewers expect your long-term career goal is to become a research professor at an R1-level institution. (R1 research institutions are those that meet benchmarks in research activity and expenditures as measured by the Carnegie Classification of Institutions of Higher Education.) Other objectives are acceptable, but may catch the reviewer's eye and require clear explanation of (1) your reasoning and motivation and (2) that you will continue to conduct research in a health-related field consistent with the goal of the NRSA.

In terms of the content of your career focus, there are several approaches to consider. One common option is for your long-term career goal to directly build upon the type of research you are pursuing for your dissertation, particularly if this is novel work that is relatively independent of your dissertation advisor's work. A second option is for your long-term career goal to build on the foundation of your dissertation work to launch you in a new direction to establish your own area of research. This would be a recommended option if your dissertation work is very close to your dissertation advisor's work. Note this clearly in your application.

The **training goals and objectives** should be uniquely suited to your current stage, being sure to take into account your previous training and research experiences. For example, F30 and F31 applicants are closer to the beginning of their career training, and therefore their goals should focus more on obtaining the broad base of knowledge and skills and that they need to develop into a strong scientist. In contrast a postdoctoral applicant for an F32 has already obtained this knowledge and, therefore, their training goals should focus more on obtaining the techniques/skills that are essential for them to transition into an independent academic position.

In other words, think of this section like a specific aims page for a research grant, in which the career goal is your overall goal, your proposed training goals are your specific aims, and the training activities are the methods you will use to achieve these specific aims.

18.4.2.1 Example Training Goals

In general, training goals for a fellowship grant encompass the following four general topics:

1. **Research fundamentals** that reviewers see as critical for up and coming researchers (e.g., statistics, experimental design, computational modeling, disease physiology, theoretical frameworks for social determinants of health)
2. **Research techniques** you seek to acquire (e.g., data collection, approaches for analysis)
3. **Career skills** (e.g., manuscript preparation, presentation skills, grant writing, networking)
4. **Responsible conduct of research**

Example Training Goals for a Postdoctoral F32 Fellowship Application

Consider an F32 applicant whose long-term career goal is to conduct independent ovarian cancer research and teach at a research-intensive university.

Training Goals
1. Gain an updated and more in-depth understanding of ovarian cancer biology and epidemiology
2. Gain additional experience in complex ovarian cancer-related data analyses such as risk prediction modeling and assessment of disease heterogeneity
3. Produce additional high-impact peer-reviewed publications
4. Improve my ability to communicate my own research, and ovarian cancer research more generally, to both scientific and nonscientific audiences
5. Develop expertise in grant writing and management
6. Maintain responsible conduct of research

18.4.3 C. Activities Planned under This Award

18.4.3.1 Training Plan

In this section, repeat each of your training goals, and below each one, list the specific training activities that correspond to that goal. Just as with writing your Research Strategy (see Chapters 8–15) in which you identified a research gap, in this section you will identify your **training gap** and what you will do to fill this gap (i.e., the specific training activities). Specifically clarify why you can't fill these gaps within your current degree program.

For F30 applications (Predoctoral MD/PhD or other Dual-Doctoral Degree), state how the training plan facilitates your transition to a residency or other program appropriate for your career goals.

For F31 and F32 applications, the training plan should state how it facilitates your transition to the next stage of your career.

Look at examples of training plans within successfully funded fellowship applications. Your university's grants office and/or your sponsor may be able to provide you with a list of former successful F-award recipients at your institution. It is considered acceptable to reach out to them to ask if they would be willing to share their application, not for the subject area content, but to get a sense of the depth and scope.

18.4.3.2 Example Training Activities

In general, training activities for a fellowship grant encompass the following general areas:

1. **Courses/workshops and journal clubs** that are *not* a standard part of your program. These can be outside of your current university.
2. **Structured mentor training** (e.g., include regular one-on-one meetings with your sponsor, co-sponsor, consultants, and collaborators).
3. **Research training** (e.g., your research training project, hands-on laboratory experiences).
4. **Professional development** (e.g., networking/collaboration building, conferences, working groups, learning laboratory management, search for an independent faculty position).

All three categories of training activities can be used to address your training goals outlined in the above section.

Tip for Success   It is important that your training activities be concrete and specific. For example, instead of stating, "I will attend a workshop in statistics," instead say "I will enroll in the Hierarchical Linear Modeling Workshop offered through the Center for Research on Families annually in June of each year, taught by Dr. XX."

Note that for F30 applications (Predoctoral MD/PhD or other Dual-Doctoral Degree), the training plan should provide opportunities to integrate clinical experiences into the training plan as well a plan for a smooth transition to the clinical training component.

18.4.3.3 Table of Training Activities over Time

Insert a table showing the planned training activities to meet each of your training goals. Organize the table by quarter and year of the award. Below each training goal, briefly describe each training activity using bullet points. Specifically, describe, by year, the activities you will be involved in during the proposed award. These different aspects of training include research training, professional development, coursework/teaching/mentoring, and clinical activities (if relevant). Professional development can encompass the writing of manuscripts and grants, presenting your work, and networking. For postdoctoral fellows, professional development should include the learning of laboratory management and the search for an independent faculty position.

TABLE 18.5   Example percent time in activities in an F32 Postdoctoral Fellowship Application

	RESEARCH (%)	PROFESSIONAL DEVELOPMENT (%)	TEACHING/MENTORING/ (%)	CLINICAL (%)	TOTAL (%)
Year 1	90	5	5	0	100
Year 2	90	5	5	0	100
Year 3	85	10	5	0	100

Include the percent time you will devote to each activity (or group of activities), being sure it totals to 100% per year. These percent efforts should change as the training period progresses and take into account that the primary role of your training is research. For example, a postdoctoral researcher may have 5% effort in professional development in the first two years; however, the final year of training will also involve the search for an independent faculty position which involves a higher level of professional development (Table 18.5).

Structure your plan so that reviewers can see how the training plan corresponds to your research plan. Reviewers will check to see that you can clearly achieve your training goals in the appropriate timeline.

Note that detailed timelines of research activities involving human subjects or clinical trials are requested in other sections of the fellowship application and should not be included here but be certain they are aligned.

Finally, take great care to ensure that your table of training activities is consistent with mentoring team roles described in the Sponsor and Co-sponsor Statements (Table 18.6).

Potential pitfall to avoid   Be sure not to omit relevant coursework, planned presentations and manuscripts, or hands-on experience in your training plan. Reviewers will focus on these areas.

Example Reviewer Comment on Training Activities in a Fellowship Grant Application
Weaknesses
No relevant coursework is planned during the proposed fellowship. The candidate could benefit from taking advanced methods courses on predictive modeling, etc. This would be a missed opportunity given the proposed length of the fellowship (i.e., three years). No planned presentations or manuscript writing are described within the scope of the proposed training plan. It is not clear how much direct hands-on experience the candidate will have on analyzing data. Proposed length of time (three years) seems too long.

18.5 RESEARCH TRAINING PLAN: SPECIFIC AIMS AND RESEARCH STRATEGY

The Research Training Plan is required for all types of fellowship awards and is a major part of the application. Note that the Research Training Plan is a training vehicle; it should be tailored to your experience level and provide an opportunity for you to acquire the necessary skills for further career advancement. It should also be well integrated with the training goals and activities you described in the prior section.

In this spirit, your mentor should be very involved in the development of your research strategy. Indeed, any reviewer concerns about the research strategy are typically ascribed to your sponsor and indicate to reviewers that inadequate mentoring may be occurring.

Remember that unlike a research grant (e.g., an R-series proposal), you can use the first person (e.g., "I") to show ownership of ideas and plans.

TABLE 18.6   Example Timeline of Fellowship Activities for an F32

TRAINING GOAL / TRAINING ACTIVITIES	YEAR 1	YEAR 2	YEAR 3
1. Gain an in-depth understanding of ovarian cancer biology and epidemiology	**15%**	**17%**	**8%**
Coursework/workshops:			
Attend Department Seminar Series	X	X	X
Take graduate-level Molecular Biology Course	X		
Take graduate-level Cancer Biology Course		X	
Structured mentored training:			
Observe in co-sponsor's lab		X	
Attend mentor meetings*	X	X	X
Professional development:			
Attend University's Office of Professional Development workshops	X	X	X
Attend two seminar series	X	X	X
Attend national conference workshops	X		
Participate in Ovarian Cancer and Pathology Working Groups	X	X	X
2. Improve my ability to communicate my own research, and ovarian cancer research more generally, to both scientific and nonscientific audiences	**2%**	**2%**	**2%**
Teaching experience:			
Guest lecture for graduate-level Cancer Epidemiology Course	X	X	X
Structured mentored training:			
Attend mentor meetings*	X	X	X
Professional development:			
Present at Biostatistics and Epidemiology Department Seminar	X	X	X
Attend/present at one to two annual scientific conferences	X	X	X
Assist mentor in mentoring undergraduate and graduate students			
3. Develop expertise in grant writing and management	**0.5%**	**0.5%**	**10%**
Structured mentored training:			
Attend mentor meetings*	X	X	X
Professional development:			
Participate in Department Grant Writing Brown Bag Lunch	X	X	X
Attend University's Office of Professional Development grant writing workshops	X	X	X
Develop K grant (K99/R00)			X
4. Gain additional experience in complex ovarian cancer-related data analyses such as risk prediction modeling and assessment of disease heterogeneity	**70%**	**70%**	**70%**
Structured mentored training:			
Attend mentor, co-mentor, consultant, collaborator meetings*	X	X	X
Research training:			
Setup data (Aims 1–3)	X		
Conduct Aim #1 analysis	X		
Conduct Aim #2 analysis	X		
Conduct Aim #3 analysis		X	
Setup data (Aim 4)		X	
Conduct Aim #4 analysis			X

(Continued)

TABLE 18.6 (CONTINUED)   Example Timeline of Fellowship Activities for an F32

TRAINING GOAL	TRAINING ACTIVITIES	YEAR 1	YEAR 2	YEAR 3
5. Produce high-impact publications		**10%**	**10%**	**10%**
Professional development:				
Participate in writing group		X	X	X
Complete manuscripts (n = 3)		X	X	X
6. Responsible conduct of research		**2.5%**	**0.5%**	**0%**
Take graduate-level Responsible Conduct of Research Course		X		
Complete CITI Biomedical Refresher			X	
Total percent effort		**100%**	**100%**	**100%**

* Mentor meetings include Primary Mentor (weekly) and Mentor Committee (at least quarterly)

TABLE 18.7   Research Strategy Outline for a Fellowship Grant

RESEARCH STRATEGY (SIX PAGES)
I. Significance and Innovation (two pages)
II. Approach (three to four pages)
A. Preliminary Studies
B. Study Design and Methods
C. Data Analysis Plan
D. Power and Sample Size
E. Alternatives and Limitations
III. Research Plan Timeline (1/4 page)
IV. Summary, Strengths of the Proposed Project, and Future Directions (1/2 page)

The **Specific Aims** for a fellowship grant should follow the same guidelines as described in Chapter 6, "Specific Aims." Of note, for fellowship grants, the Specific Aims page should describe how the proposed research will help you to achieve your training goals. Fellowship Grants typically have anywhere from two to four aims. Again, search NIH RePORTER for Fellowship abstracts to get a sense of the number of specific aims typically included. The last paragraph of your specific aims should specify how conducting this research will meet your training goals as reviewers will focus on whether your proposed research project is *well integrated with your training goals.*

As noted in the timeline at the end of this chapter, it is critical to send a draft copy of the Specific Aims page to your co-sponsors and consultants early in the process, after review by your primary sponsor.

The **Research Strategy** for a fellowship grant should follow the same guidelines as the research series (R series) grants described in Chapters 8–15 with the exception that the page length for the Research Strategy is 6 instead of 12 pages (Table 18.7). Therefore, research plans for Fellowship Grants will be more comparable to the R21 and R03 research-series grants which are also limited to six pages.

In other words, the research plan still needs to be fundamentally sound.

18.5.1 Tips for Success for the Research Strategy for a Fellowship Grant

Tip #1: Take care to make explicit **references to your training goals** within the Research Strategy section.

Tip #2: Reviewers will check that the complexity and scope of the proposed research project is **well suited to the stage** of your career development (i.e., more complex for postdoctoral F32 applicants and less complex for F31 predoctoral applicants). Pilot or preliminary studies and routine data gathering are generally not appropriate as the focus of the Research Training Plan.

Again, looking at Fellowship abstracts on NIH RePORTER will be very helpful in this respect.

Tip #3: Note that preliminary data are not required for fellowship grants but, if available, can strengthen your application. For example, include **preliminary data** collected by you or your sponsor that shows the feasibility of the approaches described in your aims. This can include pilot data. In addition, mention any related prior studies that you or your sponsor have successfully completed.

Tip #4: The research project must be **feasible** given the resources and time needed to accomplish it. Consider having a subsection titled "feasibility" to directly address this concern. Here, you can note if you have access to any specific resources that will facilitate the efficiency of data collection or other aspects of feasibility (e.g., a biostatistical core). While you will also note these in the Facilities and Resources section, it is a kindness to the reviewer to emphasize them here too.

Tip #5: On a related note, the plan should be achievable within the requested time period. For example, do not underestimate the time for data collection. Try to point to prior data when projecting the time it will take to recruit an adequate number of participants. This time commitment is often underestimated and can indicate a lack of mentorship involvement in the grant. See Chapter 11, "Study Design and Methods," for an example timeline and strategic timeline tips. Reviewers will understand that the pace of data collection for a graduate or postdoctoral student project may be slower than a faculty member's project particularly since you will be including training components in your proposal as well. The Approach section should include a **research activity timeline** that also takes into account the time needed for the training activities described in your training plan.

Tip #6: Cross check the sponsor's description of your research project in their sponsor statement with your research strategy. Reviewers will look to see that your application is **internally consistent** and well-coordinated across all the required forms of the Fellowship Grant application.

Tip #7: If you are from a **diverse background** or from a group that is underrepresented in the biomedical, behavioral, or clinical research workforce as defined by NIH, emphasize in the Significance and Innovation section that you will serve as a role model to others like you and, if relevant, that you will actively engage and support them in following your career path.

Tip #8: Finally, just as described in Chapter 8, "**Significance and Innovation**," regardless of the complexity and scope, the research project should **move the field forward**, meaning that it would be considered publishable. Therefore, view the Fellowship Grant as providing the preliminary data for your subsequent Career Award or F32.

18.6 RESPECTIVE CONTRIBUTIONS

The Respective Contributions section is limited to one page and should describe how you and your sponsor work together, how you collaborated in developing the proposal, and your sponsors' continued mentorship roles (Table 18.8).

Some key phrases that will help in the writing of this section can include, "The research plan was developed as a collaboration between Dr. X and myself," or "This plan was developed from extensive literature review and preliminary data which I performed," or "Frequent one-on-one meetings with Dr. Smith helped me to develop this plan."

TABLE 18.8   Outline for Respective Contributions Section of a Fellowship Application

A. Role of the graduate student applicant
B. Role of the sponsor and other contributors (e.g., consultants and collaborators)
C. Future contributions for the proposed work

TABLE 18.9   Example Mentorship Role Table

TEAM MEMBER	ROLE/CONTRIBUTION	CONTACT
Yourself	• I will conduct research by … • I will prepare data for dissemination by writing publications to peer-reviewed journals and presentations at conferences	My sponsor and I developed the proposed research and training plans
Primary sponsor	• Mentoring in research, provide feedback on manuscript and presentations	Weekly
Co-sponsor	• Guidance in content area of …	Weekly in person
Additional rows for consultants, collaborators, etc.		

Then, describe your mentorship team and how they contribute to each of your training goals; note their expertise in the proposed area of research and their track record of funding in this area. If you already have an **established relationship** with your primary mentor and if you are coauthors on a manuscript or presentation, emphasize this and show how you will build on this in the future. On the other hand, if you are still in the same laboratory in which you did your postdoctoral fellowship, be very clear how your proposed research will distinguish you from your primary mentor so that you can establish your independence.

Reviewers will focus on whether your research project is **significantly distinct** from your sponsor's funded research. The degree of distinction will depend on your level (i.e., greater for postdoctoral F32 applicants and smaller for F31 predoctoral applicants) but should never directly overlap. Describe how your project derived from the collaborative intellectual input of yourself and your sponsors and leverages your sponsors' projects. You don't want the reviewer to note, "while the topic is important, it appears to be an incremental extension of the primary sponsor's research; potential for developing independence is limited."

Demonstrate a clear commitment from the mentoring team to meet according to the proposed schedule. Clarify if they will be sharing materials with you that they have used in their ongoing/previous NIH-funded studies that are relevant. Or, that they are allowing you to work on these studies (e.g., conduct secondary analyses of the dataset, and contribute to manuscripts).

Consider using a table for this section. This will be a kindness to the reviewer in clearly organizing everyone's roles and has the additional benefit of serving as a space-saver as font size in tables can be a bit smaller (e.g., 10 point). The table can list each team member's role/contribution and then the approach to this contribution (Table 18.9).

Pitfall to avoid   Reviewers will focus on inadequate availability of mentors or the lack of mentoring for one or more of your specific training goals. In addition, if your mentors/co-mentors are associate professors (i.e., not full professors), this section should justify that they were selected based on their scholarly achievements, NIH funding history, and commitment to training the next generation of scholars.

18.7   SELECTION OF SPONSOR AND INSTITUTION

This section is limited to one page and should describe the rationale for why you selected your sponsor, co-sponsor (if relevant), and the institution. Specifically explain the unique *qualities* of your sponsor and

TABLE 18.10 Outline for Selection of Sponsor and Institution Section of a Fellowship Application

A. Selection of sponsor
   1. The sponsor's *research accomplishments* (awards, funding, and/or a unique tool/technique they have developed)
   2. The sponsor's *mentorship experience* (i.e., number of F awardees, postdoctoral students, doctoral students, and junior faculty they have mentored as well as their current positions)
   3. Your **fit** with your sponsor's *mentoring style*
B. Role of the co-sponsor and other contributors (e.g., consultants and collaborators)
   1. Their *research accomplishments*
   2. Their *mentorship experience*
   3. Your **fit** with their *mentoring style*
C. Selection of institution

the institution that make them ideally suited to enable you to accomplish your training goals. The goal is for the reviewer to see the exceptional nature of your choices and that your selections were mature and well informed. Therefore, you can begin each paragraph with a variation of the following phrases, "I chose to pursue my PhD at Institute X because …," "I chose to undergo my training in the department of x because …"

More importantly, describe your reasons for working with your sponsor, such as "I chose to work with Dr. Smith for multiple reasons." These can include their ability to be hands-on and provide you with extensive interactions (more important for an F30 and F31 applicant), their ability to give you more autonomy and independence (more important for an F32 applicant), their unique teaching style, their mentoring style, their mentoring experience, or the size of their lab. For example, a large lab could provide you with many opportunities to interact and learn from others, while a smaller lab could create a more nurturing environment.

Then, describe your reasons for selecting your institution. Discuss the rationale behind your selection of the specific graduate training program you are in; in other words, the assets of the program. For example, note if your area of focus is shared by more than one faculty member in the department and/or is an area of specialization. Also be sure to speak to the institution more broadly. For example, clarify if your program is affiliated with other programs across the university. Note if your institution has specific resources, centers, or core facilities (which you will describe in detail elsewhere but you might refer to here as a reason it is a good fit). Also note if the institution is situated in an ideal location to access other opportunities.

Summarize by saying how all these characteristics that are unique to your sponsor and laboratory environment are the **perfect fit** for you as an individual and your specific training needs.

This section can be divided into three sections as described in Table 18.10.

Lastly, a **track record of collaboration** between your primary sponsor and your co-sponsor(s) will be considered a strength. Collaboration can include co-mentored trainees, co-authored publications and presentations, as well as collaboration on funded grants. Be sure to describe this here and have the sponsors mention this themselves in their biosketches.

18.8 TRAINING IN THE RESPONSIBLE CONDUCT OF RESEARCH

All fellowship applicants must include a plan to obtain instruction in the responsible conduct of research (RCR). This section is limited to one page and should describe your prior formal and informal training in RCR (including the dates of last occurrence) and a proposed training plan moving forward. Also document the role of your sponsor in this instruction. A recently funded Fellowship Grant can be helpful in drafting this section as the reviewer expectations continue to evolve for this section.

Training in RCR must take place during each career stage and be appropriate for that stage and **this training must occur at least once every four years**. In other words, if you already had this training as an undergraduate student, you must gain more training as a graduate student. Reviewers will look for a mix of **formal and informal** training (e.g., individualized instruction or independent scholarly activities that will enhance your understanding of ethical issues related to your specific research activities and the societal impact of that research). Be sure that your plan is tailored to your particular career stage, for example, postdoctoral fellows may fulfill the requirement for instruction in RCR by participating as lecturers and discussion leaders.

The plan must address the following five instructional components: format, subject matter, faculty participation, duration of instruction, and frequency of instruction, as explained below.

Format: Substantial face-to-face discussions between the fellow, other individuals in a similar training status and sponsors plus a combination of didactic and small-group discussions (e.g., case studies), are highly encouraged. While online courses can be a valuable supplement to instruction in responsible conduct of research, online instruction is not considered adequate as the sole means of instruction.

Subject Matter: The following topics have been incorporated into most acceptable plans for such instruction:
- Conflict of interest (e.g., personal, professional, and financial)
- Policies regarding human subjects, live vertebrate animal subjects in research, and safe laboratory practices
- Sponsor/fellow responsibilities and relationships
- Collaborative research including collaborations with industry
- Peer review
- Data acquisition and laboratory tools; data management, sharing and ownership
- Research misconduct and policies for handling misconduct
- Responsible authorship and publication
- The scientist as a responsible member of society, contemporary ethical issues in biomedical research, and the environmental and societal impacts of scientific research

Faculty Participation: Sponsors and other appropriate faculty are highly encouraged to contribute both to formal and informal instruction. For example, informal instruction can take the form of laboratory interactions or other informal situations throughout the year. Formal instruction could be via your sponsors' roles as discussion leaders, speakers, lecturers, or course directors.

Duration of Instruction: Acceptable programs generally involve at least eight contact hours. A semester-long series of seminars/programs may be more effective than a single seminar or one-day workshop because it is expected that topics will then be considered in sufficient depth and synthesized within a broader conceptual framework.

Frequency of Instruction: As noted earlier, instruction must be undertaken at least once during each career stage, and at a frequency of no less than once every four years. It is highly encouraged that initial instruction during predoctoral training occurs as early as possible in graduate school.

Examples of Training in RCR
- A series of online training modules provided by the Collaborative Institutional Training Initiative (CITI) programs for Biomedical Responsible Conduct of Research and Human Research
- A doctoral level required course in the "Responsible Conduct of Research"
- A face-to-face workshop series (five times over the semester) offered by your University's Office of Research that involves discussion on ethical issues in research

- A "Current Issues in the Responsible Conduct of Research" course in which a faculty instructor provides case studies from history and in public health
- A doctoral level required course in the "Responsible Conduct of Research"
- One-on-one sponsor meetings, lab meetings, seminar opportunities, sessions at your scientific meetings on this topic
- Ongoing not-for-credit sessions that students and postdocs and faculty all participate in

A **table** can be included here as a kindness to your reviewer and to help keep you organized. The table should include the date/stage in your career (e.g., undergraduate, graduate), format (e.g., in person, online), subject matter (e.g., list some topics covered), faculty participation (e.g., instructors), and duration of instruction. The table should describe how your sponsor will contribute to your training. Again, remember to include an in-person course.

18.9 SPONSOR AND CO-SPONSOR STATEMENTS

The sponsor statement and co-sponsor statement should total to six pages and be written by the sponsor and/or co-sponsor themselves as one letter signed jointly. Each sponsor and co-sponsor statement must address all of the following sections (A–E) outlined in the table below. Then, the sponsor and co-sponsor statements are appended together and uploaded as a single PDF file. See NIH's Format Attachments page. The relative space within the six pages dedicated to each can vary depending on the extent of the role that the co-sponsor plays.

Note that unlike other components of the fellowship grant, this statement is written from the sponsor and/or co-sponsor's point of view (and therefore should not be written in the first person). However, writing these letters should be a joint process to ensure that it is consistent with the research plans and training goals that you outlined in the other sections of the grant application. Start working with your sponsor and/or co-sponsor on these statements at least four months prior to your submission deadline. Help them get started by sketching out a first draft for them. Table 18.11 provides the suggested outline for the Sponsor/Co-sponsor Statement.

TABLE 18.11   Outline for the Sponsor/Co-Sponsor Statement

SPONSOR/CO-SPONSOR STATEMENT

Sponsor Statement
   A. Sponsor's research support available
   B. Sponsor's previous fellows/trainees (listed in a table)
   C. Training plan, environment, and research facilities
      1. Individual training plan
      2. Training environment and research facilities
   D. Sponsor's current fellows/trainees
   E. Applicant qualifications and potential for a research career
Co-sponsor Statement
   A. Co-sponsor's research support available
   B. Co-sponsor's previous fellows/trainees (listed in a table)
   C. Training plan, environment, and research facilities
      1. Individual training plan
      2. Training environment and research facilities
   D. Co-sponsor's current fellows/trainees
   E. Applicant qualifications and potential for a research career

Note: If you are proposing to gain experience in a clinical trial as part of your research training, then the sponsor or co-sponsor should include information in the statement to document leadership of the clinical trial (in addition to the information above) as specified on the NIH instructions https://grants.nih.gov/grants/how-to-apply-application-guide/forms-e/fellowship-forms-e.pdf.

18.9.1 A. Sponsor's and Co-Sponsor's Research Support Available

The goal of this first paragraph is to describe the sponsor's research area and research accomplishments. Here, the sponsor should state their current faculty position, their overall and specific research area/ expertise, and their key contributions to the field. Be sure that they include significant awards or honors.

Your sponsor should then provide a table, listing all current and pending research and training support specifically available to you for the fellowship grant (including funding source, complete identifying number, title of the research or training program, name of the PD/PI, start and end dates, and the amount of the award.)

This statement should clarify how your research project expenses will be funded (as the fellowship only funds the student's stipend) by pointing to a particular funding source in the table. If your sponsor's research support will end prior to the end of your training period, or if multiple sources of funding will be drawn upon, your continued support should be clarified. For example, this statement should clarify how other members of the team (e.g., co-sponsor, consultants) or the department will fill any gaps.

Your sponsor should also specifically state that they will support any costs above and beyond what the grant provides support (e.g., conference travel and research costs) and point to the source of this funding (e.g., the sponsor's own research trust fund). This is particularly important as a reviewer may wonder whether your fellowship costs will be an allowable use of funding from your sponsor's grant if it is outside of the scope of their grant.

18.9.2 B. Sponsor's and Co-Sponsor's Previous Fellows/Trainees

This section addresses the sponsor's and co-sponsor's previous mentoring experience and demonstrates their commitment to supporting graduate/postdoctoral trainees via their track record of producing successful trainees who had similar goals as your own. This section requires that they include a **table of five prior mentees** including their past positions (e.g., predoctoral trainee, postdoctoral trainee), grant funding, and their current locations/positions is highly recommended. The sponsor should select prior mentees, if possible, who were at the same level as yourself (e.g., if you are applying for an F32, they should primarily list their prior F32 mentees). Most importantly, if you have stated that your goal is to be a research professor at an R1-level institution, the reviewers will look to see that either your sponsor or co-sponsor has been successful in mentoring a prior mentee to that level/position.

Your sponsor and co-sponsor can also describe in this section any other trainee/mentor roles they have held in their career or in the department (e.g., graduate program mentoring), as well as their attendance at formal workshops, classes, or courses in mentoring. If your sponsor is early in their career with a minimal track record of mentoring fellowship trainees, they can describe mentoring graduate students as a postdoctoral fellow and their access to peer-mentoring support that might help them mentor you if relevant.

18.9.3 C. Training Plan, Environment, and Research Facilities

Here, your sponsor should summarize the training plan that you described in your own section on "Applicants Background and Goals for Fellowship Training." The consistency between this section of their statement and your plan provides evidence that your sponsor was closely involved in collaborating with you on your training plan. If there are inconsistencies, reviewers will become concerned regarding the degree of mentoring.

Another common pitfall to avoid is for your sponsor to provide a generic training plan. Instead, this plan must be **individualized and tailor-made** for each applicant.

If there are more than one sponsor, this plan should describe the role of each sponsor and how they will communicate and coordinate their efforts to mentor the you effectively.

Note that for F30 applications, your sponsor should state how the training plan will provide opportunities for you to integrate clinical experiences during the training component; a plan for a smooth transition to the clinical training component, and how it facilitates your transition to a residency or other program appropriate for your career goals. For F31 and F32 applications, your sponsor should state how your training plan facilitates your transition to the next stage of your career.

In general, the training plan spans the following **technical** topics: formal education (predoctoral students), technical training, research and professional training, seminars and colloquia, and monitoring of your progress. Your sponsor can divide this section into the following subsections: individual development plan; training environment and research facilities as described below.

18.9.3.1 Individualized Development Plan

Include a plan for monitoring and evaluating your training plan. For example, consider developing an individualized development plan (IDP) with your mentors. The IDP should be **aligned directly with your research plan and goals**. Inclusion of such a plan is viewed as a strength by reviewers—see this resource: http://myidp.sciencecareers.org/.

The IDP should provide a clear communication plan—how you will communicate with your mentoring team (including your consultants) and how often. Specifically state the frequency of meetings including standard one-on-one meetings, lab group meetings, journal club meetings, and ad hoc meetings as relevant. Clarify the content of these meetings: to provide progress presentations, a list of key deliverables, and regular updates to your IDP. State that you will incorporate their feedback and work with the mentoring team to troubleshoot and develop solutions if concerns arise.

An effective training plan will also indicate how the sponsor will monitor your progress (e.g., for F30/F31 applicants, via regular one-on-one interactions or regular thesis committee meetings; for F32 applicants, via the formation of an advisory committee that meets on a regular basis).

If specific techniques are to be taught, the sponsor should clarify how will this training be accomplished, etc. This demonstrates that your sponsor has **time** to support you.

It is also important that the training plan not only focus on the technical aspects of the training but also include training in **nontechnical aspects** that a person needs to become a successful investigator. Examples of these include:

- How will the sponsor teach you to develop a sound project, experimental design, and analyze your results? For example, the sponsor could say, "I initially discuss the goal of the experiment with the applicant, after which I allow them to design and perform the experiment on their own." Or "I will provide the applicant time to analyze their own results and then we will meet and I will discuss the pros and cons of what they did."
- How will the sponsor mentor you in publication of your work? The sponsor could say, "I will discuss the purpose of each section of the manuscript/grant with the applicant, allow them to prepare the first draft, after which I will work closely with them to direct them in the development of a solid manuscript."
- What opportunities will be available for you to mentor and teach? The sponsor could point to opportunities for you to direct a summer or rotation student, assist in educational outreach programs, or serve as a teaching assistant for a course.
- How will the sponsor assist you in networking? The sponsor could say, "Postdoctoral fellows are given the opportunity to meet with invited seminar speakers providing them with valuable networking skills," and "As the applicant nears the completion of their training, I will assist them in making contacts with colleagues to obtain an appropriate position."

- Finally, for F32 applicants, the training plan should include the allowance for the applicant to develop an independent project during their training period to take with them to establish their first lab thereby allowing them to "hit the ground running." Note that this statement must be mirrored by a similar statement by yourself in the Selection of Sponsor and Institution section.

18.9.3.2 The Training Environment and Research Facilities

The training environment and research facilities section will likely reiterate points that you made in the sections on "Selection of Sponsor and Institution," "Institutional and Environmental Commitment to Training," and the "Facilities and Resources" sections, but instead of being written from your point of view, it will be written from the **point of view of your sponsor**. The sponsor should focus here on **how their laboratory (i.e., space, academic environment) stands out from others** in their more narrow field. For example, if you will be working in a sleep laboratory, the sponsor would clarify here how their sleep laboratory stands out from other sleep laboratories as a good training and research environment for your fellowship goals.

The training environment can include:

- Lab environment (e.g., lab meetings, journal clubs, one-on-one meetings)
- Departmental/program environment (e.g., courses, mentoring opportunities, or other department or graduate program opportunities)
- University environment (e.g., opportunities in grant writing, teaching skills, or other types of professional development through the university)

The research facilities can also include those on campus including:

- Lab facilities (e.g., lab space and equipment)
- Other campus facilities (e.g., core facilities, library resources)
- Reiterate any informal **research ethics training** listed in the "Training in the Responsible Conduct of Research" section (e.g., state that informal training will occur as part of one-on-one mentoring meetings)

18.9.4 D. Fellows/Trainees to Be Supervised by Sponsor

The sponsor will be asked to list the number of fellows/trainees they are currently supervising and plan to supervise over the course of the fellowship grant. Use a table which to list these fellows/trainees according to their position (e.g., undergraduate, masters, postdoctoral, other staff, etc.).

Reviewers will look for a sufficient number of fellows/trainees. If the list is short, be sure that all trainees, including undergraduate and master's students are listed. If the list seems too long, the sponsor should explain the extent of time they spend with their fellows/trainees and why your inclusion to this list would be feasible. For example, if your sponsor's laboratory involves a large number of undergraduate trainees, your sponsor could include some context as to why the undergraduates are important to making their research more efficient and how they use a **hierarchical mentoring model** to ensure that the sponsor's time is used efficiently.

18.9.5 E. Applicant Qualification and Potential for a Research Career

Because the sponsor and co-sponsor do not provide their own letter of recommendations, this section is **critical**. In other words, this section on "Applicant qualification and potential for a research career" is the sponsor's letter of recommendation. Here, the sponsor should provide their perspective on your qualifications, the importance of your proposed research plan, and your future trajectory. Most importantly, this is the place where they can make strong statements regarding your strengths.

Again, ensure that this section is consistent with your section on "Applicant's Background and Goals for Fellowship Training." The sponsor should refer to specifics in your training plan and indicate how these activities will advance your understanding of the field and techniques/skills needed for their career.

Tips for success for the sponsor and co-sponsor statements

Tip #1: A strongly written sponsor/co-sponsor statement will assert that you are extremely strong, have an excellent future trajectory, and that the Fellowship Grant will be critical in enabling this trajectory. In other words, that you are a **rising star**.

Tip #2: A strongly written sponsor/co-sponsor statement should emphasize the fit between your sponsor's research and your research interests and plan but at the same time reassure the reviewers that there is not too much **overlap**. For example, your sponsor could state that your proposed research plan builds upon their research area by going in another novel direction. As noted earlier in the chapter, the degree of distinction will depend on your level (i.e., greater for postdoctoral F32 applicants and smaller for F31 predoctoral applicants) but should never directly overlap

Tip #3: The sponsor should note that the fellowship grant will provide you with **concrete experiences** that you wouldn't otherwise get as part of your program. In addition, they should note that these experiences fit into your training plan and are relevant for your proposed research.

Tip #4: If you were **already fully funded** (e.g., via a teaching assistantship), the sponsor letter can point out that the fellowship funding will allow you not to be a teaching assistant (TA) and therefore will free up your time for more training.

Tip #5: If you had **poor academic grades** in the past or **faced other challenges**, the sponsor letter can describe how once you found your research niche, then you started to succeed. To support this assertion, the letter can point to any positive slope of graduate grades over undergraduate grades. Or, similarly an increase in grade point average (GPA) from early years in a graduate program to later years in a graduate program. On a related note, if your **timeline appears long**, for example, if it includes a sixth year of graduate school, then the sponsor letter can provide context (e.g., pandemic, equipment set-backs).

18.10 LETTERS OF SUPPORT FROM COLLABORATORS, CONTRIBUTORS, AND CONSULTANTS

Note that letters of support are *not* the same as reference letters which are described in Section 18.14. These letters are not from your sponsor and co-sponsor—they are already showing their strong support in the statement described above. The letter of support is written by all the consultants or collaborators on your fellowship grant and, in total, are limited to six pages. While these letters of support are not required, your application will be strengthened with their inclusion. For example, a consultant may be providing access to their data, their hospital records, their equipment, materials, or contributing subject area expertise if your proposed research is outside the expertise of your sponsor and co-sponsor.

Advisory committee members can also help to facilitate your research and, if you are relying upon them, reviewers will look for letters of support from them. Similarly, a non-faculty university member (e.g., a director of a core facility) can write a letter confirming rates for services or personnel support that they are providing. If your grant application is in the area of epidemiology, biostatistics, or preventive medicine, and if your sponsor(s) are not statisticians, then reviewers may look for a letter of support from a statistician.

As with any grant application, request items needed from others early in the process. Give your letter writers at least three months' notice and give them a deadline of at least a week prior to your grant submission deadline to be on the safe side. To facilitate this process, help your consultants/collaborators by sending them a draft letter which includes the details of your application (e.g., name and title of NIH office, grant title) and their expected contribution. They can then embellish and add to this letter. This is a kindness to them and avoids the accidental omission of any key items.

18.11 REFERENCE LETTERS

At least three, but no more than five, letters of recommendation are required. These letters cannot be from your sponsor and co-sponsor. Instead, reference letters are expected to be from individuals not directly involved in the application but who are familiar with your qualifications, training, and interests.

Be sure to choose reference writers who will speak highly about your strengths as a researcher and your intellect, motivation, and determination. Try to obtain letters from **full professors**. These can include those who were your undergraduate research advisors, graduate academic advisors, your graduate program director, and/or a professor from a small class who know you well.

Ideally the letters will provide unique information about you that helps you stand out among the rest of the applicants. Strong letters tend to be over a page. If you have performed research at another institute (e.g., graduate work, summer internships, undergraduate research), select your previous mentor to serve as at least one of your references. You may also select a reference writer from within your institute but from a faculty member that is outside of your present department (e.g., a thesis or advisory committee member) who will be able to comment directly on your potential as an independent researcher.

Reference writers should also be able to address **any gaps** in your record. If, as discussed above, you have a poor academic history, select a reference that can explicitly comment on this fact and why this history is not necessarily an indication of your capabilities as a scientist (e.g., it resulted from external personal issues that were beyond your control or your prior focus on an area that was not the right fit for you).

Reference writers must submit their reference letters directly to NIH. Include a link to the NIH Instructions to Fellowship Applicant Referees https://grants.nih.gov/grants/how-to-apply-application -guide/submission-process/reference-letters.htm. Again, give your letter writers at least three months' notice and give them a deadline of at least a week prior to your grant submission deadline to be on the safe side. To facilitate timely submission, send your reference letter writers a draft letter which includes the recommended items below:

- The fellow's name, eRA Commons Username, and the funding opportunity announcement (FOA) number
- The title of the application
- Description of your relationship (e.g., courses taken with them, their role on your committees, co-authored manuscripts and presentations, and/or grants written together)
- The quality of your research endeavors or publications to date that they can embellish/add to
- The adequacy of your scientific and technical background; your familiarity with the research literature
- Your written and verbal communication abilities including your ability to organize scientific data
- The evidence of originality in your Research Training Plan
- Your need for further research experience and training
- Your perseverance in pursuing goals
- Your potential for a successful career as an independent researcher (F31 and F32 applications) or physician-scientist (F30 application) in your specific area of interest.

Pitfall to avoid   Red flags can be raised by a particularly short letter from a letter writer who should know you particularly well. Alternatively, a red flag could be raised if all three letters were from writers that didn't seem to know you well. If possible, avoid reference letters from postdoctoral fellows or nonacademics. Also avoid obtaining all three reference letters from the same institute or even the department where the training is taking place. Their objectivity might be called into question.

18.12 INSTITUTIONAL ENVIRONMENT AND COMMITMENT TO TRAINING

This section is limited to two pages and is required for F30 and F31 fellowship grants, but not for F32 fellowship grants. The purpose of this section is to describe your formal graduate training program, your progress in the program, and other available opportunities that would support your training. It is typical for the graduate program director or the chair of your department to write this section, but be sure that you and your sponsor review it to be sure it is accurate and consistent with the other components of your application (Table 18.12).

TABLE 18.12   Outline for the Institutional Environment and Commitment to Training Section

INSTITUTIONAL ENVIRONMENT AND COMMITMENT TO TRAINING
A. Graduate training program
a. Structure of the program
b. Required milestones and usual timing
c. Number of courses offered
d. Any teaching commitments or clinical requirements (if relevant)
e. Doctoral qualifying exams
f. Average time to degree
g. Your progress/status in relation to the program's timeline
h. The frequency and method by which the program formally monitors and evaluates a student's progress
i. For F30 applications only: Clinical tutorials during the graduate research years and any activities to ease transition from the graduate to the clinical years of the dual-degree program. Research-associated activities during the clinical years of the dual-degree program.
B. Intellectual Environment
a. Activities of University Institutes or Centers that you and/or your mentor are affiliated with (e.g., workshops, retreats, seminars).
b. The ongoing research in your department.
c. Department and college resources: (e.g., departmental administrative staff support, seminar series, journal clubs, travel awards/funding, campus hosted conferences, program retreats).
d. Graduate school resources (e.g., travel awards/funding, career development workshops, writing support groups).
e. Facilities and other resources (i.e., only an overview here as more details will be in the standard Facilities and Resources section described below).
C. Summary and sign off

18.13 PHS HUMAN SUBJECTS AND CLINICAL TRIALS INFORMATION

Note that Chapter 17, "Submission of the Grant Proposal," provides tips and an outline for this section. It is important to note that fellowship applicants are permitted to conduct research involving human subjects; however, they are *not permitted* to lead an independent clinical trial. Instead, you can propose to **gain clinical trial research experience under a sponsor's supervision**. If so, make sure you are applying to a funding opportunity announcement (FOA) that allows clinical trial research experience (this is noted in "Section II. Award Information" of the FOA). Additionally, the sponsor or co-sponsor is required to include a statement to document leadership of the clinical trial as described in the above section on the Sponsor and Co-sponsor Statements. In this situation, even if you answered "Yes" to all the questions in the Clinical Trial Questionnaire, only certain fields of the PHS Human Subjects and Clinical Trials Information Form are required (and other fields are not allowed) because the study is not an independent clinical trial.

There is no page limit for the section on human subjects, but it is typically 1.5–3 pages. Reviewers tend to scrutinize this section of graduate student proposals in particular. If this section is not sufficiently thorough, this is interpreted as a lack of mentoring/communication with your sponsor.

18.14 FACILITIES AND OTHER RESOURCES

Note that for fellowship grants, this section should include a detailed description of the institutional Facilities and Resources *available to you as the fellowship applicant*. This information will be critical in establishing the feasibility of the goals of your Fellowship Training Plan. A potential pitfall to avoid here is by using their sponsor's generic Facilities and Other Resources description. Instead, ensure that it is tailored to your specific application and include those resources that are related to your goals stated in the Background and Goals section.

18.15 BIOGRAPHICAL SKETCHES

For your biosketch, be sure to use the fellowship format template that NIH provides https://grants.nih.gov/grants/forms/biosketch.htm. This website also provides example biosketches for both predoctoral (F31) and postdoctoral (F32) fellowships (Table 18.13).

In contrast, the biosketches for your sponsor, co-sponsor, consultants, and collaborators will follow the NIH guidelines described in Chapter 17, "Submission of the Grant Proposal." Look over the personal statements (i.e., Section A) within these biosketches to ensure that their mentoring experience is highlighted (e.g., previous mentoring of postdoctoral or predoctoral fellows, previous fellowship grant awardees, and experience with use of individualized development plans). Also look for any potential discrepancies between their personal statement and your research and training plans. As with any items that you are relying upon others to provide, request these biosketches early in the process.

Tips for each section are described below.

18.15.1 The Personal Statement

The personal statement is typically ½–¾ page—about 300–400 words. To get started, look at the NIH example (link above) which provides a nice template for this section. Keep in mind that the goal of the

TABLE 18.13 Outline for the Biosketch for the Fellowship Applicant

A. The personal statement
B. Positions, scientific appointments, and honors
C. Contributions to science
D. Scholastic performance

personal statement in the biosketch of a fellowship application is to **connect** your experience with your goals. Start by stating your long-term career goal. Follow that with a few statements on your research experiences and how these experiences make you interested and well suited for this long-term goal. Then, clearly state how the fellowship grant will facilitate your achievement of this goal. Do not use bullet points for this section. Lastly, if you also have grant-funded research support, you can note that here as well.

18.15.2 Positions, Scientific Appointments, and Honors

In this section, list your positions and employment, any other experiences and professional memberships, and honors received.

18.15.3 Contributions to Science

In this section, you are asked to list up to five contributions to science (up to ½ page), and for each contribution, up to four products (i.e., publications or conference presentations). F31 applicants typically find it difficult at this stage in their career to list contributions by a research theme, and in this case it is totally appropriate to list contributions according to career stage (i.e., undergraduate research, graduate research). Similarly, in the absence of publications or in the context of sparse publications, you can also list manuscript submitted to journals and currently under review, manuscripts in progress and their target journals, published abstracts, and poster presentations at regional, state, national, and international meetings.

For each contribution to science, list the following:

- The historical background that frames the scientific problem
- The central finding
- The influence of the finding on the progress of science or the application of those findings to health or technology
- Your specific role in the described work

18.15.4 Scholastic Performance

Predoctoral applicants/candidates (*including undergraduates and post-baccalaureates*): List by institution and year **all** undergraduate and graduate courses, with grades. In addition, explain any grading system used if it differs from a 1–100 scale; an A, B, C, D, F system; or a 0–4.0 scale. Also indicate the levels required for a passing grade.

Postdoctoral applicants: List by institution and year **all** graduate scientific and/or professional courses with grades. In addition, explain any grading system used if it differs from a 1–100 scale; an A, B, C, D, F system; or a 0–4.0 scale. Also indicate the levels required for a passing grade.

18.16 BUDGET

The budgets for Fellowship Grants are composed of stipends, tuition and fees, and institutional allowance, as described below. Overall, the budget is small but includes:

- Stipends as a subsistence allowance to help defray living expenses during the research and clinical training experiences.

- Tuition and fees (i.e., up to a specified cap/percentage). Remember to include this item even if you have completed your coursework or are only taking a few courses.
- Institutional allowance for training-related expenses:
  - Administrative support
  - Health insurance
  - Research supplies (e.g., equipment, books)
  - Travel to scientific meetings
- Childcare costs (i.e., up to a specified cap/percentage).
- On a case-by-case basis, institutional costs for accommodating disabled trainees in addition to usual costs paid by training-related expenses.

See the NIH website for the most recent details.

18.17 TIMELINE FOR WRITING

Note that Chapter 2, "Setting up a Time Frame," described a timeline for proposal writing which suggested starting four months prior to the submission due date. In the case of a fellowship grant proposal, advance work should start even earlier (Table 18.14). For example, starting six months prior to submission is reasonable due to the additional forms required in a fellowship grant application above and beyond a typical Research (R series) grant. In addition, the involvement of your sponsor, co-sponsor, and consultants is key in this work and their time to assist you may be limited. As noted earlier, it is not unusual for an F31 grant application to be over 60 pages long.

One rule of thumb is to always give your sponsor, co-sponsor, and consultants two weeks to review and documents. This should be followed by a week on your end to incorporate their comments, and then time to re-send sections to them for a second round of review and revision. The mentorship team will look askance at a request for review with no time between their response and your grant submission.

TABLE 18.14   Timeline for Submission of an NIH Fellowship Grant Application

Six Months Prior to Agency Deadline
Phase 1: Planning the Application
- Testing scope/obtaining advice: Start talking to your sponsor about your training plan and research idea to make sure your research idea is original and not already funded under the sponsor.
- Look over successful example F30/F31/F32 applications.
- Identify necessary co-sponsors, consultants, and collaborators.
- Identify 3–5 referees to write your reference letters.

Five Months Prior
Phase 2: Preparing the Application
- Start writing your *Applicant's Background and Goals for Fellowship Training* section.
- Draft Specific Aims in collaboration with your sponsor.
- Plan/start your *Research Strategy*.
- Help your sponsor write your training plan as part of their *Sponsor and Co-sponsor Statements*.

Four Months Prior
- Work on your Biosketch.
- Help your sponsor write their *Sponsor and Co-sponsor Statements*, and review their Biosketches for consistency with your *Training Plan*.
- Continue to work on your *Research Strategy* in consultation with your sponsor.
- Continue to work on your *Applicant's Background and Goals for Fellowship Training* section.

Three Months Prior
Phase 3: First Draft of Key Components
- Finalize the first draft of your *Research Strategy* and *Applicant's Background and Goals for Fellowship Training* and send them to your sponsor and co-sponsor for review.
- Send NIH reference letter instructions to your consultants and collaborators and reference letter writers.
- Work on other required forms such as *Respective Contributions*, *Selection of Sponsor and Institution*, and *Training in the Responsible Conduct of Research*.
- Contact your Graduate Program Director and help them to draft the *Institutional Environment and Commitment to Training*.

Two Months Prior
Phase 4: Revising the Application
- Have someone outside the field review your *Research Strategy* and *Training Plan*. Be sure to allocate time to make their changes and send them a revised copy.
- Incorporate comments from sponsor and co-sponsor on all the above sections and re-send to them for a final review.
- Finalize *Project Narrative* and *Project Summary/Abstract*.
- Work on other required forms such as *Human Subjects and Clinical Trials Information* and *Resource Sharing Plan*.
- Clean up the *Bibliography/References Cited*.

One Month Prior
- Final update to biosketch and other forms.
- Final reading of entire proposal to ensure consistency across all forms.

18.18 FINAL PEP TALK

In writing a grant application, it is critical to always have the reviewer's critique form in mind—see Chapter 20, "Review Process," for a list of the questions that reviewers will have to answer to complete their critique forms. Try to address each required item explicitly *using the identical subheadings in your application as in the reviewer critique form*. If you are not clear about how your application addresses the goals of Fellowship Grant, the reviewers won't do this work for you. Finally, note that few proposals are funded on the first round and rejection should always be expected and factored into your time frame. See Chapter 21, "Resubmission of the Grant Proposal," for strategic techniques on resubmitting your fellowship grant and an example Introduction page for a Fellowship Grant resubmission.

Career Development Awards*

19

This chapter focuses on **individual mentored** Career Development Awards (*K*-series awards) designed for early-career investigators (i.e., K01, K07, K08, K22, K23, K25, and K99/R00 awards): https://researchtraining.nih.gov/programs/career-development. The purpose of the Career Development Award is to **develop the research capabilities and career of the candidate** (yourself).

There are a wide range of Career Development Awards and the NIH website has an excellent tool to help you choose the appropriate one for you: https://researchtraining.nih.gov/programs/career-development. Career Development Awards provide salary support and guarantee the candidate the ability to devote at least nine person-months (typically 75% of full-time professional effort) to research career development for the duration of the award. Many of these awards also provide modest funds for research and career development costs.

The NIH website instructions for Career Development Awards are extensive and tend to require considerable time to read and navigate https://grants.nih.gov/grants/how-to-apply-application-guide/forms-f/career-forms-f.pdf. Therefore, the goal of this chapter is to present concise, useful information along with tips for success and pitfalls to avoid, as well as example reviewer comments to anticipate.

A note: Because this chapter focuses on individual mentored Career Development Awards, it does not review the K05 (Senior Research Scientist Award), K24 (Mid-Career Investigator Award in Patient-Oriented Research), K26 (Mid-Career Investigator Award in biomedical and behavioral research), and K12 (institutional career development applications) awards, among others.

Selected Individual Mentored Career Development Programs for Postdoctoral Fellows and Early-Career Investigators (Including Both Faculty and Non-faculty Researchers) (Figure 19.1):

- *K01 The Mentored Research Scientist Career Development Award:* To support postdoctoral or early-career research scientists committed to research, in need of both advanced research training and additional experience.
- *K07 Academic Career Development Award:* To support a mentored investigator to develop or enhance curricula, foster academic career development of promising early-career teacher-investigators, and to strengthen existing teaching programs.
- *K08 Mentored Clinical Scientist Research Career Development Award:* To provide the opportunity for promising clinician-scientists with demonstrated aptitude to develop into independent investigators, or for faculty members to pursue research, and aid in filling the academic faculty gap in health profession's institutions.
- *K22 Career Transition Award:* To provide support to outstanding newly trained basic or clinical investigators to develop their independent research skills through a two phase program; an initial mentored research experience, followed by a period of independent research.
- *K23 Mentored Patient-Oriented Research Career Development Award:* To provide support for the career development of clinically trained professionals who have made a commitment to patient-oriented research and who have the potential to develop into productive, clinical investigators.

---

* The author would like to acknowledge the expert contributions of Dr. Peter Lindenauer and Dr. Rebecca Spencer to this chapter.

DOI: 10.1201/9781003155140-22

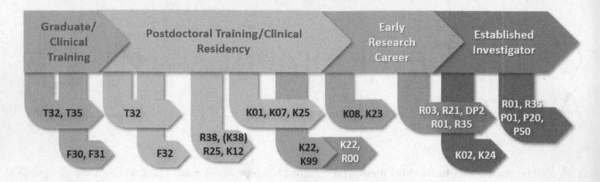

FIGURE 19.1 Career Development Awards within the timeline of your path to become an established investigator.

- *K25 Mentored Quantitative Research Career Development Award:* To support the career development of investigators with quantitative scientific and engineering backgrounds outside of biology or medicine who have made a commitment to focus their research endeavors on basic or clinical biomedical research.
- *K99/R00 Pathway to Independence Award:* To support both an initial mentored research experience (K99) followed by independent research (R00) for highly qualified, postdoctoral researchers to secure an independent research position. Award recipients are expected to compete successfully for independent R01 support during the R00 phase

19.1 ARE YOU A GOOD CANDIDATE FOR A CAREER DEVELOPMENT AWARD?

Successful candidates for an individual mentored Career Development Award are those who have demonstrated considerable potential to become independent researchers, or newly independent researchers, who need additional supervised research experience in a scientific setting. Before applying for a Career Development Award, be sure to carefully *review the NIH Funding Opportunity Announcement (FOA)* for the K award of interest—noting especially the eligibility requirements, requirements for a mentor, review criteria, and any special application instructions. These factors may all vary according to the specific NIH institute that is sponsoring your selected Career Development Award and may change over time. The NIH website will note the relevant NIH personnel to contact with questions; be sure to contact them well in advance of the submission deadline to confirm requirements. Some universities have grant writing programs or "K clubs" to provide support during this process.

19.1.1 Consider If You Have a Strong Mentorship Team at Hand

Applicants to Career Development Awards must identify a mentor at a domestic (US) institution. As with other mentored awards, mentors should be recognized as accomplished investigators in the proposed research area and have a track record of success in training and placing independent investigators. As part of the application, the mentor will be expected to provide an assessment of your qualifications and potential for a research career in addition to a plan for mentoring you and monitoring your research, publications, and progression toward independence. Therefore, highly overcommitted mentors (e.g., with too many mentees) or off-site mentors may raise a red flag for reviewers.

The mentorship team (including co-mentors and consultants) should, between all of them, have expertise in the focus areas of your training and research plan. This expertise can be individually held by respective members of your team as long as every aspect is covered. Mentors should be well-funded (ideally via NIH preferably with an R01 grant as this is widely recognized as the basic qualification of scientific independence). For grants in epidemiology and preventive medicine, reviewers may look for a statistical mentor on the team.

Primary mentors and critical co-mentors should ideally be on site. Experts that are in other institutions should best be referred to as collaborators rather than primary mentors.

19.1.2 Eligibility

By the time of appointment/award, candidates must be citizens, non-citizen nationals, or lawfully admitted for permanent residence in the US (except for selected K99/R00 awards). Awardees must have a research or clinical doctoral degree from an accredited domestic or foreign institution and a full-time appointment at the institution. They must commit to a minimum of nine person-months (75% of full-time professional effort) to research career development (some specialties permit 50%). Note that if you have already been a Principal Investigator (PI) on a major NIH research grant (e.g., an R01), another individual Career Development Awards (i.e., K awards), or the equivalent, you will not be eligible for the mentored individual Career Development Awards.

19.1.3 Consider the Benefits of a Career Development Award

The receipt of a Career Development Award is associated with a number of benefits. Because it is a competitive award, it will provide strong evidence of your success with grantsmanship, and position you well to compete for future grants. Career Development Awards provide some salary support and research support but, most importantly, provide protected time for research career development.

19.1.4 Before You Make a Final Decision

As with other funding mechanisms, it is particularly helpful to view examples of successfully funded Career Development Award applications to get a good sense of their depth and scope and whether they are appropriate for you. Search on NIH RePORTER http://projectreporter.nih.gov/reporter.cfm and limit your search to K-series awards, the institutes where your research will fall, and your key terms. You can also look up award success rates for K-series awards on the NIH website: https://report.nih.gov/funding/nih-budget-and-spending-data-past-fiscal-years/success-rates. The pay line is set for each fiscal year depending on the budget approved by congress and the number of applications received.

19.2 OUTLINE OF A CAREER DEVELOPMENT AWARD APPLICATION

Table 19.1 provides an outline of the key components required for the Career Development Award which include the candidate's background and goals and details on the career training plan. Also included are the components of a standard research grant application (i.e., R-series grants such as an R21, R03, and R01), which were described in Chapters 8–16. Therefore, the remainder of this chapter focuses on the unique sections required for a Career Development Award highlighted in bold in Table 19.1 while also *providing strategic tips* for several of the standard award sections of a grant submission.

TABLE 19.1   Outline of the Key Components of an Individual Mentored Career Development Award Application

GRANT SUBMISSION COMPONENT	CHAPTER NUMBER
I. Scientific component	
a. Title	Chapter 16
b. Project summary/abstract	Chapter 16
c. Project narrative	Chapter 16
d. Introduction to application (for resubmission applications)	Chapter 21
e. **Candidate information and goals for career development**	**Current chapter**
f. **Specific aims**	**Current chapter**
g. **Research strategy**	**Current chapter**
h. **Candidate section for career development grants (K series)**	
i. **Training in the responsible conduct of research**	
ii. **Plans and statements of mentor and co-mentor**	
iii. **Letters of support from collaborators, contributors, and consultants**	**Current chapter**
iv. **Description of institutional environment**	
v. **Institutional commitment to candidate's research career development**	
vi. **Description of candidate's contribution to program goals**	
i. PHS human subjects and clinical trials information	Chapter 17
j. Bibliography and references cited	Chapter 17
II. Nonscientific forms (selected items)	
a. SF 424 (R&R) form and other forms	Chapter 17
b. **Facilities and other resources**	**Current chapter**
d. **Biosketch**	**Current chapter**
e. **Budget and budget justification**	**Current chapter**

19.3 PROJECT SUMMARY/ABSTRACT

The Project Summary/Abstract for a Career Development Award should follow the same guidelines as described in Chapter 16, "Project Summary/Abstract," and is still limited to 30 lines of text. In addition to summarizing the research project to be conducted under the Career Development Award, **the Project Summary/Abstract** for a Career Development Award should describe the candidate's long-term career goal and training goals and activities to meet this career goal (Table 19.2). Again, searching on NIH

TABLE 19.2   Project Summary/Abstract Outline for a Career Development Award Application

  I. Significance and innovation
  II. **Career award-specific sentences**
    A. **Long-term career goal**
    B. **Career development goals for this award**
    C. **Summary of training activities**
  III. Highlights of the approach (methodology)
  IV. Specific aims and hypotheses
  V. Summary of the significance and innovation

RePORTER for K-series projects will provide you with examples of well-written Career Development Award abstracts.

Note that to meet the 30-line limit for the Abstract with these new insertions, the example below condenses the standard components of the Abstract as described for research awards in Chapter 16, "Project Summary/Abstract."

Example Project Summary/Abstract for a Career Development Award Application (Career Development Award-specific sentences are underlined)

The Institute of Medicine (IOM) has noted that Indigenous populations have been the subject of little health research and emphasized obesity and weight-related health as a critical topic that would most greatly benefit from additional study. This is an application for a K01 Career Development Award for Dr. Smith, an assistant professor at the University of Springfield. Dr. Smith has her PhD in epidemiology from Jones College, where she developed expertise in ethnic disparities in weight-related behaviors, such as physical activity, sedentary behaviors, and eating habits. Her long-term career goal is to reduce chronic disease disparities and improve the health of Indigenous youth in the US by identifying biopsychosocial pathways that contribute to disparities in diseases including type 2 diabetes. The career development goals for this award are to (1) incorporate biomarker measurement into the investigation of psychosocial, behavioral, and physiological pathways contributing to ethnic disparities in T2D risk; and (2) obtain necessary training to compete for R01 level grants to achieve her long-term goal. Training activities include a combination of formal and informal coursework in molecular epidemiology, biomarker collection and analysis, pathophysiology, endocrinology, and metabolism as well as activities to integrate acquired knowledge into understanding of health risk for type 2 diabetes among Indigenous youth. The mentorship team, is comprised of leading experts in different aspects of molecular and biomarker epidemiology, allostatic load, physiology, endocrinology, and health in Indigenous peoples. The proposed research will explore the hypothesis that compared to non-Hispanic white youth, Indigenous youth experience poorer behavioral health, which is negatively associated with physiologic stress and dysregulation (measured using AL) and contributes to greater risk for type 2 diabetes. Data from two study populations will be used: longitudinal data from the existing Arizona cohort and Indigenous youth who will be recruited to participate in a new data collection study. Findings from the proposed research will inform the development of future research on stress pathways that contribute to health disparities as well as inform evidence based public health efforts and effectively targeted intervention strategies to reduce type 2 diabetes risk among Indigenous youth.

19.4 CANDIDATE INFORMATION AND GOALS FOR CAREER DEVELOPMENT

One of the most fundamental errors encountered in Career Development Award applications is the assumption that the Career Development Plan is not as important to the application as the Research Plan. In fact, the exact opposite is probably true. As noted earlier, Career Development Awards are primarily mentored-educational grants and consequently, time spent in pursuing scholarship is more important than time spent in research. Do not underemphasize your Career Development Plan at the expense of your research plan.

The *Candidate Information and Goals for Career Development* section is limited to six pages and should include the following subsections shown in Table 19.3 (with recommended page length for each section).

TABLE 19.3 Outline for Candidate Information and Goals for Career Development

A. Candidate's background	1–2 pages
Predoctoral work	
Postdoctoral work	
Early faculty work (if relevant)	
B. Career goals and objectives	1 page
1. Long-term career goals	
2. Training goals	
C. Candidate's plan for career development/training activities during award period	2–3 pages
1. Mentorship team	
2. Training plan	
a. Training activities for Goal #1	
b. Training activities for Goal #2	
c. Training activities for Goal #3	
d. Training activities for Goal #4	
e. Table of training activities for each training aim	
3. Table of approximate person-months spent on training and research during award period	
4. Monitoring candidate's progress	

The key concept to consider here is that, unlike a research award (e.g., an R-series award such as an R21 R03, or an R01), the Career Development Award is intended to fund you, the candidate, as opposed to your research. Therefore, Career Development Award applications should be written in the first person (e.g., use "I/my" instead of "we/our"). In this section, your goal is to emphasize what makes you **unique**.

19.4.1 A. Candidate's Background

In this section, tell a narrative about your career's evolution, indicating how the award fits into your past and future career development. If there are consistent themes or issues that have guided your previous work, make these clear. Alternatively, if your work has changed direction, indicate the reasons for the change. Clearly state that your goal is to be an independent researcher pursuing distinct ideas separate from your mentor.

Clinical scientists should emphasize their commitment to pursuing research-oriented academic careers and stressing both academic and clinical accomplishments. For example, "I received excellent clinical training, but now I want to understand the scientific basis of this disease to treat the disease further. This informed the conception of my goals in pursuing laboratory-oriented research."

Key items to mention:

- The number of your publications, highlighting the number of first-authored papers and your history translating your doctoral/postdoctoral work into publications. You could also note whether the work was published in a high-impact journal.
- Any prior or current NIH funding for doctoral/postdoctoral research.
- Conference awards (e.g., best student abstract) or other awards.
- Your prior research training (this is particularly important for clinical scientists)

In this section, reviewers will be looking for your ability to translate your doctoral/postdoctoral research into **peer-reviewed publications**. They will look highly on candidates with first-authored papers in high-impact journals. Co-authored manuscripts or presentations with your mentor, although not expected, represent powerful preliminary data since these demonstrate to reviewers that you have an established mentor-mentee relationship. On the other hand, new mentor-mentee relationships are also well regarded if you can demonstrate that the relationship is a good fit.

Reviewers will also look for your experience in **leading and contributing to research**. Highlight the experience that you gained in these areas during your doctoral and postdoctoral work, and as an early-career researcher. If you collaborated on research with any members of your mentoring team, be sure to note that as well.

In an ideal world, you can point out that you are a *triple-threat*; that is, you have a track record of research, publications, and commitment to your research area of focus.

Tip for Success   If there is a gap in your career, use this section to explain clearly why this occurred. If your publication record is not strong, explain why and add this as a training goal in your Career Development Plan (see example later in this chapter).

Example Reviewer Comments on the Candidate's Background
Consider a proposal to conduct a behavioral intervention among Indigenous youth with overweight and obesity.
Strengths
"Dr. Smith has an exceptional track record of research, publications, and commitment to health disparities research as an early-career researcher.
Specifically, Dr. Smith has established expertise in social and cultural influence on health behaviors in Indigenous communities (in particular diet and activity), behavior change interventions and culturally-tailored interventions, and dyadic analysis methods. More recently, the PI has also undertaken postdoctoral research on dyadic processes among families where one child has overweight and obesity (with members of the mentoring team). This set of knowledge and skills provides a strong basis for the proposed training and research plan."

19.4.2 B. Career Goals and Objectives

Remember the purpose of the individual mentored Career Development Awards is to transition early-career faculty to research independence over a five-year period. Explicitly state this goal early in your plan and then outline how you intend to achieve this. State clearly how this award will propel you toward milestones for academic promotion.

The **training goals and objectives** should be uniquely suited to your current stage, being sure to take into account your previous training and research experiences. Think of this section like a specific aims page for a research grant, in which the career goal is your overall goal, your proposed training goals are your specific aims, and the training activities are the methods you will use to achieve these specific aims.

19.4.2.1 Example Training Goals

In general, training goals for a Career Development Award should include the following topics:

1. New/enhanced **research skills and knowledge** (e.g., expertise in rigorous research design, experimental methods, quantitative approaches and data analysis and interpretation, qualitative research methods).
2. Expertise in the concepts of **experimental design** and **hypothesis testing**.
3. Solid understanding of fundamental **statistical concepts** for proposals in epidemiology and preventive medicine.
4. Improving your **publication record** if, as commonly occurs, you are a candidate that has a low level of publications.

e g
example

Example Training Goals for an K01 Career Development Award Application
Long-term career goal: To become a productive independent researcher, advancing the science of social contributions to the prevention and management of chronic disease, conducting innovative intervention research with strong potential to reduce health disparities in Indigenous communities.
Short-term career goal: To gain expertise in designing and testing complex dyadic interventions that leverage social influences on stress among Indigenous youth with overweight/obesity.
Training Goals:
1. Develop expertise in using interventions to address health disparities
2. Gain expertise in designing effective dyadic interventions.
3. Develop expertise in developing complex behavioral interventions
4. Further develop my scientific writing and grantsmanship skills

19.4.3 C. Candidate's Plan for Career Development/ Training Activities during Award Period

Although each of these sections is crucial to success, most reviewers would agree that the Career Development Plan sets the tone; it is often the first section that is closely read by a reviewer, first impressions matter. A well-organized and carefully designed Career Development Plan reflects a candidate who has clearly identified the training skills that are critical for their eventual success as an independent investigator. And, at the same time it communicates to a reviewer that the mentor has been very actively involved in designing the grant.

19.4.3.1 Mentorship Team

Describe your mentorship team and how they contribute to each of your training goals. Consider including a mentorship table to make this clear to the reviewers (Table 19.4). Note their expertise in and track record of funding in each of the proposed areas of training and research.

If you already have an **established relationship** with your primary mentor and if you are co-authors on a manuscript or presentation, emphasize this and show how you will build on this in the future. On the other hand, if you are still in the same laboratory in which you did your postdoctoral fellowship, be very clear how your proposed research is distinct from the work that you already performed as a postdoctoral fellow in the laboratory. Just as importantly, clarify how your proposed research will distinguish you from your primary mentor so that you can establish your independence.

Demonstrate a clear commitment from the mentoring team to meet according to the proposed schedule. Clarify if they will be sharing materials with you that they have used in their ongoing/previous NIH-funded studies that are relevant. Or that they are allowing you to work on these studies (e.g. conduct secondary analyses of the dataset, and contribute to manuscripts)).

TABLE 19.4 Example Mentorship Role Table

NAME AND ROLE	MENTORING/ADVISING RESPONSIBILITIES	CONTACT
All mentors	• Responsible conduct of research • Assistance with manuscript preparation and R-level grant planning and writing	Group quarterly videoconference
Primary mentor	• Guidance in designing and implementing physical activity interventions addressing health disparities among communities with overweight/obesity	Weekly in person
Additional rows for co-mentors, scientific advisors, etc.		

Pitfall to avoid: Reviewers will focus on the potential lack of mentoring for one or more of your specific training goals, or the overall inadequate availability of mentors. In addition, if your mentors/co-mentors are associate professors (i.e., not full professors), this section should justify that they were selected based on their scholarly achievements, NIH funding history, and commitment to training the next generation of scholars.

19.4.3.2 Training Plan

In this section, repeat each of your career goals, and below each one, list the specific training activities that correspond to that goal. In other words, in this section you are identifying your training gap and what you will do to fill this gap. See this NIH resource describes a strong Career Development Plan: https://www.ninds.nih.gov/Funding/Training-Career-Awards/Mentored-Career-Awards/Suggestions-Good-Career-Development-Plan.

19.4.3.3 Example Training Activities

In general, training activities for a Career Development Award encompass the following four general areas. These training activities are then applied to each of your career development goals.

1. **Formal Didactics:** Incorporate graduate-level (or higher) coursework/workshops early into your timeline. You can also propose to obtain a formal academic degree during the award period (e.g., a Masters in Public Health or Masters in Clinical Investigation incorporate many courses critical to a Career Development Plan such as an introduction to basic statistics, epidemiology, and bioethics).
2. **Mentoring/Consultation:** Include structured mentor training (e.g., regular one-on-one meetings and possibly directed readings with your mentor, co-mentor, consultants, and collaborators).
3. **Seminars/Conferences:** Include local as well as regional/national **professional career development** seminars/courses (e.g., grant writing) early in your timeline. List planned manuscripts and target journals. Aim to publish earlier in the award period so that you can demonstrate productivity on a subsequent R01 application that you will propose to submit toward the end of your timeline.
4. **Research Activities:** Your **mentored research** plan, and manuscript preparation sometimes referred to as "experiential learning.

Pitfalls to avoid   Avoid including coursework and workshops not specific to your training goals. Note that this can be avoided by including a table (see example Table 19.5) which outlines your research and training activities *within* each training goal.

On the other hand, take care not to omit formal coursework. For example, if you would like to study the effect of nutrition on prostate cancer and you have never formally studied nutrition, rather than relying on a mentor for that expertise, include course(s) on nutrition. If you have no background in behavioral science and are proposing to collaborate on an interventional behavior trial, be sure to include courses in interventional behavior. Do not audit courses—actually take them—and at the same time, take care not to include too many courses. Clinical scientists, in particular, should clarify how they are balancing time spent clinically, in education, and in research.

19.4.3.4 Table of Training Activities with Corresponding Person-Months

Insert a table showing the planned training activities under each of your training goals; indicate the percentage of time to be dedicated to each activity by year, expressed in person-months (Table 19.6). For more information about calculating person-months, see NIH's Frequently Asked Questions on Person-Months: https://grants.nih.gov/faqs#/person-months.htm. Most typically, the percentage should total 75% or nine person-months for each year. (Note that detailed timelines of research activities are requested in other sections of the Career Development Award application and should not be included here.)

TABLE 19.5 Example Table of Training Activities for a K01

CAREER DEVELOPMENT ACTIVITIES	MENTORSHIP	Year 1	2	3	4	5
Development Goal 1: Develop expertise in using interventions to address health disparities						
Course 1	Primary mentor and scientific advisor	×				
Attend NIMHD Health Disparities Research Institute		×				
Prepare manuscript #1		×	×			
Present abstract at professional conference			×			
Development Goal 2: Gain expertise in designing effective dyadic interventions						
Course 2	Co-mentor #1	×				
Attend Professional society workshop		×				
Prepare manuscript #2		×				
Present abstract at professional conference				×		
Development Goal 3: Develop expertise in developing complex behavioral interventions						
Course 3	Co-mentor #2 and #3	×				
Course 4 (6 session online course)		×		×		
Attend workshops held by the University's Methodology Institute				×		
Prepare manuscript #3 (systematic review)				×		
Publish and present results of the proposed research and systematic review at professional conference				×	×	×
Development Goal 4: Further develop my scientific writing and grantsmanship skills						
Attend NIMHD Health Disparities Research Institute	All mentors and scientific advisors	×	×			
Center for clinical research weekly sessions		×	×	×	×	×
University's Professional Development Seminar			×			
NIH Summer Institute on Randomized Behavioral Clinical Trials				×		
Prepare R01 application				×		
University's R grant writing group					×	×

Take great care to ensure that your table of training activities is consistent with mentoring team roles described in the Plans and Statements of Mentor and Co-mentor. As noted above, the timeline should include plans to apply for subsequent grant support.

Example Reviewer Comments on the Candidate's Plan for Career Development/Training Activities during Award Period

Consider a proposal to conduct a behavioral intervention among Indigenous youth with overweight/obesity.

Strengths

"The training and career development plan logically builds upon Dr. Smith's existing skills and expertise. Specifically, her training objectives focus on developing new skills and expertise in (a) intervention design and development, (b) dyadic interventions, (c) complex intervention, (d) grant writing. This should provide the PI with the skills needed to translate her existing knowledge into well designed interventions and randomized trials. The proposed training plan is ambitious but very detailed and compelling, and includes mentoring, coursework and other professional development activities (conference workshops, etc.) for each of the key skills being developed. Dr. Smith has a well-articulated long-term plan to translate the skills and findings developed through the K, including results of the intervention evaluation, into a randomized trial of this optimized intervention (R01 grant application)."

TABLE 19.6   Distribution of Effort during the Award Period for a K23

Distribution of effort during award period, by year	1	2	3
Research activities (analyses, manuscript preparation)	40%	45%	45%
Formal coursework	20%	10%	5%
Meeting with mentors, conferences, and seminars	5%	5%	5%
Grant writing workshops and preparation of R01	10%	15%	20%
Total K23 effort	**75%**	**75%**	**75%**
Clinical work and teaching	25%	25%	25%

19.5 RESEARCH PLAN: SPECIFIC AIMS AND RESEARCH STRATEGY

The Research Plan is required for all types of individual Career Development Awards and is a major part of the application. In this section, it is critical to relate your proposed research plan to your career goals. Describe how the research, coupled with other developmental activities that you outlined above will: (1) build logically on your existing skills and expertise, (2) provide you with the experience, knowledge, and skills necessary to achieve your training objectives, and (3) ultimately enable you to reach your long-term career goal of conducting an independent research career.

Although it must be independently written, the specific aims and research strategy should be designed with the mentor and time should be given for the mentoring team to comment extensively on the working drafts before submission. It is often clear to reviewers when research plans have not been reviewed by your mentors, and this reflect poorly on the mentoring team. Ensure that your research plan is not overly ambitious and that it is achievable within the requested time period.

The **Specific Aims** for a Career Development Award should follow the same guidelines as described in Chapter 6, "Specific Aims." Of note, for Career Development Awards, the Specific Aims page should describe how the proposed research will be a vehicle for you to achieve your training goals. Again, see NIH RePORTER to view the abstracts of successfully funded career awards. This will help you get a sense of the ideal scope of the research plan for a career award.

The **Research Strategy** for a Career Development Award should follow the same guidelines as the research series (R series) grants described in Chapters 8–15 with the exception that the page length for the Research Strategy is 6 instead of 12 pages. Therefore, research plans for Career Development Awards will be more comparable to the R21 and R03 research-series grants which are also limited to six pages. In other words, an exciting, creative research idea is important even for a K award.

Include any **preliminary data**, collected by you or your mentor, to demonstrate the feasibility of the approaches described in your aims. Remember that these data will support the feasibility of your methods, and are not designed to answer your research questions. Unlike a research grant, when you are referring to a study you have done in your lab with your research team, use the pronoun "I" to show ownership of ideas and plans. Clarify which preliminary data are results of your own work and which have resulted from your mentor's work.

As noted in Table 19.7, The Approach section can include a **research activity timeline**. Be sure this timeline takes into account the time needed for the training activities described in the prior section on "Candidate Information and Goals for Career Development."

Tips for Success

Tip #1: Explain the relationship between your proposed research and your mentor's ongoing research program. Reviewers will focus on whether your research project is *significantly distinct* from your mentor's funded research. Remember that your goal is to be an independent researcher pursuing distinct ideas separate from your mentor.

TABLE 19.7 Research Strategy Outline for a Career Development Award

RESEARCH STRATEGY (SIX PAGES)	RECOMMENDED PAGE LENGTH
Significance	1.5 pages
Innovation	0.5 pages
III. Approach	3–4 pages
A. Preliminary studies	
B. Study design and methods (including a short research plan timeline)	
C. Data analysis plan	
D. Power and sample size	
E. Alternatives and limitations	
IV. Brief summary, strengths of the proposed project, and future directions	0.25 pages

Tip #2: Reviewers will check that the complexity and scope of the proposed research project is consistent with your *stage* of career development. View it as providing the preliminary data for your subsequent R01 award. On the other hand, proposals for routine collection of data or for small pilot studies are not usually considered sufficient as the sole component of the research plan for a career award. Your mentor should be able to help you with this. Again, viewing Career Development Award abstracts on NIH RePORTER will be very helpful in this respect.

Tip #3: When listing specific aims, one rule of thumb is to, at most, list three or four. A common error is to list three specific aims and then subdivide them into four or five sub-aims which can look overly ambitious. Similarly, take care not to include three time-consuming specific aims, such as three randomized multicenter clinical trials, all to be completed over the course of the grant. In general, even a single center randomized clinical trial may not be well received given the modest research funding provided by the career award. A pilot trial would be more acceptable.

Tip #4: Just as described in Chapter 8, "Significance and Innovation," regardless of the complexity and scope, the research project should move the field forward, meaning that it would be considered publishable.

Tip #5: The research project must be feasible given the resources and time needed to accomplish it. Consider having a subsection titled 'feasibility' to directly address this concern. Here, you can note if you have access to any specific resources that will facilitate the efficiency of data collection or other aspects of feasibility (e.g., a biostatistical core). While you will also note these in the *Facilities and Other Resources* section, it is a kindness to the reviewer to emphasize them here too.

Tip #6: On a related note, do not underestimate the time for data collection. Try to point to prior data when projecting the time it will take to recruit an adequate number of participants. This time commitment is often underestimated and can indicate a lack of mentorship involvement in the grant. See Chapter 11, "Study Design and Methods," for an example timeline for the Research Strategy and strategic timeline tips.

Tip #7: Cross check the mentor's description of your research strategy in their statement with your research strategy. Reviewers will look to see that your application is internally consistent and well-coordinated across all the required forms of the Career Development Award application.

Example Reviewer Comments on the Research Strategy

Consider a proposal to conduct a behavioral intervention among Indigenous youth with overweight/obesity.

Strengths

"The proposed research is innovative, well justified, and likely to provide significant insights and useful preliminary data for a future randomized trial that incorporates dyadic 'social support' components into interventions specifically tailored to Indigenous communities with overweight/obesity, to decrease stress, and to improve health outcomes."

19.6 TRAINING IN THE RESPONSIBLE CONDUCT OF RESEARCH

Mentored Career Development Award applications should describe a plan to acquire instruction in the responsible conduct of research (RCR). This section is limited to one page and should document prior instruction or participation in RCR training during your current career stage (including the date instruction was last completed). This section should also propose plans to either receive instruction or provide instruction (e.g., to participate as a course lecturer). Instruction must occur during each career stage and **at least once every four years**. Reviewers will look for a mix of **formal and informal** career stage-appropriate training (e.g., individualized instruction or independent scholarly activities to enhance your understanding of ethical issues related to your specific research activities and the societal impact of that research).

The plan must address the five instructional components, format, subject matter, faculty participation, duration of instruction, and frequency of instruction, as outlined below.

Format: Substantial face-to-face discussions between the candidate, other individuals in a similar training status and mentors plus a combination of didactic and small-group discussions (e.g., case studies), are highly encouraged. While online courses can be a valuable supplement to instruction in responsible conduct of research, online instruction is not considered adequate as the sole means of instruction.

Subject Matter: The following topics have been incorporated into most acceptable plans for such instruction:

- Conflict of interest (e.g., personal, professional, and financial)
- Policies regarding human subjects, live vertebrate animal subjects in research, and safe laboratory practices
- Mentor/candidate responsibilities and relationships
- Collaborative research including collaborations with industry
- Peer review
- Data acquisition and laboratory tools; data management, sharing, and ownership
- Research misconduct and policies for handling misconduct
- Responsible authorship and publication
- The scientist as a responsible member of society, contemporary ethical issues in biomedical research, and the environmental and societal impacts of scientific research

Faculty Participation: Mentors and other appropriate faculty are highly encouraged to contribute both to formal and informal instruction in responsible conduct of research. Informal instruction can occur in the course of laboratory interactions and in other informal situations throughout the year. Name the individual and include their degree.

Duration of Instruction: Acceptable programs generally involve at least eight in-person contact hours. A semester-long series of seminars/programs may be more effective than a single seminar or one-day workshop because it is expected that topics will then be considered in sufficient depth and synthesized within a broader conceptual framework.

Frequency of Instruction: Reflection on responsible conduct of research should recur throughout a scientist's career: at the undergraduate, post-baccalaureate, predoctoral, post-doctoral, and faculty levels. As noted earlier, instruction must be undertaken at least once during each career stage, and at a frequency of no less than once every four years. To meet the above requirements, instruction in responsible conduct of research may take place, in appropriate circumstances, in a year when the career award recipient/scholar is not actually supported by an NIH grant.

Examples of Training in RCR
- A series of online training modules provided by the Collaborative Institutional Training Initiative (CITI) programs for Biomedical Responsible Conduct of Research and Human Research
- Leading a face-to-face discussion in a seminar course related to human subjects research and research misconduct
- Completion of at least one graduate-level course on the RCR
- Weekly meetings with your primary mentor and biweekly meetings with your co-mentors on RCR
- A face-to-face workshop series (five times over the semester) offered by your University's Office of Research that involves discussion of ethical issues in research

19.7 PLANS AND STATEMENTS OF MENTOR AND CO-MENTOR(S)

A detailed mentor letter is often seen by the reviewers as one of the most important markers of success of a Career Development Award. The mentor statement and co-mentor statement should total to six pages and be written by the mentor and/or co-mentor themselves as one letter signed jointly. Each mentor and co-mentor statement must address all of the following sections (A–F) outlined in the table below. Then, the mentor and co-mentor statements are appended together and uploaded as a single PDF file. See NIH's Format Attachments page. The relative space within the six pages dedicated to each can vary depending upon the extent of the role that the co-mentor plays.

Unlike other components of the Career Development Award grant, this statement is written from the mentor/co-mentor's point of view (and therefore should not be written in the first person). However, writing these letters should be a joint process to ensure that it is consistent with the Research Plan and Training goals that you outlined in the other sections of the grant application. Start working with your mentor/co-mentor on this statement at least four months prior to your submission deadline. Help them get started by sketching out a first draft for them. Table 19.8 provides

TABLE 19.8 Outline for the Mentor/Co-Mentor Statements

MENTOR/CO-MENTOR STATEMENTS
Mentor Statement
A. Candidate's qualifications
B. Plan for the candidate's training and research career development
C. Mentor's qualifications and experience
D. Nature and extent of supervision and mentoring
E. Source of anticipated support for candidate's research project/candidate's anticipated teaching load
F. Plan for transitioning the candidate to an independent investigator
Co-mentor Statement
A. Candidate's qualifications
B. Plan for the candidate's training and research career development
C. Mentor's qualifications and experience
D. Nature and extent of supervision and mentoring
E. Source of anticipated support for candidate's research project/candidate's anticipated teaching load
F. Plan for transitioning the candidate to an independent investigator

the suggested outline for the Mentor/Co-mentor Statement; use these items as subheadings in the statement to be kind to your reviewers.

Note: If you are proposing to gain experience in a clinical trial as part of your research training, then the mentor or co-mentor should include information in the statement to document leadership of the clinical trial (in addition to the information above) as specified on the NIH instructions: https://grants.nih.gov/grants/how-to-apply-application-guide/forms-f/career-forms-f.pdf.

The mentor should start their statement by describing your **qualifications** and expertise while clearly stating the need for additional training. Then the mentor should describe the proposed research along with the other **training activities** that you described in your candidate's training plan.

They can then transition to describing their **own expertise** that will enable them to mentor you. For example, "regarding my own background relevant to this application ..." As part of this section, they should describe their previous experience as a mentor, including type of mentoring (e.g., graduate students, career development awardees, postdoctoral fellows), number of persons mentored, and career outcomes. The mentors/co-mentors should demonstrate that their prior mentees have been successful through a **table of prior mentees** including their current positions and grant funding and current locations/positions. Ideally, previous mentees have been successful in a career path similar to your stated career goal.

The letter should go on to describe the **nature and extent of supervision** and mentoring, and commitment to your development that will occur during the award period. The frequency of face-to-face meetings with the primary mentor is reviewed very carefully in study sections. Weekly face-to-face meetings are usually the accepted norm. The mentoring group should also meet together as a group once per month or quarterly with the candidate. Reviewers are critical when candidates downplay the importance of these weekly or monthly meetings. Often candidates write that the primary purpose of the meeting is "to monitor progress." Be more specific and detailed, and encourage your mentors to do the same in their mentor letter. For example, the mentor can specify expectations for publications over the entire period of the proposed project.

The mentor should describe the anticipated **source of support** for your research project. For example, a K01 award is often received early in a faculty position and support would therefore come from your start-up package. The mentor should also describe your **anticipated teaching load** for the award period (number and types of courses or seminars), clinical responsibilities (if relevant), committee and administrative assignments, and the portion of protected time available for research. Lastly, the mentor should present a **plan for transitioning** you from the mentored stage to the independent investigator stage by the end of the project period of the award. They can define what aspects of the proposed research project you will be allowed to continue to pursue as part of your independent research program.

Note for co-mentor statements: Co-mentors must also address each of the above areas. They should specify their role in your Career Development Plan and how they will share responsibility with the primary mentor. They should describe their area of expertise and how it will complement/expand upon the primary mentor's expertise to enhance your career development. A track record of collaboration between your primary mentor and your co-mentor(s) will be considered a strength (e.g., previous co-mentored trainees, co-authored publications and presentations, as well as collaboration on funded grants).

Potential Pitfalls to Avoid: Take great care to ensure that the mentoring team roles described in this section are consistent with the table of training activities that you presented in the Candidate's Plan for Career Development/Training Activities. This is consistently checked by reviewers and any ambiguities are often viewed as a lack of communication between mentor and mentee and a harbinger of a failed mentoring relationship. Note that in the example below, weaknesses in the Research Strategy are attributed to the mentoring team and not to the candidate.

Example Reviewer Comments on the "Mentor, Co-mentors, Consultants, Collaborators" Criteria

Consider a proposal to conduct a behavioral intervention among Indigenous youth with overweight/obesity.

Strengths

- The Primary mentor (Dr. X) has expertise in diabetes related interventions and policy, as well as social determinants of health and community-based health interventions. The mentoring team provides appropriate expertise in behavior change interventions (Dr. Y), social support (Dr. Yi), research methods to evaluate and optimize interventions (Dr. X; the leading expert on this approach), behavioral intervention component design (Dr. Z), interventions for Indigenous communities (Dr. Q), and biostatistics (Dr. S).
- The Principal Investigator has established a successful working relationship with Dr. X (primary mentor) and co-mentor (3 co-authored publications).
- Mentors have strong research support that will enable them to provide mentoring and resources to the PI.
- Mentoring responsibilities for specific aspects of training are clearly defined; aligned with their expertise, and include input from all mentors in responsible conduct of research and scientific writing and project planning.

Weaknesses

- Although Dr. S has expertise in biostatistics, and analytic methods for intervention evaluation (in addition to an existing working relationship with the PI), it is not evident that she will be able to provide mentoring and training on the complex statistical analyses required for most factorial designs, with the added complexity of dyadic data.
- Some weaknesses and missing detail are noted in the analytic approach, that I believe could be resolved with input from the mentoring team.

19.8 LETTERS OF SUPPORT FROM COLLABORATORS, CONTRIBUTORS, AND CONSULTANTS

While letters of support are not required, your application will be strengthened by including them. Note that letters of support are *not* the same as reference letters which are which are required for some Career Development Award applications and are described in Section 19.9. The letter of support is written by all collaborators and consultants on your Career Development Award grant, and in total, it is limited to six pages of the application. These letters are not from your mentor and co-mentor—they are already showing their strong support in the statement described above.

The letters should describe the research materials, data, guidance, or advice each person will provide. Letters from consultants should include rates/charges for consulting services.

For example, a consultant may be providing access to their data, their hospital records, their equipment, materials, or serving as subject area expertise if your proposed research is outside of the expertise of your mentor and co-mentor. Letters are not required for personnel (such as research assistants) not contributing in a substantive, measurable way to the scientific development or execution of the project.

Tip for Success   Ensure that your collaborators and consultants do not copy and paste large sections from your primary mentor's letter especially if the latter is well written. Multiple letters with the same language are easily recognized and discredited. Note that for grants in epidemiology, preventive medicine, and health services research, if your mentor or co-mentors are not statisticians, reviewers may also look for a statistical mentor on the team. Consider including them as a consultant.

As with any grant application, request items needed from others early in the process. Give your letter writers at least three months' notice and give them a deadline of at least a week prior to your grant submission deadline to be on the safe side. To facilitate this process, help your collaborators/consultants by sending them a draft letter that they can embellish/add to. This is a kindness to them, and by including the required information for this section, you help avoid the accidental omission of any required items.

19.9 REFERENCE LETTERS

The individual mentored Career Development Awards require at least 3, but no more than 5, letters of recommendation. These letters cannot be from your mentor and co-mentor. Instead, reference letters are expected to be from individuals not directly involved in the application but who are familiar with your qualifications, training, and interests.

Be sure to choose reference writers who will speak highly about your strength as a researcher and your intellect, motivation, drive, persistence, determination, and potential to become a leader in your chosen field. They should also be able to address **any gaps** in your record. Try to obtain letters from **full professors** and avoid reference letters from postdoctoral fellows or nonacademics if possible.

Ideally the letters will provide unique information about you that helps you stand out among the rest of the applicants. Strong letters tend to be over a page.

Reference writers must submit their reference letters directly to NIH. Include a link to the NIH Instructions to Career Development Award Referees: https://grants.nih.gov/grants/how-to-apply-application-guide/submission-process/reference-letters.htm. Again, give your letter writers at least three months' notice and give them a deadline of at least a week prior to your grant submission deadline to be on the safe side. To facilitate timely submission, send your reference letter writers a draft letter which includes the recommended items below:

- The candidate's (your) name, eRA Commons Username, and the FOA number
- The title of the application
- Description of your relationship with the reference writer (e.g., courses taken with them, their role on your committees, co-authored manuscripts and presentations, and/or grants written together)
- The quality of your research endeavors or publications to date, if applicable, that they can embellish/add to
- The adequacy of your scientific and technical background, your familiarity with the research literature
- The importance of the topic of your Career Development Award proposal
- The evidence of originality in your Research Training Plan
- Your need for further research experience and training
- Your commitment to health-oriented research
- Your potential to develop into an independent investigator

Pitfall to avoid   Red flags can be raised by a particularly short letter from a letter writer who should know you particularly well. Strong letters tend to be over a page.

19.10 INSTITUTIONAL COMMITMENT TO CANDIDATE'S RESEARCH CAREER DEVELOPMENT

This section is limited to one page and describes the institution's commitment to you and your career development, independent of the receipt of the Career Development Award. While it is signed by the institution's representative (e.g., the department chair or an associate dean) on institutional letterhead, it is **highly recommended that you draft this letter yourself**. In this manner, you will avoid the submission of a boilerplate letter that is not tailored to your specific career development goals.

The letter should describe the institution's commitment to your retention, development, and advancement during the period of the award. Clarify that there is a strong, well-established research program related to your area of interest, including the names of key faculty members and other investigators relevant to your proposed developmental plan and capable of productive collaboration with you. Describe opportunities for intellectual interactions with other investigators, including courses offered, journal clubs, seminars, and presentations. The letter can also refer to the resources described in the "Facilities & Other Resources" section of the application (see Chapter 17, "Submission of the Grant Proposal").

The letter should also document the institution's agreement to provide adequate time, support, equipment, facilities, and resources to you for research and career development activities. Note that any institutional commitment must be careful not to imply that your position or faculty appointment is contingent on receiving the Career Development Award. Institutional commitment is important especially for a clinician applicant who is contemplating protecting more than 75% of their time in profitable clinical activity. Lastly, reviewers will check to see if the Career Development Award alone has the adequate resources for the activities in your Research Plan or if there the need for supplemental funding.

Tip for Success   Be sure to take advantage of the infrastructure of your institution when designing the research plan. For example, reviewers will wonder why a candidate did not use the full resources of his institution especially if the university has been designated a "Center of Excellence" in a particular area.

19.11 DESCRIPTION OF CANDIDATE'S CONTRIBUTION TO PROGRAM GOALS

This section is included only in applications for diversity-related Career Development Awards (e.g., diversity-related K01 and diversity-related K22s). In this document, the sponsoring institution explains how your participation will further the goals of the career development program to promote diversity in health-related research. For NIH's Interest in Diversity, see the Notice of NIH's Interest in Diversity: https://grants.nih.gov/grants/guide/notice-files/NOT-OD-20-031.html.

19.12 PHS HUMAN SUBJECTS AND CLINICAL TRIALS INFORMATION

It is important to note that Career Development Award applicants are permitted to conduct research involving human subjects, however are *not permitted* to lead an independent clinical trial although a pilot trial is acceptable. Instead, you can propose to **gain clinical trial research experience under a mentor's supervision**.

In this situation, even if you answered "Yes" to all the questions in the Clinical Trial Questionnaire, only certain fields of the PHS Human Subjects and Clinical Trials Information form are required (and other fields are not allowed) because the study is not an independent clinical trial. You will generally follow the standard instructions to complete the PHS Human Subjects and Clinical Trials Information form, but follow relevant Career Development instructions where they are given: https://grants.nih.gov/grants/how-to-apply-application-guide/forms-f/career-forms-f.pdf.

For example, you will not follow the standard instructions for a data and safety monitoring plan) and instead only provide the names of the individual(s) or group that will be responsible for trial monitoring (i.e., the lead investigator of the clinical trial) and the name of an independent safety monitor or a data and safety monitoring board. Note that Chapter 17, "Submission of the Grant Proposal," provides tips and an outline for this section.

19.13 FACILITIES AND OTHER RESOURCES

This section is described in Chapter 17, "Submission of the Grant Proposal," and the same guidelines and tips should be followed. Your mentor likely has a boilerplate for this section already written. However, note that for Career Development Award grants, this section should include a detailed description of the institutional facilities and resources *available to you*.

19.14 BIOGRAPHICAL SKETCH

The Biographical Sketch is described in detail in Chapter 17, "Submission of the Grant Proposal."

For all Career Development Award applications, the candidate is considered the Principal Investigator. Career Development Award applicants should complete Section D "Research Support" section but skip the "Scholastic Performance" section. Biosketches are limited to five pages.

19.15 BUDGET

The budgets for Career Development Awards are composed of salary and other program-related expenses. The awards typically provide the following:

- Salary and fringe benefits for the award recipient (up to a specified cap depending upon the type of K award)
- Research development support for the award recipient:
  - Tuition and fees related to career development
  - Research-related expenses, such as supplies, equipment, and technical personnel
  - Travel to research meetings or training
  - Statistical services including personnel and computer time

Note that salary for mentors and administrative assistants is not allowed.

See the NIH website for the most recent details.

19.16 TIMELINE FOR WRITING

Note that Chapter 2, "Setting up a Time Frame," described a timeline for proposal writing which suggested starting four months prior to the submission due date. In the case of a proposal for a Career Development

TABLE 19.9 Timeline for Submission of an Individual Mentored NIH Career Development Award Application

Six months prior to agency deadline
Phase 1: Planning the Application
- Testing scope/obtaining advice: Start talking to your mentor about your training plan and research idea to make sure your research idea is original and not already funded under the mentor
- Look over successful example Career Development Award applications
- Identify necessary co-mentors, consultants, and collaborators
- Identify three to five referees to write your reference letters

Five months prior
Phase 2: Preparing the Application
- Start writing your *Candidate's Information and Goals for Career Development* section
- Draft specific aims in collaboration with your mentor
- Plan/start your *Research Strategy*
- Help your mentor write your training plan as part of their *Plans and Statements of Mentor and Co-mentor*

Four months prior
- Work on your Biosketch
- Help your mentor write their *Plans and Statements of Mentor and Co-mentors* and review their Biosketches for consistency with your plan for career development/training activities
- Continue to work on your *Research Strategy* in consultation with your mentor
- Continue to work on the *Candidate's Information and Goals for Career Development*

Three months prior
Phase 3: First Draft of Key Components
- Finalize the first draft of your *Research Strategy* and *Candidate's Information and Goals for Career Development* and send them to your mentor and co-mentor for review and present them at a K club if available to you
- Send NIH reference letter instructions for *Letters of Support from Collaborators* and *Reference Letter* writers
- Work on other required forms such as *Training in the Responsible Conduct of Research*, and *Description of Institutional Environment*
- Contact your Department Chair and help them to draft the *Institutional Commitment to Candidate's Research Career Development*

Two months prior
Phase 3: Revising the Application
- Have someone outside the field review your *Research Strategy* and *Candidate's Information and Goals for Career Development*. Be sure to allocate time to make their changes and send them a revised copy
- Incorporate comments from your mentoring team on all the above sections and resubmit to them for a final review
- Finalize *Project Narrative* and *Project Summary/Abstract*
- Work on other required forms such as *Human Subjects and Clinical Trials Information* and *Resource Sharing Plan*
- Clean up the *Bibliography/References Cited*

One month prior
- Final update to biosketch and other forms
- Final reading of entire proposal to ensure consistency across all forms

Award, advance work should start even earlier (Table 19.9). For example, starting six months prior to submission is reasonable due to the additional forms required in a Career Development Award application above and beyond a typical research (R series) grant. In addition, the involvement of your mentor, co-mentor, and consultants is key in this work and their time to assist you may be limited.

It is considered appropriate to give your mentor, co-mentors, and consultants 2 weeks to review and documents. In addition, you will want to factor in sufficient time to have others outside your field read your application for comments. This should be followed by a week on your end to incorporate their comments. The mentorship team will look askance at a request for review with no time between their response and your grant submission).

Note that the above timeline may not apply directly to a K99/R00 *Pathway to Independence Award* which is designed to facilitate the transition of postdoctoral researchers or clinician-scientists from mentored research positions to tenure-track faculty positions. In this case, the timeline should take into account time dedicated to the transition (e.g., searching for the faculty position). See more details on the NIH website: https://grants.nih.gov/faqs#/New-Investigators-Program.

19.17 FINAL PEP TALK

In writing a grant application, it is critical to always have the reviewer's critique form in mind – see Chapter 20, "Review Process," for a list of the questions that reviewers will have to answer to complete their critique forms. Try to address each required item explicitly *using the identical subheadings in your application as in the reviewer critique form.* If you are not clear about how your application addresses the goals of the Career Development Award, the reviewers won't do this work for you. Finally, note that few proposals are funded on the first round. See Chapter 21, "Resubmission of the Grant Proposal," for strategic techniques on resubmitting your Career Development Award and an example Introduction page for a Career Development Award resubmission.

Review Process

20

After passing the hurdle of submitting your grant proposal, the next stage is the grant review process. Part I of this chapter describes the review process for Research Grants (R series), Fellowship (F series) Awards, and Career Development (K series) Awards. Part II provides tips for how to proceed after the review, including how to interpret your summary statement as well as issues that influence the potential funding of your award. The Appendix provides the specific review criteria for Research Grants, Fellowship Grants, and Career Development Awards, respectively.

Given today's economic challenges and corresponding lower NIH pay lines, it is important to anticipate that your first submission will not be funded. Therefore, Chapter 21 follows up with *Resubmission of the Grant Proposal*.

20.1 PART I: REVIEW PROCESS

20.1.1 Immediately after Submission: eRA Commons Confirmation

After you (the *applicant*) complete your grant proposal according to the grant application instructions, your institution's office of grants and contracts submits the application to NIH (Figure 20.1). At this point, you will be notified that you can log onto the NIH website (Electronic Research Administration (**eRA**) **Commons** [https://commons.era.nih.gov/]) to check for any errors within two business days.

Typically two weeks after submission, you will be notified that your application it has been assigned to both of the following:

1. A Scientific Review Group (*study section*) at the Center for Scientific Review (CSR)
2. A primary NIH institute and possibly one or more secondary NIH institutes (e.g., NHLBI, NCI)

First, double check that these assignments match the requests that you submitted as part of the via the PHS Assignment form. If they do not match, contact the assigned officials as noted on the eRA Commons website.

20.1.2 Scientific Review Group (Study Section)

The first stage of your grant review is performed by the Scientific Review Group (more familiarly termed "study section"), which evaluates the application in terms of its **scientific and technical merit only**.

Study sections are based at the Center for Scientific Review (CSR) within the NIH Office of the Director. It is a common **misconception** to believe that your grant is first reviewed by the NIH institute which would ultimately award your grant if it were funded. Instead, science trumps NIH institute priorities during the **initial** stage of peer review. In other words, grants are reviewed first for their scientific

DOI: 10.1201/9781003155140-23

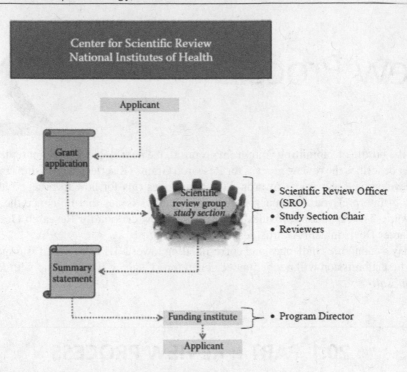

FIGURE 20.1 Where does my application go once I submit it?

merit by study sections organized according to scientific discipline (e.g., epidemiology, behavioral interventions, genetics) by study sections which focus on those areas. Indeed, study sections usually review applications assigned to a variety of NIH institutes and it is not until **after** this first stage of peer view that your application makes its way to the institute (Figure 20.1).

A complete list of study sections can be found on the NIH CSR website: http://www.csr.nih.gov/committees/rosterindex.asp. The three types of study sections that are most relevant for early-career faculty are listed in Table 20.1.

20.1.3 Role of the Scientific Review Officer

Each study section is led by a **Scientific Review Officer (SRO)**, an extramural staff scientist at NIH. Once you have submitted your application, the SRO is your NIH point of contact until the study section meets. Make sure to avoid communicating directly with study section members about your application and do

TABLE 20.1 Types of NIH Scientific Review Groups (Study Sections)

	TYPES OF STUDY SECTIONS
Regular standing study sections	These study sections review most of the investigator- initiated Research Awards including R01, R03, R21, and Career Development Awards (K series) among others. They are typically made up of 20–30 members.
Fellowship Grant study sections	These study sections review Fellowship Grant (F series) applications including F30, F31, F32, and F33s.
Special emphasis panels	These *one-time* meetings are composed of temporary members only who are selected for their expertise regarding the applications under consideration. They are usually used to review specific RFAs.

not contact the program officials (e.g., Program Directors [sometimes called Program Officers]) at the assigned NIH institute(s).

Instead, direct any questions you may have to the SRO. Typically, the only questions you may have are after the review is conducted (more on that in Part II below).

20.1.3.1 SRO's Roles and Responsibilities

Overall, the SRO is responsible for ensuring that each application receives an objective and fair initial peer review and that all applicable laws, regulations, and policies are followed.

The SRO:

- Recruits qualified reviewers based on scientific and technical qualifications
- Assigns applications to specific reviewers
- Documents and manages conflicts of interest
- Ensures that proper review criteria are used during the review
- Prepares summary statements of the review, which are made available to you after the review is completed

20.1.4 Study Section Reviewers

Study section reviewers are either permanent or temporary members of their study section. They are scientists who are chosen as members due to their:

- Appropriate expertise for that review panel
- Authority in their scientific field
- Dedication to high-quality, fair, and objective reviews
- Ability to work collegially in a group setting
- Experience in research grant review

The **study section chair** is also a study section member who also serves as a moderator of the discussion.

The names of the specific SRO, study section chair, reviewers, and their institutional affiliations and titles are all public information and are posted on the NIH CSR website (www.csr.nih.gov/) in advance of your review.

Tip for Success   The **NIH Early-Career Reviewer (ECR) Program** is a highly recommended program which aims to help early-career faculty become more competitive as grant applicants through firsthand experience with peer review and to enrich and diversify CSR's pool of trained reviewers. Assistant Professors with at least one year of full-time faculty experience are eligible to apply if they show evidence of an active, independent research program and have not served on an NIH study section in the past (aside from as a mail reviewer). They must not have held a large R-series grant (R01 equivalent) but must have submitted a grant proposal as a Principal Investigator and received the associated summary statement. This program provides an insider's view of the grant review process and also has the side-benefit of allowing you to network with scientists.

20.1.5 How the Study Section Members Review Your Grant Application

The SRO typically assigns each grant application to three reviewers—a primary, secondary, and tertiary reviewer (sometimes termed *discussant*).

Prior to the study section meeting, each reviewer/discussant reads their assigned applications and completes a critique form. The critique form asks for bullet points regarding **strengths and weaknesses** as well as **preliminary scores** in five specific review criteria and in terms of the application's overall impact. See the Appendix of this chapter for review criteria for Research Grants, Fellowship Grants, and Career Development Awards, respectively.

It is important to note that when the reviewer is writing their critique, they are not provided with access to view other reviewer's critiques assigned to the same application. In this manner, reviewers are not influenced by other opinions during their first reading of your application. Once the critiques are all posted, the reviewers are provided with anywhere from several days or up to a week to view each other's critiques in advance of the study section meeting. During this time, reviewers assigned to the same application are expected to read each other's critiques and determine if they agree/disagree with the other remarks. Because each reviewer brings a different set of expertise to your application, they will typically each have unique comments, and at the same time, may also share some of the same comments with the other reviewers (see Chapter 21, "Resubmission of the Grant Proposal," for how to view the relative weights of comments held in common by several reviewers).

If a reviewer feels strongly favorable about your application and continues to feel strongly favorable about your application after reading the other critiques, they may attempt to "champion your grant" by preparing rebuttals or counter arguments to respond to the other assigned reviewers' comments in advance of the meeting.

20.1.6 Scoring: The NIH Rating Scale

Study section members assigned to your application are asked to provide preliminary scores in addition to their written critiques. Scores are on a 9-point rating scale (1 = exceptional; 9 = poor) (Figure 20.2) for five specific review criteria and in terms of the application's overall impact. The preliminary overall impact scores are used to determine which applications will be discussed by the entire panel of reviewers at the study section meeting (see Section 20.1.7). Note that the overall impact score is not necessarily the arithmetic mean of the scores for each individual review criteria. Instead, reviewers are instructed to consider each of the review criteria but are not told how to *weigh* them. Other factors may affect the score (e.g., a human subject concern).

Finally, it is important to note that these scores relate to the application's scientific and technical merit only, not whether the grant should be funded by the NIH. In a sense, these scores are a "grade" for the grant.

Impact	Score	Descriptor	Additional Guidance on Strengths/Weaknesses
High	1	Exceptional	Exceptionally strong with essentially no weaknesses
	2	Outstanding	Extremely strong with negligible weaknesses
	3	Excellent	Very strong with only some minor weaknesses
Medium	4	Very good	Strong but with numerous minor weaknesses
	5	Good	Strong but with at least one moderate weakness
	6	Satisfactory	Some strengths but also some moderate weaknesses
Low	7	Fair	Some strengths but with at least one major weakness
	8	Marginal	A few strengths and a few major weaknesses
	9	Poor	Very few strengths and numerous major weaknesses
Minor weakness: An easily addressable weakness that does not substantially lessen impact Moderate weakness: A weakness that lessens impact Major weakness: A weakness that severely limits impact			

FIGURE 20.2   NIH 9-point rating scale.

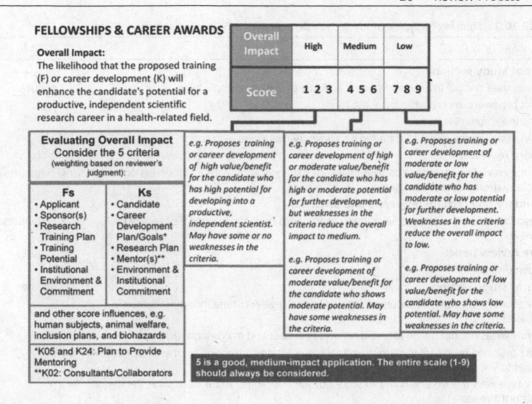

FIGURE 20.3   NIH rating scale for Fellowship Grants and Career Development Awards.

Note that scoring considerations differ for Fellowship Grants and Career Development Awards and can be found on the NIH website and are summarized in Figure 20.3: https://grants.nih.gov/grants/peer/guidelines_general/scoring_guidance_training.pdf.

20.1.7 During the Study Section Meeting

Based on the reviewers and discussants' submitted written comments and preliminary scores, if all the reviewers agree in advance that an application for a Research Award (R series) is noncompetitive, the study section may choose not to discuss the application. These applications typically have preliminary scores in the bottom half (i.e., below the median) of the applications. This process is termed **streamlining** or **triaging**. In general, approximately half of the applications reviewed by a study section in advance of the meeting are streamlined and therefore not discussed at the study section meeting.

For applications that are discussed at the meeting, the assigned reviewers will lead the discussion, presenting their impressions of the strengths and weaknesses of the application in terms of the review criteria (Table 20.2). The discussion is then opened up to comments from all the study section members (without conflicts of interest). After this discussion (generally limited to 10–20 min), each study section member including the assigned reviewers provides an overall impact score as described in the prior section.

Tip for Success   The Center for Scientific Review has produced a series of webinars and videos to give you the inside look at how the NIH review process works. I highly recommend viewing these before you submit your proposal: https://public.csr.nih.gov/NewsAndPolicy/PeerReviewVideos. For example, see a mock NIH study section: https://www.youtube.com/watch?v=lzBhKeR6VIE.

TABLE 20.2 Format of a Typical Study Section Discussion of a Grant Application

STUDY SECTION ROLE	TIME
Chair of study section	
Reads the Principal Investigator's name and title of the grant application	1 minute
Asks reviewers in conflict to leave the room	
Lists the three reviewers	
Asks assigned reviewers to state their preliminary overall impact scores	
Primary reviewer	
Primary reviewer presents a concise review of the application with an emphasis on its impact, strengths and weaknesses	4–5 minutes
Secondary and tertiary reviewers and discussant	
Describes additional score-driving items and/or adds or expands upon Reviewer #1's review	3–4 minutes
Entire review panel	6 minutes
Open discussion	
Chair of study section	2 minutes
Asks for any comments/concerns re the additional review criteria including human subjects research	
Summarizes the discussion focusing on overall impact and major score-driving issues	
Asks assigned reviewers to state their final scores. States this range for the entire review panel to vote within	
Ask reviewers if anyone is going to score outside this range, and if so to state the reason (but not the score)	
Entire review panel	
Reviewers enter scores	1 minute
Chair of study section	
Asks if there are concerns regarding non-scoreable issues (e.g., budget, data sharing plan, foreign institution) All of these categories do not influence the score	1 minute
Total time	20 minutes

A rigorous discussion of a grant will not involve a word-by-word reading of the critiques verbatim but will highlight key issues for the entire review panel.

Note that funding is never discussed in the study sections and there is a long-standing joke among study section reviewers that *funding* is considered a *four-letter word*!

20.1.8 After the Study Section Meeting

The SRO will derive the **final overall impact score** for each discussed application by calculating the mean score from all the study section members' (without conflicts of interest) impact scores and multiplying the average by 10. Thus, the final overall impact score ranges from 10 (high impact) to 90 (low impact).

Numerical impact scores are not reported for applications that are not discussed (e.g., streamlined applications). Although not discussed, you will receive the written critiques of your assigned reviewers/discussants as well as their individual criterion scores.

Rarely, an application may be designated Not Recommended for Further Consideration (NRFC) by the study section if it lacks significant and substantial merit, presents serious ethical problems in the protections for human subjects from research risks, or in the use of vertebrate animals, biohazards, and/or select agents. Applications designated as NRFC do not proceed to the second level of peer review (i.e., the NIH institute).

20.1.9 Tips for a Successful Review

Many of these tips have been mentioned throughout this text, but bear repeating here.

Tip #1: Volunteer to Serve on a Study Section

One of the best ways to get a sense for how a review is conducted is to volunteer to serve on a study section or participate in the NIH Early-Career Reviewer (ECR) Program. You will learn firsthand which aspects of an application lead to a strong score and which lead to the application being triaged. In addition, you will be exposed to the experiences of senior reviewers on the panel. At a minimum view the mock NIH study section meeting https://www.youtube.com /watch?v=lzBhKeR6VIE as well as the peer-review videos published by NIH https://public.csr .nih.gov/NewsAndPolicy/PeerReviewVideos.

Tip #2: Find Out Who the Study Section Members Will Be

Determine your target study section(s) in advance to review their list of members. In this way, you can obtain a sense of their expertise. It will also ensure that you do not omit to cite a relevant reference published by one of these members!

Tip #3: Be Kind to Your Reviewers: Subheadings Should Match Review Criteria

Reviewers on a study section are assigned a large number of applications to read and discuss. This task is in addition to their own responsibilities as a researcher themselves. So, a happy reviewer should be one of your top goals. The most effective way to make a reviewer happy is to help them complete their review forms. As mentioned above, NIH reviewers are required to comment on the strengths and weaknesses of your application according to five specific review criteria (i.e., significance, investigators, innovation, approach, and environment) and its overall impact. Include these key terms as subheadings in your application to make it easier for the reviewers to complete their forms

Tip #4: The Abstract and Specific Aims Page Should Include a Synopsis of the Significance and Innovation

The reviewers assigned to your application will need to introduce it to the rest of the members of the study section. They have very limited time to do so. By including a synopsis of the significance and innovation of your proposal on the Abstract and Specific Aims pages, you increase the odds that the most important aspects of your application will be heard by the entire panel.

Tip #5: Include a Brief Synopsis of Your Overall Approach

Another way of being kind to the reviewers is by inserting a brief summary paragraph at the very beginning of your Approach section that encapsulates all the key features of the study design. This paragraph would give the sample size, study population, study design, the key assessment tools to be used, and any other key features of your study methods. This will help the reviewer to concisely present your study to the rest of the study section. Examples of such summaries are provided in Chapter 11, "Study Design and Methods."

20.2 PART II: ONCE YOU RECEIVE YOUR SCORES

20.2.1 Step #1: Read the Summary Statement

Shortly after the study section meeting, your overall impact score or an explanation that your application was streamlined (*not discussed* [ND]) will be posted on the NIH website (eRA Commons https:// commons.era.nih.gov/). If you receive a numerical score, you are probably in the top half of applications reviewed by that section.

Wait for the summary statement from the study section meeting to also be posted—this usually occurs within 30 days or even sooner for new investigator applications. Do not call the Program Director at NIH until you receive this summary statement.

The summary statement will include the reviewers' critiques of your application and numerical scores for each of the individual review criteria. All discussed applications also include a *resume and summary of the discussion* written by the SRO that highlights the major factors in the discussion that drove the final scores.

Even an application that was not discussed (streamlined) at the review meeting will still receive a summary statement with the written critiques and preliminary criterion scores from each of the assigned reviewers.

20.2.2 If Your Application Was Streamlined (Unscored)

Do not despair because you are in good company. I advise my mentees to always plan for the need to resubmit and include this in their timelines. When your summary statement is available, read it quickly, then put it aside for a few days. Then, take it out and go through it carefully with your coinvestigators and mentors. See Chapter 21, "Resubmission of the Grant Proposal," for the next steps to take.

There are *two categories of streamlined applications*:

1. The most troubling is when there is low perceived scientific importance that may not be addressable. Alternatively, this may be due to the need to better clarify the *Significance and Innovation* of the proposal.
2. However, usually there are weaknesses that are addressable.

Responses to reviewer comments for **both** these categories of streamlined applications are described in Chapter 21, "Resubmission of the Grant Proposal."

Common reasons for poor scores:

- Lack of original idea and/or scientific rationale, or lack of clarity in conveying this to reviewers
- Diffuse, superficial, or unfocused research plan
- Questionable methodology
- Lack of important details
- Lack of experience in methodology
- Lack of generalizability of findings or methods
- No attention to human subjects issues
- Unrealistically large amount of work
- No apparent translatability of research into practice or policy
- Insufficient statistical power
- No or insufficient statistical support

20.2.3 Step #2: Contact Your Program Director

After the study section meeting is complete, your priority scores and corresponding percentile rankings are transmitted to the assigned NIH institute. The **Program Director at the assigned institute(s) now becomes your NIH contact** and it is no longer appropriate to contact your SRO.

After reading the summary statement, make an appointment to discuss the critiques and your options with the Program Director assigned to your application. The Program Director can help you in interpreting your summary statement as he or she may have listened to or attended the review meeting.

The Program Director may also be able to provide guidance on the following issues:

- Further discussion and interpretation of the reviewers' comments
- The likelihood of NIH funding the application in light of your overall impact score and the institute's current funding pay line
- What to address in your resubmission application, if this is your first submission
- How to develop a new application, if your resubmission was not successful
- The acceptable basis for appealing the peer-review process

20.2.4 Appeal

Sometimes comments by reviewers in your summary statement might seem unfair or might indicate that the reviewer misunderstood your application. Usually, the best strategy is to diplomatically address all of the reviewers' comments in the Introduction to your resubmission application as described in Chapter 21, "Resubmission of the Grant Proposal."

However, you may appeal the review process if there is evidence of bias or conflict of interest on the part of one or more of the reviewers, lack of appropriate expertise within the study section, and/or substantial factual errors made by one or more of the reviewers that could have altered the outcome of the review substantially. Note that a difference in scientific opinion is not grounds for appeal. The decision to appeal should be discussed with your Program Director. However, while your appeal is making its way through the system, use the appeal memo you wrote as a basis for the Introduction section of the resubmission and start writing.

20.2.5 Funding: What Determines Which Awards Are Made?

The Program Director will make funding recommendations to the institute's National Advisory Council which conducts a second level of review (after the Study Section review) and makes the final funding decision. You will see the date of the assigned NIH institute's Advisory Council Review on the NIH commons website.

The pay line is set for each fiscal year depending on the budget approved by congress and the number of applications received. Some institutes publish their pay lines and/or funding policies on their websites. You can look up award success rates for on the NIH website: https://report.nih.gov/funding/nih-budget-and-spending-data-past-fiscal-years/success-rates. Again, the Program Director may be able to provide information on the likelihood (not a guarantee) of funding.

Generally, if you have an overall impact score or percentile ranking less **than or equal to the pay line**, this is a good indication, but not a guarantee, of funding. It is important to note that some institutes may choose not to fund some applications within their pay line or, alternatively, may reach beyond the pay line to fund an application to maintain mission focus, balance portfolios, or limit redundancy. However, these latter examples are unusual.

Issues that may impact the institute's funding decision are:

- Program considerations
- Existing portfolio balance
- Anticipated impact of research
- Availability of funds

20.2.6 "Bubble Grants"—on the Cusp of the Pay Line

Grants which fall directly on or slightly above are unofficially termed "bubble grants" as they fall on the "bubble" of the pay line. In these circumstances, if you listed a secondary NIH institute on your PHS

Assignment Request form, and you see this institute listed on your eRA Commons page, check their pay line as well. If you see that you fall above their pay line (e.g., it is more favorable), it is essential that you first contact the Program Director at your primary institute to discuss the possibility of re-assigning that application to the secondary institute. Only at their suggestion, should you reach out to the Program Director at the secondary that institute to ascertain whether your application is a good fit for their priorities. Note that this type of transfer seldom occurs, and that communication should be handled delicately. However, if all parties approve, then your primary institute will request that the application be transferred to the secondary institute and the referral and receipt office will accept and assign your application to the appropriate branch in that secondary institute.

20.3 APPENDIX: REVIEW CRITERIA

20.3.1 Review Criteria for Research Grants (R Series)

The review criteria for Research Awards (R series) are listed on https://grants.nih.gov/grants/peer/guidelines_general/Review_Criteria_at_a_glance.pdf and in Table 20.3. Each of these important criteria is discussed in the subsections below.

There are five specific review criteria for Research Grants: Significance, Investigators, Innovation, Approach, and Environment, which are **all scored individually** and considered by the reviewers in determining an overall impact score. Additional criteria that are not scored individually, but **considered in the overall impact score** are: protections for human subjects, inclusion across the lifespan, vertebrate animals (if relevant), and biohazards (if relevant). For clinical trial applications, the timeline is also considered. Lastly, there are additional review considerations which are not scored individually and **not considered in the overall impact score**. These include the budget, resource sharing plans, and several other items.

Note that NIH Research Enhancement Awards (R15 applications) which supports small-scale research projects at educational institutions that have not been major recipients of NIH support) have some additional/alternative review criteria which are not discussed here.

TABLE 20.3 Review Criteria for Research Awards (R Series: R01, R03, R21, R34)

Scored Review Criteria
Overall impact
  1. Significance
  2. Investigators
  3. Innovation
  4. Approach
  5. Environment
Additional scored criteria (selected items)
Protections for human subjects
Inclusion across the lifespan
Resubmission/renewal/revision (see Chapter 21, "Resubmission of the Grant Proposal")
Not scored (selected items)
Applications from foreign organizations
Resource sharing plans
Authentication of key biological and/or chemical resources
Budget and period of support

20.3.1.1 Overall Impact

The overall impact score reflects the reviewer's assessment of the project's ability to exert a sustained, powerful influence on the research field(s) involved. However, it is important to note that an application does not need to be strong in all five individual review criteria to still be judged likely to have a major scientific impact. In other words, the overall impact score is not an average of the scores for each of the five individual review criteria.

20.3.1.2 Significance

In scoring the application's **Significance**, reviewers are asked to consider the following questions:

- Does the project address an important problem or a critical barrier to progress in the field?
- Is the prior research that serves as the key support for the proposed project rigorous?
- If the aims of the project are achieved, how will scientific knowledge, technical capability, and/ or clinical practice be improved?
- How will successful completion of the aims change the concepts, methods, technologies, treatments, services, or preventative interventions that drive this field?

See Chapter 8, "Significance and Innovation," for tips on justifying the significance of your proposal.

20.3.1.3 Investigators

In scoring the application's **Investigators**, reviewers are asked to consider the following questions:

- Are the Principal Investigators, collaborators, and other researchers well suited to the project?
- If the applicant is an early-stage investigator (ESI) or in the early stages of their independent career, do they have appropriate experience and training?
- If the applicant is an established investigator, have they demonstrated an ongoing record of accomplishments that have advanced their field?
- If the project is collaborative or multi-Principal Investigator, do the investigators have complementary and integrated expertise? Are their leadership approach, governance, and organizational structure appropriate for the project?

See Chapter 17, "Submission of the Grant Proposal," for tips on choosing your investigative team.

20.3.1.4 Innovation

In scoring the application's **Innovation**, reviewers are asked to consider the following questions:

- Does the application challenge and seek to shift current research or clinical practice paradigms by utilizing novel theoretical concepts, approaches or methodologies, instrumentation, or interventions?
- Are the concepts, approaches or methodologies, instrumentation, or interventions novel to one field of research or novel in a broad sense?
- Is a refinement, improvement, or new application of theoretical concepts, approaches or methodologies, instrumentation, or interventions proposed?

See Chapter 8, "Significance and Innovation," for tips on justifying the innovation of your proposal.

20.3.1.5 Approach

In scoring the application's **Approach**, reviewers are asked to consider the following questions:

- Are the overall strategy, methodology, and analyses well-reasoned and appropriate to accomplish the specific aims of the project?
- Have the investigators included plans to address weaknesses in the rigor of prior research that serves as the key support for the proposed project?
- Have the investigators presented strategies to ensure a robust and unbiased approach, as appropriate for the work proposed?
- Are potential problems, alternative strategies, and benchmarks for success presented?
- If the project is in the early stages of development, will the strategy establish feasibility and will particularly risky aspects be managed?
- If the project involves human subjects and/or NIH-defined clinical research, are the plans to address (1) the protection of human subjects from research risks, and (2) inclusion (or exclusion) of individuals on the basis of sex/gender, race, and ethnicity, as well as the inclusion or exclusion of individuals of all ages (including children and older adults), justified in terms of the scientific goals and research strategy proposed?

See Chapters 11 through 15 for tips on writing the Approach section of your proposal.

20.3.1.6 Environment

In scoring the application's **Environment**, reviewers are asked to consider the following questions:

- Will the scientific environment in which the work will be done contribute to the probability of success?
- Are the institutional support, equipment, and other physical resources available to the investigators adequate for the project proposed?
- Will the project benefit from unique features of the scientific environment, subject populations, or collaborative arrangements?

See Chapter 17, "Submission of the Grant Proposal," for tips on writing the environment section.

20.3.2 Review Criteria for Fellowship Grants (F Series)

The review criteria for the Fellowship Grants (F series) differ from the review criteria for Research Awards (R series) and are listed on https://grants.nih.gov/grants/peer/guidelines_general/Review_Criteria_at_a _glance.pdf and in Table 20.4. Each of these important criteria are discussed in the subsections below.

20.3.2.1 Overall Impact/Merit for a Fellowship Grant

The overall impact reflects the reviewer's assessment of the likelihood that the fellowship will enhance the candidate's potential for, and commitment to, a productive independent scientific research career in a health-related field, taking into consideration the criteria below in determining the overall impact score.

See Chapter 18, "Fellowship Grants," for tips on writing a fellowship grant and choosing an appropriate mentor.

20.3.2.2 Fellowship Applicant

In scoring the application's section on **Fellowship applicant**, reviewers are asked to consider the following questions:

TABLE 20.4 Review Criteria for Fellowship Grants (F Series)

Scored review criteria

Overall impact

1. Fellowship applicant
2. Sponsors, collaborators, and consultants
3. Research training plan
4. Training potential
5. Institutional environment and commitment to training

Additional scored criteria (selected items)

Protections for human subjects

Inclusion across the lifespan

Resubmission (see Chapter 21, "Resubmission of the Grant Proposal")

Not scored (selected items)

Training in the responsible conduct of research

Resource sharing plans

Budget and period of support

- Are the candidate's academic record and research experience of high quality?
- Does the candidate have the potential to develop into an independent and productive researcher?
- Does the candidate demonstrate commitment to a research career in the future?
- Does the research project reflect a significant contribution of the candidate to the originality of the project idea, approach, and/or hypotheses relative to the career stage of the applicant?

20.3.2.3 Sponsors, Collaborators, and Consultants

In scoring the application's section on **Sponsors, collaborators, and consultants**, reviewers are asked to consider the following questions:

- Are the sponsors' research qualifications (including recent publications) and track record of mentoring individuals at a similar stage appropriate for the needs of the candidate?
- Is there evidence of a match between the research and clinical interests (if applicable) of the candidate and the sponsors?
- Do the sponsors demonstrate an understanding of the candidate's training needs as well as the ability and commitment to assist in meeting these needs?
- Is there evidence of adequate research funds to support the candidate's proposed research project and training for the duration of the research component of the fellowship?
- If a team of sponsors is proposed, is the team structure well justified for the mentored training plan, and are the roles of the individual members appropriate and clearly defined?
- Are the qualifications of any collaborators and/or consultants, including their complementary expertise and previous experience in fostering the training of fellows, appropriate for the proposed project?
- If the candidate is proposing to gain experience in a clinical trial as part of his or her research training, is there evidence of the appropriate expertise, experience, resources, and ability on the part of the sponsors to guide the candidate during the clinical trial research experience?
- Does the sponsor's research and training record, as well as mentoring statement, indicate that the candidate will receive outstanding training in the proposed research area and have the opportunity to publish high-quality papers and present research data at national meetings as the project progresses?

20.3.2.4 Research Training Plan

In scoring the application's section on **Research training plan,** reviewers are asked to consider the following questions:

- Is the proposed research project of high scientific quality, and is it well integrated with the proposed research training plan?
- Is the prior research that serves as the key support for the proposed project rigorous?
- Has the applicant included plans to address weaknesses in the rigor of prior research that serves as the key support for the proposed project?
- Has the applicant presented strategies to ensure a robust and unbiased approach, as appropriate for the work proposed?
- Has the applicant presented adequate plans to address relevant biological variables, such as sex, for studies in vertebrate animals or human subjects?
- Based on the sponsor's description of his/her active research program, is the candidate's proposed research project sufficiently distinct from the sponsor's funded research for the candidate's career stage?
- Is the research project consistent with the candidate's stage of research development?
- Is the proposed time frame feasible to accomplish the proposed training?
- Does the training plan provide adequate opportunities to present and publish research findings and meet with scientists in the community at national meetings as the work progresses?
- Will the training plan provide the professional skills needed for the candidate to transition to the next stage of his/her research career?
- If proposed, will the clinical trial experience contribute to the proposed project and/or the candidate's research training?

20.3.2.5 Training Potential

In scoring the application's section on **Training potential,** reviewers are asked to consider the following questions:

- Are the proposed research project and training plan likely to provide the candidate with the requisite individualized and mentored experiences in order to obtain appropriate skills for a research career?
- Does the training plan take advantage of the candidate's strengths and address gaps in needed skills? Does the training plan document a clear need for, and value of, the proposed training?
- Does the proposed training have the potential to serve as a sound foundation that will clearly enhance the candidate's ability to develop into a productive researcher?

20.3.2.6 Institutional Environment and Commitment to Training

In scoring the application's section on **Institutional environment and commitment to training**, reviewers are asked to consider the following questions:

- Are the research facilities, resources (e.g., equipment, laboratory space, computer time, subject populations, clinical training settings) and training opportunities (e.g. seminars, workshops, professional development opportunities) adequate and appropriate?
- Is the institutional environment for the candidate's scientific development of high quality?
- Is there appropriate institutional commitment to fostering the candidate's mentored training?

20.3.2.7 Additional Review Considerations: Training in the Responsible Conduct of Research

Reviewers are asked to state whether the proposed training is "Acceptable" or "Not Acceptable" taking into account the level of experience of the candidate, including any prior instruction or participation in responsible conduct of research (RCR) as appropriate for the candidate's career stage and in relation to the following five required components:

- *Format*—the required format of instruction, i.e., face-to-face lectures, coursework, and/or real-time discussion groups (a plan with only on-line instruction is not acceptable)
- *Subject Matter*—the breadth of subject matter, e.g., conflict of interest, authorship, data management, human subjects and animal use, laboratory safety, research misconduct, research ethics
- *Faculty Participation*—the role of the sponsors and other faculty involvement in the fellow's instruction
- *Duration of Instruction*—the number of contact hours of instruction (at least eight contact hours are required)
- *Frequency of Instruction*—instruction must occur during each career stage and at least once every four years

20.3.3 Review Criteria for Research Career Development Awards (K Series)

The review criteria for the Research Career Development Awards (K series) differ from the review criteria for Research Awards (R series) and are listed on https://grants.nih.gov/grants/peer/guidelines_general/Review_Criteria_at_a_glance.pdf and in Table 20.5 Each of these important criteria is discussed in the subsections below.

In general, the primary focus of the review for Career Development Awards is on the candidate and the career development plan, with less emphasis on the research plan although that is still important.

There are a variety of Career Development Awards depending upon your training and stage of career (as described in Chapter 4, "Choosing the Right Funding Source," and the review criteria differ slightly

TABLE 20.5   Review Criteria for Career Development Awards (K Series)

Scored review criteria

Overall impact

1. Candidate
2. Career development plan/career goals and objectives
3. Research plan
4. Mentor, co-mentor, consultants, collaborators
5. Environmental and institutional commitment to the candidate

Additional scored criteria (selected items)

Protections for human subjects
Inclusion across the lifespan
Resubmission (see Chapter 21, "Resubmission of the Grant Proposal")

Not scored (selected items)

Training in the responsible conduct of research
Resource sharing plans
Budget and period of support

across these awards. Therefore, it is important to consult the specific program announcement to which you are applying (https://researchtraining.nih.gov/programs/career-development). Because the **individual mentored** Career Development Awards are the most typical awards for early-career investigators, this section focuses on review criteria for the NIH Mentored Research Scientist Development Award (K01).

20.3.3.1 Overall Impact for a Career Development Award

The overall impact reflects the reviewer's assessment of the likelihood that the proposed career development and research plan will enhance the candidate's potential for a productive, independent scientific research career in a health-related field, taking into consideration the criteria below in determining the overall impact score.

See Chapter 19, "Career Development Awards," for tips on writing a career development award and choosing an appropriate mentor.

20.3.3.2 Candidate

In scoring the **Candidate**, reviewers are asked to consider the following questions:

- Does the candidate have the potential to develop as an independent and productive researcher?
- Are the candidate's prior training and research experience appropriate for this award?
- Is the candidate's academic, clinical (if relevant), and research record of high quality?
- Is there evidence of the candidate's commitment to meeting the program objectives to become an independent investigator in research?
- Do the reference letters address the above review criteria, and do they provide evidence that the candidate has a high potential for becoming an independent investigator?

20.3.3.3 Career Development Plan/Career Goals and Objectives

In scoring the application's **career development plan/career goals** and objectives, reviewers are asked to consider the following questions:

- What is the likelihood that the plan will contribute substantially to the scientific development of the candidate and lead to scientific independence?
- Are the candidate's prior training and research experience appropriate for this award?
- Are the content, scope, phasing, and duration of the career development plan appropriate when considered in the context of prior training/research experience and the stated training and research objectives for achieving research independence?
- Are there adequate plans for monitoring and evaluating the candidate's research and career development progress?
- If proposed, will the clinical trial experience contribute to the applicant's research career development?

20.3.3.4 Research Plan

In scoring the application's **Research plan** reviewers are asked to consider the following questions:

- Is the prior research that serves as the key support for the proposed project rigorous?
- Has the candidate included plans to address weaknesses in the rigor of prior research that serves as the key support of the proposed project?
- Has the candidate presented strategies to ensure a robust and unbiased approach, as appropriate for the work proposed?

- Has the candidate presented adequate plans to address relevant biological variables, such as sex, for studies in vertebrate animals or human subjects?
- Are the proposed research question, design, and methodology of significant scientific and technical merit?
- Is the research plan relevant to the candidate's research career objectives?
- Is the research plan appropriate to the candidate's stage of research development and as a vehicle for developing the research skills described in the career development plan?
- If proposed, will the clinical trial experience contribute to the proposed research project?

20.3.3.5 Mentor, Co-Mentor, Consultants, and Collaborators

In scoring the application's section on **mentor, co-mentor, consultants, and collaborators**, reviewers are asked to consider the following questions:

- Are the qualifications of the mentor(s) in the area of the proposed research appropriate?
- Does the mentor(s) adequately address the candidate's potential and his/her strengths and areas needing improvement?
- Is there adequate description of the quality and extent of the mentor's proposed role in providing guidance and advice to the candidate?
- Is the mentor's description of the elements of the research career development activities, including formal course work adequate?
- Is there evidence of the mentor's, consultant's, and/or collaborator's previous experience in fostering the development of independent investigators?
- Is there evidence of the mentor's current research productivity and peer-reviewed support?
- Is active/pending support for the proposed research project appropriate and adequate?
- Are there adequate plans for monitoring and evaluating the career development awardee's progress toward independence?
- If the applicant is proposing to gain experience in a clinical trial as part of his or her research career development, is there evidence of the appropriate expertise, experience, and ability on the part of the mentor(s) to guide the applicant during participation in the clinical trial?

20.3.3.6 Environment and Institutional Commitment to the Candidate

In scoring the application's **Environment and institutional commitment to the candidate** reviewers are asked to consider the following questions:

- Is there clear commitment of the sponsoring institution to ensure that a minimum of nine person-months (75% of the candidate's full-time professional effort) will be devoted directly to the research and career development activities described in the application, with the remaining percent effort being devoted to an appropriate balance of research, teaching, administrative, and clinical responsibilities?
- Is the institutional commitment to the career development of the candidate appropriately strong?
- Are the research facilities, resources and training opportunities, including faculty capable of productive collaboration with the candidate adequate and appropriate?
- Is the environment for the candidate's scientific and professional development of high quality?
- Is there assurance that the institution intends the candidate to be an integral part of its research program as an independent investigator?

Resubmission of the Grant Proposal

21

A critical factor in success in grantsmanship is to plan on the fact that your first submission of any proposal will be rejected. Rejection on the first submission is so common, that it is almost the norm. Reviewers will want to make their mark on your proposal and even the most famous scientists have had their grant proposals rejected. In light of current NIH policies that only a single resubmission of an original application will be accepted, strategies for making your resubmission as strong as possible are critical. Note that following an unsuccessful resubmission, you may submit the same idea as a new application for the next appropriate new application due date.

Thus, your overall grantsmanship timeline should take into account the time to revise and resubmit even before you first submit the proposal. This is not to say that you should submit a version that is not the absolute best of your abilities, but that grit and persistence are more predictive (or just as predictive) of ultimate success.

Therefore, this chapter describes the resubmission process along with strategic tips for how to be highly responsive to reviewer concerns—the key criterion in a successful resubmission. Part I describes the pathway to resubmitting your grant proposal. Part II goes on to provide strategic tips for the Introduction to the resubmission, the most critical aspect of the resubmission. Part III describes issues in revising the remainder of the body of the application. The chapter ends with three examples of Introductions to resubmission applications for a Research Award (R01), Fellowship Award (F31) and a Career Development Award (K01).

21.1 PART I: PATHWAY TO RESUBMITTING

21.1.1 Whether to Resubmit

There should almost never be a question as to whether to resubmit your grant proposal. Once you receive your summary statement, sit down with a nice beverage of your choice and read the reviewers' comments. You are likely to feel sad and angry—sad regarding the amount of work that you put into the submission and angry at the reviewers for not understanding what you meant.

However, it is important to remember that the reviewers were selected due to their substantial track record of NIH funding as well as expertise in peer review. If, as scientists, they misinterpreted your writing, then it is likely that many more people would make a similar misinterpretation. Therefore, any errors in their comprehension are ultimately due to the need for you to more clearly convey your points.

Wait a few days to calm down and then reread the reviews as well as your application. Ask your coinvestigators and mentors to read the reviews as well. Consider the reviewers' suggestions for change and their requests for more preliminary data, if applicable. Determine what parts of your application might have confused them. Then decide in conjunction with your mentor whether your application is fatally flawed or fixable. More often than not, the latter is the best decision. A mentor skilled in reading

DOI: 10.1201/9781003155140-24

NIH reviews will be invaluable. They can read between the lines to assess whether the flaws should be considered *fatal* or largely addressable (more on this in the rest of the chapter) and whether the reviewers showed any enthusiasm for your study.

21.1.2 If Your Application Was Streamlined (Unscored)

Do not despair because you are in good company. I advise my mentees to always plan for the need to resubmit and include this in their timelines. When your summary statement is available, read it quickly, then put it aside for a few days. Then, take it out and go through it carefully with your coinvestigators and mentors.

There are *two categories of streamlined applications*:

1. The most troubling is when there is low perceived scientific importance that may not be addressable. Alternatively, this may be due to the need to better clarify the *Significance and Innovation* of the proposal.
2. However, usually there are weaknesses that are addressable.

Responses to reviewer comments for **both** these categories of streamlined applications are described in the sections below.

21.1.3 Contact Your Program Director

After reading the summary statement and discussing with your mentors/colleagues, make an appointment to discuss the critiques and your options with the program director at the institute assigned to your application. The Program Director's name is listed on the upper left of the ERA Commons website. Note that the Program Director is different from the Scientific Review Officer (SRO) whom you may have contacted prior to your review.

The program director can help you in interpreting your summary statement as he or she may have listened to or attended the review meeting. They may also be able to provide guidance on what to address in your resubmission application. Lastly, they can also give you a sense of the institute's payline, and whether your application falls above or below that line.

21.1.4 Timing of a Resubmission

Resubmitting as soon as possible after you receive the summary statement is preferable to ensure that you maximize your chances of obtaining the same review panel. As noted above, reviewers like to make their mark on your proposals, and if your resubmission is reviewed by a new reviewer, this will be their first chance to make their own mark. Resubmissions (termed "A1" applications by NIH) must be submitted within 37 months of your original application. Note that resubmission dates differ slightly from the standard due dates for original submissions as noted on the NIH website: https://grants.nih.gov/grants/how-to -apply-application-guide/due-dates-and-submission-policies/due-dates.htm.

The primary reason for delaying a resubmission would be in response to a reviewer request that you provide additional pilot data. Often, but not always, this takes more time than the approximately three months between receiving your summary statement and the next upcoming resubmission due date. In an ideal world, you may have already anticipated this request and started a pilot while your original submission was under review. If so, you will be well positioned to submit these new data as part of your resubmission by the next submission due date.

Example Response to Reviewer Comment Regarding More Pilot Data

Consider a reviewer comment that you should conduct a small pilot study to support the feasibility of your proposal. In the Introduction to the resubmission, you could state:

Since the time of the original submission, we have been in the field with a pilot feasibility study, "Healthy Heart Pilot" (Faculty Research Grant; PI: yourself). The goal of this pilot is to evaluate the feasibility and acceptability of the proposed intervention. The pilot has randomized 47 men to date and is on track for its goal of 66 men. Participants endorsed the interest and utility of the study materials (86%), ability to access a telephone for telephone interviews (100%), and the amount of time spent on the study (appropriate: 86%, sometimes too much time: 14%). Recruitment and retention rates from this pilot have been used to inform the revised power calculations.

21.1.5 Not All Reviewer Comments Are Equal

Reviewer comments will correspond to the criteria for Research (R series) awards as presented in Chapter 20, "Review Process" (Table 21.1).

Weaknesses that fall under *Overall Impact* and *Significance* should be considered the most serious. These comments may mean that the reviewers are not fully convinced as to the need for your proposal. However, before deciding to shift the grant's focus, consider whether these comments reflect a failure on your part to clearly convey the (1) research gap, (2) clinical significance, and (3) public health implications of your study findings. Typically, there is great potential to improve the persuasiveness of these sections (see more tips below).

In contrast, concerns about *approach* are typically more addressable as they may reflect logistic concerns about your ability to pull off the actual study.

Parts II and III of this chapter provide examples of responding to concerns pertaining to each of the review criteria.

TABLE 21.1   Review Criteria for Research Awards (R Series: R01, R03, R21, R34)

Overall impact
1. Significance
2. Investigators
3. Innovation
4. Approach
5. Environment

21.1.6 How Much Revision Is Necessary

A general rule of thumb is that the amount of revision should be **proportional** to the score of the application. In other words, significant revisions are required if your application was triaged (i.e., not discussed). In contrast, if the application was scored, the number of revisions should decrease as the score decreases. In fact, if you have a low score, be careful not to make dramatic revisions—just a few tweaks may be sufficient to respond to the reviewer comments.

This advice, however, assumes that the score is congruent with the content of the reviews. This is not always the case. While all reviewers are instructed to justify their numerical scores with appropriate text, variability exists among reviewers in the extent to which they describe the strengths and weaknesses of the scored criteria. If one of the critiques provided little justification for a poor criterion score, try checking the corresponding comments on the other critiques. These can provide you with multiple viewpoints on that criterion.

In addition, check the *Resume and Summary of Discussion* section of the summary statement (included on all discussed applications). This summary may have additional information on the content and emphasis of the verbal discussion on your proposal. Your NIH program director also can help you to interpret this summary, and he or she may have listened to or attended the review meeting.

21.1.7 Study Section Review of Resubmission

In an ideal world, your resubmitted application will be assigned to the same study section reviewers who reviewed the first submission. However, in reality, often the same reviewers (or at least some of them) are no longer available due to the ending of their study section term, the ad hoc nature of their involvement, and/or other conflicts. These reviewers will evaluate the application as now presented, taking into consideration your responses to their prior comments and corresponding changes made to the proposal. If new reviewers are assigned to your grant review for the first time, they will also be focused on ascertaining how responsive you were to the prior reviewer's concerns.

Note that all these reviewers will *not* reread/have access to your original submission and will only have access to your resubmission and the prior reviewer comments. Therefore, take care not to omit key sections in order to meet the page limitations. Just as in the review of your first submission, the entire study section will score your application and not just your assigned reviewers (see Chapter 20, "Review Process," for more details on scoring). Thus, the entire study section will consider whether your responses to comments from the previous study section are adequate and whether substantial changes are clearly evident.

21.2 PART II: INTRODUCTION TO THE RESUBMISSION

Just as the Specific Aims page was the most important page of your original application, the Introduction is the **most vital part** of the resubmission. Approximately half of your time revising your application should be spent on this **one-page** Introduction. Early drafts of the Introduction should be sent to your co-investigators/mentors well in advance of the resubmission date with plenty of time for you to revise and re-send them updated drafts.

The reviewers of resubmissions will **focus primarily on your responsiveness to their critiques** as summarized in your Introduction. Specifically, they will cross-check each of their prior comments against your response in the Introduction as well as with the corresponding changes in the body of the proposal.

Even new reviewers who are assigned to your resubmission will often defer to the expertise of the prior reviewers and therefore will focus primarily on how responsive you are to the prior reviewers' comments.

Below are **strategic tips** for writing the Introduction. You will see that the **overall theme** is "If at all possible, try to take the advice of the reviewers."

21.2.1 General Format of the Introduction Page

Table 21.2 outlines the typical format for the Introduction page.

21.2.1.1 First Paragraph of the Introduction

Resubmission applications should normally have the same title as the previous grant or application; however, if the specific aims of the project have significantly changed, choose a new title.

TABLE 21.2   Outline for the Introduction Page of a Grant Resubmission

	ITEM	LENGTH
1.	Specify the title and NIH assigned number of the grant proposal Thank the reviewers Quote several positive remarks from the reviews Clarify how revisions are highlighted in the body of the proposal	First paragraph

2.	Point-by-point response to most important reviewer comments
	   a. Option 1: Organize by importance of comment
	   b. Option 2: Organize by review criterion
		Bulk of the page

3.	Brief summary of response to more minor comments (one to two sentences)	Second to last paragraph
4.	Final positive summary (one to two sentences)	Last paragraph

Thank the reviewers for their review and quote several of the most positive remarks from the review. Focus on those remarks that relate to *Significance and Innovation*. Lastly, clarify how revisions are highlighted in the body of the proposal (see Section 21.3.1, "How to Identify Revisions to a Grant Proposal").

Example Paragraph #1 of the Introduction Page
This is a resubmission of DKxxxxx-01 "An Exercise Intervention to Prevent Diabetes" to test the hypothesis that an exercise intervention is an effective tool for preventing diabetes. The comments of the review panel were very helpful in revising this proposal. As the reviewers noted, "The application addresses a highly significant area in women's health that may have a lasting impact in a high-risk population for development of obesity and diabetes." "Using moderate intensity exercise to diabetes is innovative and could easily be translated into clinical practice." Changes made to the proposal are highlighted in blue throughout the text.

21.2.1.2 *Bulk of the Introduction*

The majority of the Introduction will be made up by a point-by-point response to the major reviewer concerns.

How to determine which concerns are major?

- Concerns that reviewers noted in the *Resume and Summary of Discussion* section
- Concerns shared by more than one reviewer
- Concerns that reviewers noted in the *Overall Impact* section

There are **two ways to organize your responses**, as noted in Table 21.2:

- Option 1: organize responses according to the importance of the reviewer comment.
- Option 2: organize responses according to the review criteria: Significance, Investigators, Innovation, Approach, and Environment.

The advantage of Option 2 is that it gives you a chance to comment on a section that received poorer scores but few or no specific reviewer comments. Reviewers will all see clearly that each section of your application was changed (assuming that each section did not receive scores of 1 from all reviewers!).

Regardless of which option you choose, clearly connect your responses to specific reviewer concerns. While it is important to be brief in summarizing reviewer concerns to save space in the Introduction, be sure that the reviewer(s) can clearly find their concerns and your corresponding response in the Introduction.

How to connect your responses to reviewer concerns:

1. Start by listing which reviewers share this concern according to reviewer number (i.e., R1, R2, R3).
2. Then, paraphrase their concern in bold.
3. Describe the revision you made in response, using active voice and being sure to repeat some of the identical phrasing used by the reviewers.

Citing the reviewer number when listing the reviewer concern is a way of being kind to your reviewers. This will not only reassure the reviewers that you have covered their points but also help you to be sure that you have not missed any reviewer comments.

Example Connecting Responses to Reviewer Concerns
R1, R3: Statistical analyses, particularly causal inference methods, lack detail. We have added Dr. Smith, a biostatistician with expertise in causal inference as a co-investigator. All analyses will be informed by the Causal Roadmap, a formal framework for causal inference, to transparently represent relationships between study variables, including potential sources of bias and unmeasured factors. We have revised the statistical analysis plan (see 3.10) to provide extensive details on this approach including the use of inverse probability weighting[1] and targeted maximum likelihood estimation (TMLE)[2] to estimate adjusted associations.
R2, R3: Given the limitations of clinic BP, ambulatory blood pressure monitoring would be better. We have revised the proposal to now use ambulatory BP monitoring in conjunction with actigraphy.

21.2.1.3 Last Paragraph of the Introduction

The last paragraph of the Introduction should end on a positive note by providing a summary of all the changes made in response to the reviewer comments.

Example Final Positive Summary on the Introduction Page
In summary, since the original submission, we have been in the field with three pilot studies. We have utilized information gleaned from these studies to make cultural modifications to our intervention materials, ensuring that the materials will be efficacious in Hispanics, the ethnic group with the highest rates of diabetes, as well as the other ethnic groups represented in the study population, while being sure to retain the integrity of our evidence-based intervention approach.

21.2.2 Tip #1: Resist the Urge to Defend Yourself

If you are a new investigator, your first instinct may be to try to *prove* yourself to the reviewers. The natural tendency is to defend yourself against their concerns by spending time justifying your original decisions.

This approach tends to backfire because the reviewers' top priority is to see that you have been **responsive** to their concerns. They don't want you to spend time showing that you are smart, well-educated, and/or never make errors. Instead, they will be going through each item in your Introduction and *checking off* in their notes whether or not you have made the changes they suggested.

Therefore, the most tactical approach is to set aside any need to prove yourself. Instead, if the suggested revision is feasible and does not seriously detract from your goals, then simply make the change. In the Introduction, simply state that you have made this change—there is no need to waste space by providing a rationale for why you originally did it another way.

21.2.3 Tip #2: Avoid Disagreeing with a Reviewer

It is almost never effective to not be responsive to a reviewer comment in some fashion. Even a small revision is better than no revision. That is, you need to show that you are doing something in response to a reviewer concern.

If you are unable to be fully responsive to reviewer concerns,

1. Acknowledge the reviewer concern.
2. Describe the revision you made in response (even if it is a slight alternative to the reviewer's suggestion).
3. Describe what you are unable to address and why.

This approach avoids the common pitfall of starting your response by sounding nonresponsive or, at worst, argumentative. Instead, start out by saying that you recognize the reviewers' concern, followed by the positive change that you have made to the application in response to the reviewer comments (even if this is an alternative way to satisfy their concern), followed by any caveats regarding what you are unable to address.

Example Response to Reviewer Comment
Original Version Needs Improvement
R1. Add a six-month follow-up study to ascertain if the effect persists after the structured intervention.
Response: We chose not to conduct a follow-up study as our primary focus in this application was to determine whether the intervention could be effective in real time.

Improved Version
R1. Add a six-month follow-up study to ascertain if the effect persists after the structured intervention.
Response: The reviewer raises an important point. Therefore, we have added a three-month postintervention focus group that will assess whether the family continues to dance together, how often, and in what format. We are unable to follow the participants for six months due to the fact that recruitment is rolling over the first two years of the grant, leaving insufficient time to follow the last recruited family. However, we will also perform a six-month focus group in a subgroup of the first 50 recruited families.

In the above example, it was not feasible to follow the reviewer's recommendation of a six month follow-up exactly. However, instead, the investigator recognized the underlying rationale behind the reviewer's concern and came up with two alternative approaches to address this concern—specifically, both a shorter term follow-up and a focus group. Both these approaches get to the heart of the reviewer's concern and would therefore satisfy most reviewers.

21.2.4 Tip #3: If You Must Disagree with a Reviewer, Focus on the Science

It is okay to disagree with reviewer concerns if you explain your decision in a way that will engage the reviewer scientifically. Do not write to the reviewers; write to the science. However, even in this situation, it is important to still try to be somewhat responsive to at least a part of their concern if at all possible. Two options to consider include:

1. Propose **an alternative approach** to address the reviewers' concern instead of the reviewers' specific suggestion.
2. Make the reviewers' suggested changes **and** also follow your original approach in a sensitivity analysis.

Example Response to Reviewer Comment
Original Version Needs Improvement
R1: It is unclear why the proposed data analysis plan will only adjust for family history of diabetes and not history of preterm birth.
Response: The dataset that we will be using does not include information on history of preterm birth.

Improved Version
Response: While our dataset does not include information on history of preterm birth, we will address the threat of confounding by history of preterm birth by repeating the analysis among nulliparous women. We will compare the findings from this sensitivity analysis to the primary analysis to evaluate the degree of potential confounding by this variable.

The example above follows the first option above in that it provides an alternative approach to address the reviewer's concern. Thus, it gets to the heart of the concern (i.e., confounding) and acknowledges it, while simply providing an alternative method to address it. In other words, it does not diminish the reviewer's concern.

Example Response to Reviewer Comment
R2: The investigators should consider defining physical activity using three cut points instead of two cut points.
Response: In response to the reviewer's suggestion, we have added an additional analysis utilizing three cut points. However, because prior validation studies support the use of two cut points,[1,2] we also propose to retain our analysis using two cut points. This will facilitate comparisons with the prior literature that has, in general, utilized this approach. We will present findings from both approaches.

The example above follows the second option by making the reviewers' suggested changes **and** also following the original approach.

21.2.5 Tip #4: Avoid Using Cost or Logistics as a Rationale for Not Being Responsive to a Reviewer Comment

It is important to try to avoid cost or logistics as a rationale for why the reviewer's advice was not taken. Ideally, try to refer to a scientific rationale in addressing reviewer comments as displayed in the example below.

Example Response to Reviewer Comment
Original Version Needs Improvement
R1. Concern that dropout rates may be high—monetary incentives should be considered.
Response: The reviewer's valid point about possible attrition without monetary incentives concerns me also. However, our budget cannot afford such incentives.

Improved Version
R1. Concern that dropout rates may be high—monetary incentives should be considered.
We agree with the reviewer. We have added a modest monetary incentive and will also partner with the school/community to incorporate nonmonetary ways to incentivize the participants.

21.2.6 Tip #5: Multiple-Bullet-Point Response to Major Concerns Is Highly Responsive

The space dedicated to each response should be in proportion to the importance of the reviewer concern. As mentioned earlier, the most serious concerns are those that fall under *Overall Impact* were mentioned by multiple reviewers or were mentioned in the *Resume and Summary of Discussion*. In these situations, a bulleted list of multiple responses to this concern is recommended.

Example Response to Reviewer Comment
R1, R3. Need for data to demonstrate the efficacy of the physical activity intervention among pregnant Hispanic women.
Response: In response to this important concern, our investigative team has been in the field with three pilot studies since the time of the original submission:
  • Pilot #1 is our focus group work among Hispanic women led by Dr. Smith (new coinvestigator). We have revised the intervention to address the themes from these six focus groups (Sections C.1 and D.3).
  • Pilot #2 is our ongoing exercise intervention among eight pregnant women that provides strong support for the efficacy of our exercise intervention (Section C.2).
  • Pilot #3 is our completed pilot of acceptability/feasibility among 40 prenatal care patients that showed that the stage-matched manuals were feasible and acceptable in our population of Hispanic pregnant women (Section C.3).
Finally, since the time of original submission, a small vanguard pilot study has been published[1] supporting the efficacy of an exercise intervention in pregnant women at risk for GDM.

21.2.7 Tip #6: Acknowledge Your Mistakes or Lack of Clarity

At times, reviewers will make **basic errors of understanding** in their interpretation of your proposal. This may simply be due to the fact that they are facing a heavy load of proposals to review with a tight deadline, in combination with your proposal's failure to present something clearly.

In this case, it is important to be humble and apologize for your lack of clarity—even if you feel that the original proposal was already clear and the reviewer was mistaken. Resist the temptation to point out that the first submission already described this point. Remember, you are not trying to prove to the reviewer that you are *smart*; instead, you are trying to prove to the reviewer that you are responsive to their comments.

Example Response to Reviewer Comment
Consider that you proposed to conduct a matched case-control study with age, being your matching criteria. The reviewer missed the fact that you already included age as a matching criterion and asks you to do so in their comments.
Original Version Needs Improvement
Response: We already included age as a matching criterion as noted on page 18 of the original application.

Improved Version
Response: We apologize for our lack of clarity in describing the study design. We will include age as a matching criterion. Specifically, cases and controls will be matched on age<18, age≥18 (see Section C.4. Study Design).

21.2.8 Tip #7: Don't Skip Any Reviewer Comments

Address each reviewer comment, if not individually, then at least in a summary paragraph near the end of the Introduction. The reviewers have each spent a lot of time reviewing your original application and will therefore carefully check whether you have addressed all their comments.

21.2.9 Tip #8: Avoid Collapsing Too Many Reviewer Concerns into One Bullet Point

This tip falls under the concept of being kind to your reviewer. In the example below, you can see how collapsing multiple concerns can lead to reviewer confusion. Instead, by listing the reviewer comments separately, your response to the reviewer comments can be more targeted.

Example Summary of Reviewer Comments
Consider a proposal to conduct focus groups among girls.
Original Version Needs Improvement
R1, R2, R3. Aim 1 unclear; measurement of fun; control group.

Improved Version
R1, R2: Aim 1 is unclear.
R2, R3: Clarify how "fun" will be measured.
R1, R3: Concern that the control group has less contact time.

21.2.10 Tip #9: What about Areas That Reviewers Did NOT Comment On?

It is important to check all subsection scores regardless of content. In other words, in addition to reading the reviewer comments, also look at their scores for each of the review criteria (i.e., Significance, Investigators, Innovation, Approach, Environment). You may face the situation in which one or more of these criteria areas had poorer scores (e.g., 3 or greater) but did not receive any (or few) specific reviewer comments.

Even if the reviewers don't give you much reasoning for a poorer score within any of the five review criteria, it is still critical to highlight in the Introduction how you've enhanced that particular section. For example, if the reviewers scored a "3" for *Innovation* but provided minimal comments, it is still critical to highlight in the Introduction how you've now enhanced the innovation of the proposal. In other words, if the reviewers think the *Innovation* section has remain unchanged from the original submission, their score for *Innovation* will be unchanged. This is one argument for organizing the Introduction section by scoring area. The reviewers who gave innovation a poorer score without any reasoning will clearly see how you enhanced the *Innovation* section. This approach also works well if one reviewer (e.g., Reviewer #2) had a specific concern about an area, but the other reviewers (e.g., Reviewers #1 and #3) did not list concerns but also scored this area poorly.

Example Response in the Absence of Reviewer Comments but a Poor Score Enhanced Innovation. Although reviewers had few comments on these sections, scores suggested that the Innovation was not sufficiently clear. As such, we now provide stronger evidence that this work is theoretically and translationally significant and is an excellent fit with the NIH definition of Innovation.

In the absence of reviewer comments, but poorer scores, for the Significance section, another approach is to delineate how your proposal meets the funding opportunity announcement (FOA), that is, the Program Announcement (PA) or Request for Application (RFA). Specifically quote from the FOA and clarify how you are meeting that call.

If you find that you don't have space in the Introduction, by highlighting this in the body of your resubmission (e.g., in blue font), the reviewers will more clearly see the significance even if you don't mention it in the Introduction.

Example Response in the Absence of Reviewer Comments but a Poor Score Enhanced Significance. Through the development of a high-impact lifestyle intervention for at-risk Hispanic women, this RO1 application meets the NIH criteria of "having a sustained and powerful impact on the field."

21.2.11 Tip #10: Be Sure to Make Changes to the Body of the Proposal

In general, all responses to reviewer comments should refer to a section in the body of the proposal—so that the reviewer will be assured that you made the change to the protocol itself. The only exception would be items that reviewers suggested that you delete (however, sometimes even these are worth mentioning in the *Alternatives and Limitations* section).

Avoid the mistake of simply stating that you made a change in the Introduction and then leaving the body of the proposal unchanged. Reviewers will check this.

21.2.12 Stylistic Tip #1: Use Active (Not Passive) Voice

Just as with writing of the body of the grant proposal, the use of the active voice in writing the Introduction to a resubmission further highlights your responsiveness to reviewer comments.

Example Response to Reviewer Comment:
Original Version Needs Improvement
R2. The intervention should incorporate a social support component based on recent findings supporting the efficacy of this approach.
Response: Changes were made to the proposal to incorporate a social support component.

Improved Version
Response: We agree with the reviewer and have now revised the intervention to incorporate a social support component.

21.2.13 Stylistic Tip #2: Avoid Use of the First Person

Just as with writing of the body of the grant proposal, in Research Award applications (R series) it is also best to avoid use of the first person when writing the Introduction to a resubmission. You will almost always be submitting an application with a team of coinvestigators, collaborators, consultants, or mentors. The use of the term *we* always sounds more impressive than *I*, which can inadvertently come off as sounding like your own personal opinion.

Example Response to Reviewer Comments
Original Version Needs Improvement
R1, R3: Lack of rationale for choosing the Facial Affective Scale.
Response: I selected the Facial Affective Scale in light of the lower validity which I believe the other scales face.

Improved Version
R1, R3: Lack of rationale for choosing the Facial Affective Scale.
Response: We selected the Facial Affective Scale based on published findings that show higher overall validity for this scale (r=0.75–0.88) as compared to alternative scales (r=0.33–0.66).[1,2]

Note that the improved version, in addition to using the term "we," also cites prior studies to support the assertion of validity.

21.2.14 Stylistic Tip #3: Don't Waste Too Much Space Apologizing

Space in the Introduction is at a premium as you are limited to one page. Your primary emphasis will be on highlighting the changes you have made in response to reviewer concerns, as opposed to apologizing.

Example Response to Reviewer Comments
Original Version Needs Improvement
R1. Application fails to address alternatives if aim #1 is not successful.
Response: We apologize for not explaining what will happen if we do not successfully establish the methodology. Since the time of the application, the methodology has been developed and validated as now described in Section C.3

Improved Version
R1. Application fails to address alternatives if aim #1 is not successful
Response: We apologize for this omission. Since the time of the application, the methodology has been developed and validated as now described in Section C.3.

21.3 PART III: BODY OF THE RESUBMISSION

21.3.1 How to Identify Revisions to a Grant Proposal

NIH has recently removed the requirement to identify "substantial scientific changes" in the text of a Resubmission application by "bracketing, indenting, or change of typography." Instead, is sufficient to outline the changes made to the Resubmission application in the Introduction. However, it is important to note that NIH will continue to accept applications that contain these specific mark-ups and they are often considered a kindness by reviewers. These marks often include highlighting, coloring, bolding, or italicizing changes in Research Strategy.

Take care that if your original application used bolding and italics to emphasize points, that you don't use these styles to mark revisions to your application. If your reviewer comments and your corresponding revisions were fairly focused, consider using a different font color or brackets for revisions. This simple change in font color (e.g., blue) can be a kindness to the reviewers paging through your application to identify your revisions.

In the situation where the revisions are substantial, it is best not to mark them, as this would be distracting for the reviewer and make it difficult to read. Instead, the Introduction can state that every section of the proposal was rewritten and therefore that revisions are not highlighted.

Example First Paragraph of the Introduction

Over the past eight months since the initial proposal submission, we have continued to develop the research outlined in the original proposal and hence can be more specific about the next steps that need to be undertaken. This has resulted in extensive changes in the proposal, including a change in the proposal's title to more appropriately reflect the central theme of the research. Every section of the proposal has been rewritten; new sections are not highlighted.

Be sure to cross-check the body of your revised proposal with your Introduction. Check that all revisions that you mentioned in the Introduction are not only made but also indicated, if relevant, in the body of the proposal. Similarly, be sure that any changes to the body of the proposal are also summarized, even briefly, in the Introduction.

21.3.2 Review the Published Literature for Recent Relevant Publications

Reviewing the literature for new relevant publications is a critical task in the resubmission process as there will be a time lag between your first submission and your resubmission. Assess whether the new data answer or inform your specific aims. If they do, refine your goals and specific aims and inform the reviewers about these new findings. At a minimum, add relevant citations to your *Significance and Innovation* section.

21.3.3 Obtain Revised Letters of Collaboration

Given the time lag between the original submission and the resubmission, it is important to obtain new letters of collaboration with a recent date for the purposes of the resubmission. The use of original letters will raise reviewer concerns that these collaborators may no longer be available to your proposed study.

21.3.4 Update Biosketches: Both Your Own and Those of Your Coinvestigators

Again, due to the time lag, be sure that all biosketches are revised to include any recent relevant publications as well as newly funded, or completed, grants.

21.4 RESUBMISSION OF A FELLOWSHIP GRANT

For Fellowship Grants, follow the same advice as described above with the following additional considerations.

Before resubmitting a Fellowship Grant, take care to look at the potential timing of the award within the context of the number of years left in your program. Some reviewers consider the date by which the funds would be received, compare them to the time remaining in the training program, and decide that the applicant should be nearing the end of their training and no longer requires funding to complete this process. At the same time, they may expect more publications due to the elapsed time.

For example, if your original F31 Predoctoral Fellowship Grant submission was for a three-year fellowship, and your resubmission is still for a three-year fellowship then, given the lag in submission/resubmission due dates, this will result in a six-year doctoral program. Reviewers may look askance at this time frame if it is not typical. One alternative is to shorten the timeline in your resubmission to be a two-year fellowship or to clarify that it is typical that your doctoral program takes six years to complete due to the type of research conducted (e.g., relying upon human subjects).

21.5 RESUBMISSION OF A CAREER DEVELOPMENT AWARD

For Career Development Awards, follow the same advice as described above with the following additional considerations.

If at all possible, prior to your grant resubmission, publish at least one piece of work with your mentor. Even a small clinical case report or a short review article that only marginally relates to your proposed research demonstrates a mentee's diligence and a mentor's commitment to your progress. Again, at this stage in career development, it is critical to demonstrate shared goals and obligations of the mentee and the mentor.

21.6 EXAMPLES

21.6.1 Example Introduction to the Resubmission of an R01 Proposal to Conduct a Randomized Trial of a Postpartum Diabetes Prevention Program

Note that this Introduction follows the format of option 2, that is **organizing responses according to review criteria**: Significance, Investigators, Innovation, Approach, and Environment.

INTRODUCTION TO REVISION

This is a resubmission of R03 DK12345 "Randomized Trial of a Postpartum Diabetes Prevention Program for Hispanic Women" (16th percentile score) to test the efficacy of a culturally and linguistically modified, individually tailored lifestyle intervention to reduce risk factors for type 2 diabetes and CVD among postpartum Hispanic women with a history of abnormal glucose tolerance during pregnancy. We thank the reviewers for noting, "Innovative proposal from an experienced team of investigators targeting a high-risk population." "Finding effective, culturally relevant ways to reduce risk of developing T2D among Hispanic women with GDM or glucose intolerance has substantial public health significance." The comments of the review panel were very helpful in revising the proposal. Changes are highlighted in blue throughout the text.

Significance. Weight loss not included as an intervention target (R1). As recommended by the reviewer, we have revised the protocol to focus on weight loss as a key intervention target in addition to the exercise and dietary targets. Consistent with this revision, we now utilize dietary intervention materials found to be efficacious in our recent WIC Postpartum Pilot Study[1] that focused on *reduction in total caloric intake* (C.2. and Appendix II). We also provide our prior weight loss findings to support our ability to achieve these goals (C.2. Preliminary Studies).

Investigators. No expert in dietary assessment is included (R1). We have added Dr. Taylor, professor of nutritional epidemiology and an expert in Hispanic dietary assessment, to lead the dietary assessment. Dr. Taylor and the PI have a track record of collaboration (C.1. *Progress Report* and Biosketches). We now describe the training and certification of the diet assessors in the Methods section (C.3. *Measure of Adherence with Diet*).

Innovation: Others have studied weight loss interventions in this group (R1). Prior studies are few; intervention studies that do exist had small samples of predominantly non-Hispanic white women. **No prior study has targeted at-risk Hispanic women.** We now clarify innovative aspects of our work relative to existing studies (see Significance Innovation).

Approach. Dietary intervention is not sufficiently developed nor described (R2). We have revised the Methods section to carefully describe the dietary intervention in detail (C.3. and Appendix II). We now clarify how quality control procedures ensure that stage of change and social cognitive constructs are consistently represented in all intervention materials. Our systems-based pilot study ensures that all mailings of physical activity and dietary intervention materials are synchronized such that participants receive them at the same time (C.3. *Lifestyle Intervention*; Table 1). We provide revised power calculations for the expected reduction in total daily caloric intake based on prior postpartum interventions. **Conduct a small feasibility study prior to the evaluation study (R2).** Since the time of the original submission, we have been in the field with a pilot feasibility study, "Healthy Pilot" (Faculty Research Grant; PI: yourself). The goal of this pilot is to evaluate the feasibility and acceptability of the proposed intervention. The pilot has randomized 47 women to date and is on track for its goal of 66 women. Participants endorsed the interest and utility of the study materials (86%), ability to access a telephone for telephone interviews (100%), and the amount of time spent on the study (appropriate 86%, sometimes too much time 14%). Recruitment and retention rates were used to inform the proposed power calculations (C.3. *Power Calculations*). **Initiate intervention during pregnancy after GDM diagnosis (R1).** We have revised the proposal to now initiate the intervention in pregnancy immediately after GDM diagnosis and the baseline assessment (randomization at ~29 weeks gestation) to capitalize on the fact that pregnant women with abnormal glucose tolerance receive counseling during that time period (C.3. *Usual Care*) and are motivated to make behavioral changes

Environment. Details regarding data reduction/sharing across sites is lacking (R1). We now provide a clear plan for data reduction and sharing across sites (see Facilities and Data Safety Monitoring Plan.)

Other. Comments on Budget/Appendix (R1). We have revised the Methods section and budget to identify the participant incentive value. We have removed photos from the stage-matched manuals that depicted parents swinging toddlers and now use more appropriate photos (Appendix II).

R3: No concerns.

SUMMARY OF CHANGES TO REVISED PROPOSAL

In summary, since the original submission we have substantively revised the intervention to target weight loss through reduction in total caloric intake and increase in physical activity based on our efficacious program in postpartum women; added an expert in dietary assessment in Hispanics; and have been in the field with a pilot study which supports the feasibility and acceptability of the proposed lifestyle intervention as a complete unit.

21.6.2 Example Introduction to the Resubmission of a Career Development Award (K01) Proposal to Conduct a Web-Based Intervention Study to Prevent Weight Gain in Men

Note that this Introduction follows the format of option 1: **organizing responses by the importance of reviewer comment**.

INTRODUCTION TO RESUBMISSION

We are pleased that the reviewers noted strengths of our original application including "a candidate with a good publication record and positive letters of support; an outstanding team of mentors with specific and varied expertise that is ideally suited to the proposed training and research plan; and an excellent research and training environment." We believe the application is significantly improved by our efforts to address the reviewers' comments. Major additions are in blue throughout the application and are summarized below.

R1, R2. Concern that characterization of weight gain patterns will not add to known determinants of excessive weight gain nor be a fruitful approach to intervening to prevent excessive weight gain. In response to these concerns, we have refocused the research and training plans on intervention development and testing feasibility and acceptability (Approach section). We feel these changes have considerably strengthened the application and better reflect training and mentored research experiences needed to accelerate the candidate's research program in the area of weight gain and long-term cardiometabolic health.

R3. Suggest eliminating unwieldy stratification of focus groups. We have revised the application to conduct four focus groups of "all comers" as suggested by the reviewer (Focus Groups section).

R1, R3. Need for a more detailed description of proposed intervention including specific behavioral strategies. We now provide a more detailed description of our theory-driven web-based intervention to prevent excessive weight gain that uses evidence-based strategies to help men achieve the recommendations for weight gain, nutrition, and physical activity (Intervention section).

R2. Add a pilot randomized controlled trial (RCT) to evaluate intervention feasibility and acceptability. We have added a pilot trial to evaluate intervention feasibility and acceptability (Section RCT), which will provide critical data to support an R01 application to conduct a large RCT to evaluate efficacy (Future section).

R1, R2. The candidate does not list publications directly related to proposed research topic. Since the time of the original submission, the candidate now has two papers in the area of weight gain published or accepted for publication and an additional three under review (Candidate and Preliminary Studies sections).

R1, 2, 3. Need for additional preliminary data. We now highlight the work we have done in direct support of this application since the time of the original submission (Preliminary Studies section).

R1. Replace the semester-long statistical courses with didactic training in obesity biology. We have added didactic training obesity biology and clinical shadowing; the revised training plan now better aligns with the revised research plan (Training section).

R2. Clarify how mentors will monitor progress, including yearly team meetings. See Section Mentors.

R3. Clarify manuscripts and grant applications to be submitted during award period. See Dissemination section.

Summary: We are pleased that the reviewers recognized the importance of the research topic. We have refocused the research plan to develop and test the feasibility and acceptability of a theory-driven web-based intervention to prevent excessive weight gain that uses evidence-based strategies to help men achieve recommendations for weight gain, nutrition, and physical activity.

21.6.3 Example Introduction to the Resubmission of a Fellowship Grant (F31) Proposal to Conduct a Cohort Study of Physical Activity (PA) and Neonatal Anthropometric Measures

Note that this Introduction follows the format of option 1: **organizing responses by the importance of reviewer comment**.

INTRODUCTION TO RESUBMISSION

This is a resubmission of my NIH NRSA F31 application titled "**Physical Activity Across Pregnancy and Neonatal Anthropometric Measures in African American Women**" (Impact Score: 50, 60%). We thank the reviewers for noting that the project addresses "a novel and important research topic involving prenatal physical activity and childbirth weight outcomes", "a compelling need in the field" and that "the applicant has a strong interest and track record in reproductive epidemiology and this project will allow the applicant to expand their work to incorporate physical activity" with "a strong mentor team". We have made substantial modifications to address reviewer comments indicated in blue.

R1, R2, R3. Research Plan lacks rigor and critical details (i.e., does not address sensitive timepoints of PA and lacks a description of covariates). Physical activity is aggregated into a final total volume metric thus the details around the dimensions are lost. We have revised the Research Strategy to leverage the multi-dimensional aspects of physical activity longitudinally throughout pregnancy using the following methods: 1) group-based trajectory analysis to indirectly capture sensitive windows of PA exposure, and 2) time-specific analysis to address PA timing in pregnancy. These two analytical approaches will capitalize on the ability of the In addition, we note that the Pregnancy Physical Activity Questionnaire was designed to capture domain-specific PA for ethnically diverse pregnant populations. This revision provides specific information on covariates for multivariable modeling (Aims 1–3).

R2, R3. The statistical plan is vague, lacks information on mediation, trajectory, and how to model relationships with birthweight and it is unclear how applicant will disentangle the impact of PA on associations between race/ethnicity on birth outcomes. We now provide a detailed statistical plan for Aims 1–3 and description of specific hypotheses (see Research Strategy, Figure 2, 3, 4a-b). We have also added an *Outcome and Interpretation* section for each Aim, to clarify how we will disentangle the impact of PA on associations between race/ethnicity on birth outcomes,.

R1, R3. The mentorship team has somewhat weak expertise in dietary assessment, does not include a strong biostatistician, nor expertise in behavioral/health psychology. We have added Dr. Jones, health behavior consultant and a longtime collaborator with my co-sponsor on physical activity interventions, as a consultant. We apologize for not noting that my co-sponsor is a leader in dietary assessment and developed the first pregnancy dietary questionnaire[1] which is now used in over 50 countries with 21 years of continual NIH funding in this area. We also failed to note that the biostatistician, Dr. Smith, has led the statistical analyses for Project Health for 20 years—and is an integral statistician with the Springfield Center for Disease Prevention.

R1, R2, R3. The training plan does not include sufficient training in physical activity epidemiology, health behavior change, and advanced epidemiologic methods. We have revised the proposal to include hands-on training in my consultant's physical activity epidemiology lab specifically focused on physical activity assessment (i.e., accelerometers) and cohort recruitment and management using data from his R21 (R21HD1234). We have added mentored training and coursework in the areas of health behavior change and racial/ethnic disparities, and causal inference, as well as workshops and short courses in advanced epidemiologic methods (Background and Goals, Respective Contributions).

R1, R3. Concerns about mentorship team. We now highlight a 15-year track record of collaboration between the sponsor and co-sponsor, which include: > 15 publications and presentations, six co-mentored fellows, and five co-mentored doctoral students. We have added (1) clear description how the mentorship team will work together (Table 2, Background and Goals), (2) details on yearly training evaluation of candidate's progress on fellowship, and (3) additional opportunities for the candidate to receive professional development with mentor involvement.

R1, R3. Other Changes: We have added detail clarifying the unique suitability of the dataset for the proposed research, including on cohort recruitment, missingness, and drop out (Research Strategy), additional detail regarding professional development of the candidate, and plans for dissemination of findings to the scientific community (Table 1, Background and Goals).

In summary: This study will advance our understanding of which etiologic factors play a role in racial/ethnic disparities, and which aspects of fetal development may be impacted by PA. This important work will provide the first step towards future epidemiologic and community-based research which will inform culturally tailored PA interventions that incorporate considerable disparities in PA access throughout the pregnancy period.

Index

Printed in the United States
by Baker & Taylor Publisher Services